LET YOUR ORGANS BREATHE

Dr. Jayanto (Jay) Das (Ph.D.)
Former Fellow of the Royal Society of Health (FRSH, London)
&
Royal Australian Chemical Institute (RACI, Australia)

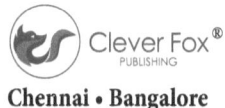

Chennai • Bangalore

CLEVER FOX PUBLISHING
Chennai, India

Published by CLEVER FOX PUBLISHING 2025
Copyright © Dr. Jay Das 2025

All Rights Reserved.
ISBN: 978-93-67075-64-7

This book has been published with all reasonable efforts taken to make the material error-free after the consent of the author. No part of this book shall be used, reproduced in any manner whatsoever without written permission from the author, except in the case of brief quotations embodied in critical articles and reviews.

The Author of this book is solely responsible and liable for its content including but not limited to the views, representations, descriptions, statements, information, opinions and references ["Content"]. The Content of this book shall not constitute or be construed or deemed to reflect the opinion or expression of the Publisher or Editor. Neither the Publisher nor Editor endorse or approve the Content of this book or guarantee the reliability, accuracy or completeness of the Content published herein and do not make any representations or warranties of any kind, express or implied, including but not limited to the implied warranties of merchantability, fitness for a particular purpose. The Publisher and Editor shall not be liable whatsoever for any errors, omissions, whether such errors or omissions result from negligence, accident, or any other cause or claims for loss or damages of any kind, including without limitation, indirect or consequential loss or damage arising out of use, inability to use, or about the reliability, accuracy or sufficiency of the information contained in this book.

Dr Jay immigrated to Australia from India in July 1971 to undertake his PhD studies in biochemistry. He then joined the pharmaceutical industry via multinational corporations, Fisons and 3M, where he successfully developed a broad range of pharmaceutical products and researched their medical application.

After meeting with the late Bob Lucy, one of the pioneers in advancing the use of nutritional supplements in Australia, Dr Jay successfully transitioned to natural therapies working across research and development, manufacturing and quality control. He retired from commercial assignments as a General Manager at the age of 52 and started his own company with various interests. He still continues to be involved in the industry but in a much less involved way.

Now at the age of 75, Dr Jay intends to share the knowledge he has gained from over 40 years of experience in the health and wellness industry. His writing is based on the firm belief that good nutrition and a healthy mind, body and soul are the key to living long and meaningful lives.

To my family for their patience and understanding and to put up with my busy schedule during my working life.

Writing a book on any subject matter is not an easy task. There are many considerations that need to be assessed and finalised for inclusions. There are several issues which need to be resolved before the manuscript is put together for the first reading. Also, many people in the background who must be acknowledged as the task I have undertaken could not have been made possible without their help. There are a few people who have encouraged me throughout this process; my family even my little grandsons played an important role by asking me: "Dadu, what are you writing?" Dadu means Grandpa.

Some of my colleagues, especial mention to David Woolcott, who is a natural therapies practitioner and one of the best in his chosen profession and still practicing in Perth region in Western Australia has been a continued source of inspiration. My two nieces firstly Dr. Anjana Poddar who did the first reading of the manuscript and provided valuable suggestions and my other niece Dr Suranjana (Su) Guha-Agashe who provided me with her biochemistry knowledge for which I am so, so grateful; they did it out of love and respect and did not expect or want any returns. To my son Sandeep Das for his expert comments on nutrition and also on movements and exercises.

Clever Fox Publishing who helped me with the editing, layouts, designing, printing and publishing of the book; they have done a wonderful professional job.

Finally, to Millenium Pharmaceuticals for their sponsorship even though I am an integral part of the company and have a vested interest in it.

But most of all, to all the readership, who I hope will read the book not as a textbook but as a fun read. My sincere wish and hope is that people who read this book will gain some health awareness and consciousness to live a long, healthy and happy life. Please read the book and enjoy the journey as I have enjoyed writing for you.

Table of Contents

Preface xi
About the Book xiii
Chapter 1: The Philosophy of Keeping Well 1
Out of Africa: 3
Chapter 2: Pranayama and the Concept of 'om' (the Philosophy of Keeping Well) 16
Origin: 16
The Concept of 'OM': 21
Our Energy Chakras: 26
Chapter 3: Preparedness, Commitment and Planning (the Philosophy of Keeping Well) 34
Mental Preparedness and Planning 34
What to Do Then? 38
Your Daily Routine Set Up 43
Risks and Hazards of Daily Living 52
Chapter 4: Food Categories and Diet 55
Food Contamination and Factors Affecting Quality of Food: 59
Risk minimisation should be practiced as best as possible: 61
People Who Are at High Risk of Getting Infected: 64
Water 67
Some Popular Test Parameters Indicative of Health Status 71
Liquid Water: 72
Water Toxicity: How Much Water Is Too Much? 74
Seniors and Water Consumption 75
Sugar, a Modern-Day Villain or a Myth? 77
Common Table Salt, Is It Good for You or Bad? 82
Food Categories 84
Carbohydrates and Diabetes 86
Fruits and Vegetables 91
Fats and Proteins in Our Diet 94

Nuts, Cereals and Seeds in Our Diet: 96
Dietary Considerations 99
Food Selection and Choices 100
Food and Energy 101
Good Diets and Bad Diets 107
Palaeolithic Diet 114
High Energy Diets 116
Low Energy/Weight Management Diets 117
Vegetarian/Vegan Diets 118
Diabetic Diet 119
The Australian Diet 120

Chapter 5: Basic Human Anatomy 122
Let's Start with Our Heart 127
Our Blood Pressure Control (BP) 128
Our Lungs 130
Our Liver 132
Anatomy of Our Liver 134
Love Your Liver 136
Our Brain 137
Tips on How to Enhance Your Brain Function and Capacity 138
Pituitary Gland 139
Our Pituitary Gland Hormones and Their Main Function 140
Our Kidneys 141
Our Skin 143
Layers of the Skin 144

Chapter 6: Vitamins in Our Health and Wellbeing 148
What Are Vitamins? 148
Water-Soluble Vitamins: 149
Fat-Soluble Vitamins 150
Vitamin Nomenclature 153
The Era of Vitamin Discovery 153
Vitamin D 155
Discovery and Time Line for Vitamin D 159
Discovery and Time Line for Vitamin E 162
Mechanism of Blood Clotting: 164
Vitamin Safety and Risk Factors 165
The Great Vitamin Controversy 172
Vitamins and Nobel Prizes 175

Vitamin Deficiency Is Not Rare *180*
Vitamin-Derived Co-Enzymes and Co-Factors in Nutrition *194*
Vitamin B-Complex *197*
Vitamin B-Complex in Our Body *198*

Chapter 7: Vitamin C: the Spark of Life 202
Vitamin C: The Spark of Life *202*
Historical Progression *204*
Vitamin C and Some Other Milestones since 1937 .... *210*
Vitamin C and Requirement *212*
Vitamin C and Stress *214*
Vitamin C's Distribution in Our Body: *215*
Benefits of Vitamin C (and Its Derivatives) in Topical Dermatology *216*

Chapter 8: Minerals And Herbs 217
Minerals in Our Health and Well-Being *217*
Mineral Chart *221*
Metal-Enzymes Complexes *225*
Schuessler's salts: *227*
Health Benefits of Commonly Used Herbs *229*
Herb/Drug Interactions *240*
Early History of Herbs *241*

Chapter 9: Movements, Energy Expenditure and Some Basic Exercise Guides 245
Why do we need to do exercises? *246*
Exercise with Equipment *253*
Illustrations of Some Skipping Positions *259*
Seniors and Stretching Exercises *264*
Grading of Daily Activity levels *270*
Body Mass Index (BMI) *272*
Waist Hip Ratio (WHR) *276*

Chapter 10: Senior's Nutrition 279
Seniors in Our society? *279*
Sensory Changes *282*
Cognitive Health *283*
Under-Nutrition, Malnutrition and Nourishment *284*
Loss of Balance and Physical Injuries *285*
Mental Issues *286*
Seniors and Their Dietary Requirements *286*

Seniors and Their Medicinal and Supplement Requirements.......................... *295*
Self-Affirmations..*298*
Chapter 11: Covid Crisis **300**
World Health Organisation (WHO) and Coronavirus................................ *300*
So, What Is COVID-19?...*302*
Variants of COVID-19...*306*
Anatomy of COVID-19 Virus (Simplified)...*307*
COVID-19 and Nutrition *307*
COVID-19 and Prognosis...*315*
How Covid-19 has changed our lives *319*

Preface

For several years, various people have asked me to write a book on human nutrition, a subject very near and dear to my heart. I did not venture then as I felt that there was something missing from my thought process which was preventing me from writing. Could it have been my inexperience as an author, although, I have in the past written thesis and several articles both in scientific journals and newsprints but as I say something was missing then?

Or simply, I was not ready.

I started writing this book around Christmas 2020 and this is my first book, and being experienced in this subject for a number of years, 40 years and counting I decided to put pen to paper. This I felt was the appropriate time and my inner guidance approved of it. A semi-retired life and time to reflect on my long career and the conducive situation with COVID-19 lock-downs and restrictions around were the driving forces which spurred me on. I now have something permanent to give back to the community and industry, which I have served diligently and with utmost respect and care. I have also received so much goodwill and positive vibes from everyone around me and the very opportunity to bring all of this together for which I am ever so grateful.

Writing on any subject matter is not an easy task, especially on human nutrition. It is a topic of current interest and very relevant to our modern society as we strive for good health and well-being. It is also very dynamic as new theories, postulations and guidelines are being put forward as a result of continued research into human nutrition.

In writing this book, I am making a few assumptions that, all of us need to be more vigilant about our health and general well-being, more so, the more venerable members of our community e.g., senior citizens and also above 50s who, sub-consciously are thinking of making the transition into the senior years. Being a senior citizen myself, what better time than now. The aim is to promote nutritional awareness, good health and well-being.

I have long held the view that philosophy is the key to every quest in life unlocking the complexity and understanding the real meaning of life and our relationship with nature and all living beings around us. Application of philosophy has a special significance to our health and well-being as it tries to seek clarification of the ethics and practices which bind us and draws a way forward to realise our ability to harness our own potential in managing our own health, well-being and destiny.

In moving forward and searching for the answer to the question, what is health; we can look to both our biological existence and holistic state, with philosophy being the conduit.

With this in mind, I have introduced elements of the philosophy of keeping well where I could entertain the idea that our physical being and mental state are the two most vulnerable areas for exploration.

I have tried to keep scientific jargon out as much as possible, introduced several available postulations and theories that I have backed up with scientific references and have tried to make the content as simple and easily accessible to the community at large.

Whether we believe in our creation or evolution, we are here now and acknowledge that philosophy is the common thread that unites Science and Nature, and it is this environment of co-union that we inhabit in. Earth, Water, Fire, Sky and Air the five universal elements are the basic manifestation of all that is in our constitution, in our makeup. We are an indivisible part of Mother Nature; *from ashes to ashes, dust to dust.*

About the Book

This book is written in simple easily understandable chapters which will serve to enhance better awareness of the importance of human nutrition. Human Nutrition is a defined Science; a new and dynamic field which allows us to know ourselves from our general health and well-being perspective.

It is also an emerging topic of discussion.

After all, why should it not be? We all are very conscientious of our health and looking for that extra awareness which will provide us with healthy living and wellness in our advancing years.

Introducing philosophy has a great bonus which goes hand in hand with the understanding of wellness. I believe that our WELLNESS is the accomplishment of our health and general well-being in relation to our spiritual being as a part of our greater cosmic existence.

Philosophy combines two Greek words *Philein* and *Sophia* and means Love of Wisdom and helps us to guide our destiny in life for the common understanding of the broader issues we are likely to face through our life's journey.

This book should not serve as a text book, far from it; but should be viewed as an informal read offering many interesting and helpful pieces of information which often remain in the background from the main texts in nutrition and related text books.

It is my sincere wish and desire that readers will develop a taste and curiosity to learn more by reading other books and publications on the broader subject of human nutrition. I have tried to put the context into simple everyday language without losing sight of the actual subject matter and where possible and appropriate have introduced elements of spirituality to make reading more pleasant and engrossing.

I have developed and extended simple ideas to make the subject matter more informative by incorporating many views that are contained in many scientific publications entering into various search engines and surfing the internet. My attempts and motivations are derived from many life stories that I have heard and partaken in conversations with people whom I have served as a consultant during my many years of involvement in the industry.

This book is by no stretch of the imagination complete, as there are so many entries that could have been considered worthy of inclusion; but there is a limit to all, and all good things must come to an end. If I am successful in stimulating young and old minds alike, then I am so grateful for all your readership and consider myself lucky to have done my job. I welcome readers to further their readership and explore new chapters in health and nutrition and become more nutritionally aware.

I also wish that many seniors in our community who are vulnerable due to age and or socio-economic constrains may be able to read this book and take something good from it and follow simple nutritional habits and exercises which are very basic, easy to do and inexpensive; but always remember to have a medical appraisal to know your abilities and limitations before you get stuck into it.

Also, remember that every movement that is happening within and outside of our body expends energy which must be compensated for or burned depending on our dietary habits and needs and also on our physique. Please read the book and enjoy the journey as I have enjoyed writing for you.

Disclaimer: This book is written in good faith as a fun read and not as a text book. The author has attempted to verify all facts used in the book but does not guarantee its validity; readers must use their own discretion when using any part of the book. For all references used, the author is grateful and no copyright infringement is intended.

If the author has forgotten to acknowledge any reference then it is not intentional and seeks apology for such omissions.

Finally, never neglect medical advice given to you; read the book enjoy and be nutritionally aware.

Since writing this book to its completion into a completed work, several years have elapsed and several information presented may have been outdated specially COVID-19 related topics. For the latest information readers must refer to relevant updated texts.

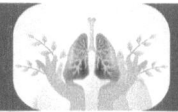

Chapter 1

THE PHILOSOPHY OF KEEPING WELL

Wellness is the apex of our body, mind and soul combined, which encompasses all that is good in us.

– Jay Das, 2020

Health and wellness are states of our consciousness that are reflected in our body, mind and soul. To enhance our state of consciousness where we can appreciate Life and Nature, we need to keep our body fit and healthy; our mind sharp and vigilant; and our soul free. As organic beings we are composed of trillions of cells; each cell is like a reactor carrying out biochemical processes that release energy for us to sustain life. For this to happen, the cells use nutrients from the foods we eat and oxygen from the air we breathe in. If our diet is not adequate in nutrient content and the quality of air is not of a minimum standard of purity, then the body does not get the required level of energy for good health and well-being.

Our state of consciousness suffers which is reflected in our body, mind and soul in varying degrees. Perhaps, we become tired and irritable, breeding discontentment, negativity and rebellion, which may lead us to engage in unpleasant conduct or even show aggression towards our fellow humans.

Wellness is the glue which holds our body, mind and soul together and keeps us focused. Any loosening of this glue can basically manifest itself as a deviation from normality in life and in our physical, mental and spiritual, cognitions. This can cause an imbalance in our many faculties that make us human, thus affecting our daily lives and activities.

In my many years on planet Earth, I have witnessed or personally experienced the effect of such imbalances. So, wellness has a profound effect on our lives and the activities we perform as human beings on a daily basis.

In my early days of consulting as a young nutritional biochemist, I was once asked, "What, if any, is the relationship between wellness and lifestyle?"

Although simple, the question took me by surprise as it reflected a deep nutritional awareness or perhaps a lack of it, and, took on a greater meaning for me. I cannot exactly recall the answer I gave then but in the many years that have passed since, I have thought about it long and hard. "What is the true answer?" I still seek for answers.

Has spirituality got anything to do with it?

While a relationship between wellness and lifestyle would be easier to explain from a physical and mental perspective, adding a third dimension of spirituality, makes it more complex.

Wellness as I reflect on, is the encompassment of all that is good in us. However, for all to be good, we need to look after our physical and mental health, as well as summon our spiritualism hidden deep in our inner soul to complete us as human beings. Hence, we develop strong feelings for the life around us, including fellow humans, our religious practices and most importantly our intellect.

As a highly developed societal species, we have dominated this planet sheerly through our intellectual capacity which has endowed us with many complex characteristics and essential survival instincts. Perhaps that is why humankind has survived on the highest rung of the evolutionary ladder when more than 95% of other species including birds and insects have become extinct over that time.

But there are certain very interesting flaws in this evolution of ours which we will touch upon in its relevant context in a later chapter.

How humankind has managed to survive this long is truly an admirable feat.

A six-million-year story in the making. We have battled with environmental factors, with other species threatening our existence in the early stages of our being and with ourselves. Some say we are still being challenged by other forms of life; bacteria, viruses, etc.; a case in point being COVID-19 in our recent history; and not to mention with ourselves and fellow beings. Case in point is the war and destruction we cause ourselves; will this, or, can this lead to our eventual demise?

You may have noticed I refer to battling with ourselves. Yes, this is in our psyche starting from our early existence and still continuing. Look at the two World Wars I and II we have had followed by Vietnam War, war in Afghanistan and more recently the war in Ukraine which still rages on.

We have not learned.

Since over a million years or so ago there were several species of humans dominated by *Homo sapiens*, the true ancestors of the modern human; we competed with several other species of hominins like *H. naledi*, *H. erectus*, Neanderthals, Denisovans and others who cohabited the earth at similar geological times.

Was it for survival, dominance or supremacy over other like species, or the *Homo sapiens* were more adaptable to the climatic changes and the development of their brain structure? I don't quite know. But it may seem that the evil seeds of mistrust and intolerance towards those who are different from us could have been sown in the human psyche from those very early days of evolution. It still raises its ugly head often in the form of hatred, violence and racism in modern society; an example of the evolution of our negative traits alongside that of all the uniquely positive qualities that distinguish our species. Sadly, enough it is not limited to this and recent war and catastrophic destruction amongst ourselves is a classic example.

Out of Africa:

It is now a commonly held view that our cradle of evolution is East Africa where it is believed we evolved some 2 million years ago as a refinement of our tree-dwelling ancestors and developed as *Homo habilis* the handyman. Earlier if you consider a few other species of hominins such as *Australopithecus afarensis* who were believed to be one of the very early species who lived around 4 million years ago and walked upright on two legs; many of us must have heard about Lucy the most famous preserved fossilised find who was believed to have lived 3.2–3.5 million years ago.

If we go back further in time around 5.5 to 6 million years ago, it is believed that the species *Orrorin tugenensis* was one of our earliest ancestors which walked on 2 legs. It is indeed fascinating that palaeontologists and anthropologists can infer and predict so much about our early ancestry from pre-historic fossilised bone fragments.

It is now certain that the species *Homo sapiens* our closest anatomical relatives started an orderly and mass migration from East Africa roughly 350–315 thousand years ago, give or take a few thousand years.

The timeline of the human evolutionary pathway is very interesting and depending on which way you want to lean; I think if we go back to 4 million years ago, we may be pretty certain of the following facts:

3.9–2.8 million years ago the appearance of Australopithecus and similar other species collectively known as Australopithecines evolved in Africa.

2.5–2.0 million years ago *Homo habilis* appeared, and are credited to be the first known species who had human-like features with larger brain capacity than their fore-bearers. They are also the first known species who started using stone tools thus they became known as 'The handyman'.

2.1–0.5 million years ago the evolution of *Home erectus* started the chain reaction into human evolution and refinement.

Although, *Home erectus* was not directly related to the early ancestors of modern man this particular species travelled widely and believed to have intermated with other species of that time. They are thought to be the first of their kind to have learned the controlled use of fire and began to modify the earlier stone tools used by *Homo habilis*. This species of early humans is believed to have survived the longest and is thought to have started migrating into the other parts of the world.

600,000–100,000 years ago Neanderthals evolved in Africa like all other human species but migrated to Europe and Asia long before the *Homo sapiens*. Neanderthals also had large brain cavities and had learned the controlled use of fire. They were predominantly hunters and gatherers and had many attributes of humans such as burial rituals. Although they are not supposed to be directly related to modern *Homo sapiens* (modern man), they had left an indelible mark on modern society.

Their fossilised remains have been found in many places of Africa, Asia and Europe. According to the Natural History Museum, the Neanderthals lived as recently as 130,000 to 40,000 years ago. It is also theorised that as late as 5000 years ago Neanderthals and modern humans existed and also inter-bred. But they all died out soon after.

300,000–160,000 years ago *Homo sapiens* appeared to evolve and started to move out of Africa and transformed into our modern cousins. It is still debatable the actual timeline for the *Homo sapiens* as to when transformation into modern humans began. Anatomically it is believed that the transformation or evolution into modern Homo sapiens began around 130,000 years ago. The size of their brain cavity was around the size of today's modern humans, they were quite agile moving from one place to another searching for food, water and shelter. It is further believed that the transformation from *Homo sapiens* to modern man happened inside Africa and that modern migration did not start until much later perhaps around 100,000 years ago. The cause of this later migration is also worth noting, given the earlier migrations happened around 2 million years ago by our ancestral species *Homo erectus*.

Around 100,000 years ago the prevailing conditions of our planet Earth may not have been conducive to facilitate the migratory population. The land mass may not have been connected 100,000 years ago as may have been 2 million years ago. Active volcanoes and constant eruptions which gave rise to several extreme conditions (tsunamis, etc.) may have made, the then human species more co-operative among each other which resulted in the development of many skills such as shelter building, families taking shape and tribal or societal and collective decision making which thought to have taken place to develop their sense of security and safety. Due to these added skills, our modern ancestors found it much easier to migrate out of Africa and colonise; sorry wrong word, spread out into the whole new world and establish new habitats and permanent homes.

A Map below showing human migration out of Africa.

Image credit: Genome Research Limited (Gratefully referenced: Evolution of modern humans—Your Genome: https://www.yourgenome.org/stories/evolution-of-modern-humans/)

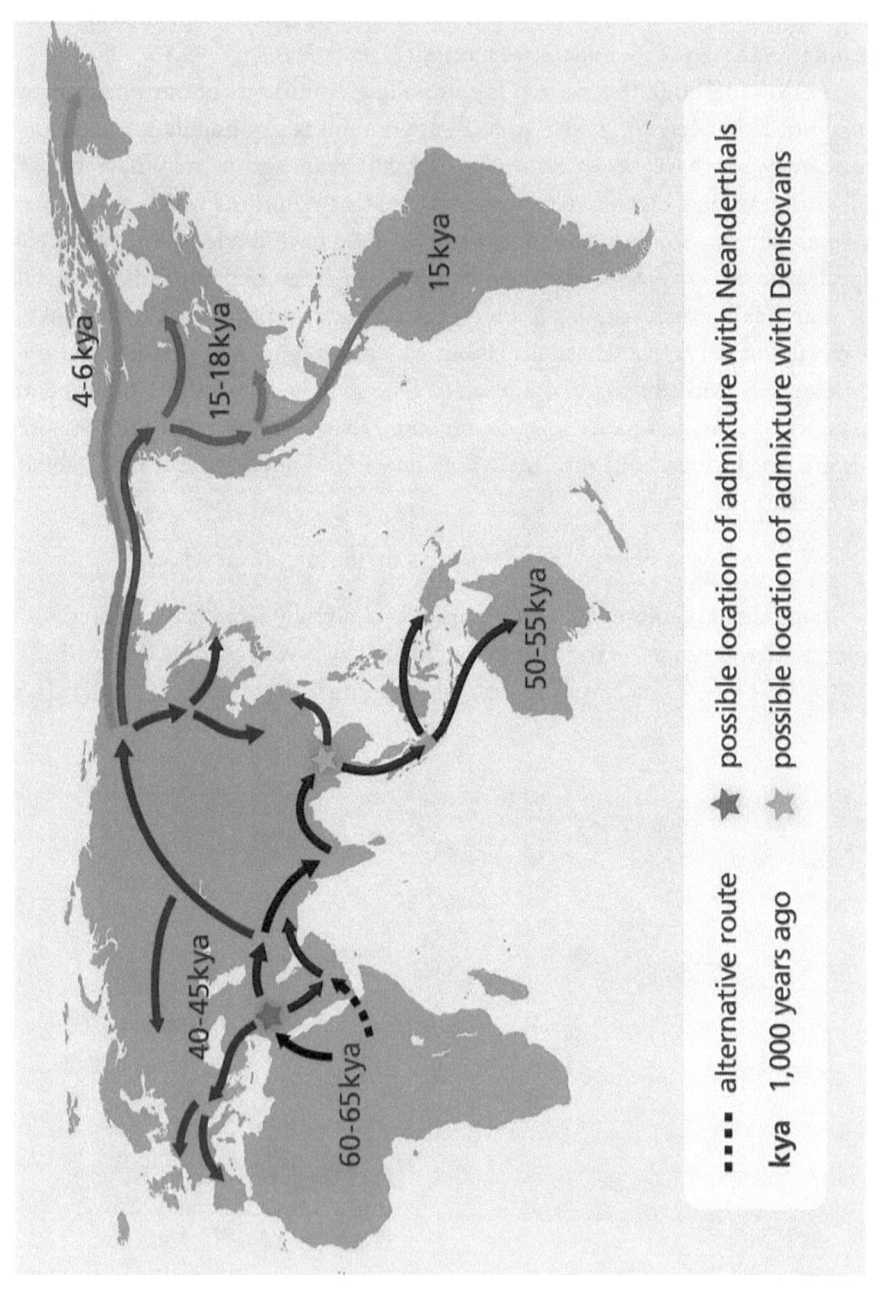

This route seems to be quite feasible in context to a group of *Homo sapiens* migrating from Africa probably by canoes, and some walking their way from the Indian sub-continent and populating Australia around 50–65 thousand years ago.

Fossilised remains and DNA studies suggest that with continued evolution and refinement of our recent ancestors came technological advancements as evident from tools, artefacts, cave paintings and other archaeological finds that our recent ancestors were truly on their way to modernisation. This transformation was more recently around 50,000–65,000 years ago. According to various publications it was not until 10,000 or so years ago that we became us, true societal creatures involved in farming and domesticating animals for food and companionship.

My only concern about this timeline is when we take the Australian First Nations People 'The Australian Aborigines' into the equation, who may have settled on this continent around 60,000 years ago and still inhabit this great southern land. It is quite certain that the present population of the Australian first nation's people had descended from the earlier group of migrants out of Africa, but this must have happened more than 50-55 thousand years ago as reported. Science has already endorsed, that all modern humans share the same genetic makeup with only minute differences contributing to our appearance and health. It does not matter where we are from or what is the colour or our skin and constitutional makeup is, we humans currently residing on this planet Earth are all related. At the risk of inviting controversy, I ask, if this is not enough reason for practicing tolerance and equality in modern society then what is?

From the very early time of our civilisation, soon after we had learned to communicate, we started using our minds to communicate long distances by way of telepathy and thought waves.

These practices are now long gone or may even be extinct as they are no longer needed in our society due to the advent of modern communication and innovations.

Even before the word meditation was coined, a primitive form of meditation was practiced by ancient tribes of men and women who alerted the clans of imminent danger or adverse situations and made them prepared of the impending danger. It has been suggested that as early 200,000 years ago the early humans practiced shamanistic meditation for healing processes (Ref: Rossano, Meditate on It | Science | Smithsonian Magazine https://www.smithsonianmag.com › science-nature › medi…)

I found an interesting publication 'A Timeline of Meditation's History' which gives quite a bit of detailed reference of modern meditation practices and origins. The reference is quite credible and worth the read.

(Ref: The History and Origin of Meditation—PositivePsychology.com https://positivepsychology.com › history-of-meditation)

Timeline	Development	Practices	Origin
5,000 BC–3,500 BC	Early development	The oldest documented evidence of the practice of meditation is wall art in India.	India
1500 BC	Hindu meditation	The Vedas, a large body of religious texts, contains the oldest written mention of meditation.	India
6th–5th century BC	Early development	Development of other forms of meditation in Taoist China and Buddhist India.	China, India
6th century BC	Buddhist Meditation	Siddhartha Gautama sets out to reach Enlightenment, learning meditation in the process.	India
8th century BC	Buddhist Meditation	The expansion of Japanese Buddhism meditation practices spreads into Japan.	Japan
10th–14th century	Christian Meditation	Hesychasm, a tradition of contemplative prayer in the Eastern Orthodox Church, and involves the repetition of the Jesus prayer.	Greece
11th–12th century AD	Islamic Meditation	The Islamic concept of Dhikr is interpreted by various meditative techniques and becomes one of the essential elements of Sufism.	**(Present day Middle East)?**
18th century	Buddhist Meditation	The study of Buddhism in the West remains a topic mainly focused upon by intellectuals.	Europe, America
1936	Western Research	An early piece of scientific research on meditation is published.	America
1950	Buddhist Meditation	The Vipassana movement, or insight meditation, start in Burma.	Burma (Now Myanmar)

1950s	Transcendental Meditation	Maharishi Mahesh Yogi promotes transcendental meditation.	America
1955	Western Research	The first piece of scientific research on meditation using EEGs is published.	**1955?**
1960s	Transcendental Meditation	Swami Rama becomes one of the first yogis to be studied by Western scientists.	America
1970s	Western Research	Jon Kabat-Zinn begins developing a mindfulness program for adults in clinical settings. He calls it mindfulness-based stress reduction (MBSR).	America
1970s	Western Research	Herbert Benson shows the effectiveness of meditation through his research.	America
1977	Western Research	James Funderburk publishes an early collection of scientific studies on meditation.	America
1979	Medical Application	Jon Kabat-Zinn opens the Centre for Mindfulness and teaches mindfulness-based stress reduction to treat chronic conditions.	America
1981	Vipassana Meditation	The first Vipassana meditation centres outside India and Myanmar are established in Massachusetts and Australia.	America, Australia
1996	Modern Meditation	The Chopra Centre for Wellbeing is founded by Deepak Chopra and David Simon.	America
2000	Medical Application	The first major clinical trial of mindfulness with cancer patients is conducted, with results indicating beneficial outcomes for the mindfulness-based stress reduction programs.	America

So, you may ask what the link between meditation and human evolution is. With available theories and views, it can now be inferred that ancient humans practiced some form of rituals around a ring of fire singing, dancing and chanting to connect with each other. Can this be the prelude to the modern form of meditation?

It is now firmly established that our early ancestors *Homo erectus* had invented the controlled use of fire during the early stone ages (Archaeological evidence; Fire Good. Make Human Inspiration Happen—Smithsonian; https://www.smithsonianmag.com › science-nature › fire).

According to Rossano of South-eastern Louisiana University, the shamanistic rituals practiced by our ancient ancestors may have had a positive psychological effects (Ref: Rossano's theories were published in the February Cambridge Archaeological Journal). He also suggested from the available fossil records that anatomically modern humans split from Neanderthals about 200,000 years ago and predicts it was about this time early humans practiced meditation to help heal their sick. Rossano also inferred that the deep focus achieved during such rituals strengthened parts of the brain involved in memory.

Rossano's theories were subsequently studied scientifically by neuroscientist Sara Lazar of Harvard University in 2005 and found that it does have some credibility.

So, a wider inference can be drawn from this that early meditation in the form of shamanistic meditation as practiced by our ancient ancestors may have really helped in the evolution of the complex brain structure of modern humans and helped in attempting to control over their minds.

The power of meditation on our health and well-being has long been known to Indian yogis; several wall art depictions around 5000 BCE shows yogis in a seated posture with eyes closed, as if in a trance, focusing on their inner self: the classic meditative posture as we know it today.

In the Buddhist period around the 6th century BCE, yoga and meditation were well advanced and practiced in daily life. Buddhism is credited for the spread of the modern form of meditation through its doctrines to Far East via the silk route into China, Japan and other trade destinations along the way. Transcendental Meditation Practices became immensely popular in the West in the 1970s when members of the Beatles Band (George, Paul, John and Ringo) became followers of Maharishi Mahesh Yogi who through Transcendental Meditation preached world peace and inner harmony.

Prior to Maharishi Mahesh Yogi it is believed that an Indian yogi Paramhansa Yogananda in 1920s travelled to America and founded Self-Realisation Fellowship. But in my view, it was Swami Vivekananda who defined meditation to the Western World in his first trip to America in 1893. His preaching of philosophy through meditation was simple and remains a guideline to this day. He preached to question our inner self, and an appraisal as to who we are and to practice meditation according to Vedanta and Yoga as a means of enlightening our realisation of the Supreme Being. Swami Vivekananda between 1893 and 1897 had a wide audience both in America and United Kingdom and conducted many lectures both public and private and established yoga, meditation and the teachings from Vedas and Upanishads the ancient Indian philosophical texts.

Meditation was originally thought to have been practiced by the Indian Yogis many thousands of years ago (around 5000 BCE) in a more involved and earthy way. The difference between now and then is that now we practice in the comfort of our homes and meditation studios as a group and at the conclusion it becomes a social event where mingling and exchanges of social pleasantries are a ritual. While the original yogis practiced their meditation in isolation and harsh conditions under a tree or somewhere in caves or ashrams where they could be one with nature and channel their energies and focus on achieving their ultimate goal of attaining Moksha or liberation from the worldly life and become one with the Creator.

Yoga is a form of ancient physical exercise. Many believe that yoga exercises are the meeting point of mind body and soul. By practicing a series of simple body postures in yogic tradition provides us the discipline needed to move forward and unblock any mental blockages.

Anecdotal evidences complimented by some speculative research data generated have found that modern yoga concepts share many common roots with the ancient traditional yoga concepts, and so it seems that the surge of interest in Eastern Philosophy through Eastern yoga techniques in the West in recent times have gained greater traction and popularity.

Also, yoga and yogic postures and practices enhance body flexibility and improve our capacity to control our minds from multidimensional wondering thus promoting a soothing effect on our body mind and soul.

A meeting ground of ancient wisdom and modern psychology.

The word yogi comes from yoga and therefore a yogi is a practitioner of yoga. Yoga and Meditation are like two sides to a coin. The main purpose of yoga is to bring discipline to the body while meditation attempts to discipline the mind. What a strong combination, and imagine if we conquered our physical excesses and the ever-wondering mind, and channelled both powers into the body then we will be able to attain the ever-lasting peace and harmony. Something to aspire for; it takes years of discipline and practice to get to that state of self-realisation.

So, what are the benefits of yoga and meditation?

As you read below you will find many health benefits from regular practice of yoga and meditation; but please keep in mind, that as many mental and physical conditions are medical in nature, they may need medical intervention. Stress is the biggest killer in our modern society; as I see it, living is a health hazard. Too many of us are moving at a rapid pace to keep up with our fast-moving societal needs and changes which many of us find hard to cope with. Money worries, health issues, lack of job satisfaction and peer pressure can lead to instability in family life and aggravate our stress levels which if not controlled can be devastating leading to both mental and physical complications and in extreme situations may cause death.

Stress symptoms: Effects on your body and behaviour—Mayo Clinic: (Ref: www.mayoclinic.org › in-depth › art-20050987)

Effect on our body	Effect on our mood	Effect on our behaviour
Headache	Anxiety	Over and/or under eating
Muscle tension or pain	Restlessness	Angry outbursts
Chest pain	Lack of motivation or focus	Drug or alcohol misuse
Fatigue	Feeling overwhelmed	Tobacco use
Change in sex drive	Irritability or anger	Social withdrawal
Stomach upset	Sadness or depression	Exercising less often

Sleep problems can also be a manifestation of stress. Lack of sleep, restlessness and frequently waking up at night without an underlying health issue must be read as emanating from either a minor disturbance or a deep-seated cause leading to stress-related factors.

Young people sadly are also not spared, and are vulnerable. In a highly competitive society, where there is a constant push and pressure on young people to perform or otherwise be left behind has in many instances resulted in tragedy, some young people taking their own life. We as a society are fully to blame. I really cannot understand the logic behind parents putting insurmountable pressure on their children. In recent times, every parent wants their child to become a lawyer, a doctor or a very highly paid public servant.

What is wrong in letting your child choose his or her own destiny, and who knows that if given a free and clear passage some can become elite in their chosen profession. Not everybody can be a doctor or a lawyer or someone higher up. It is better to have a healthy happy child contributing to the happiness of the family. This will cause less stress on parents who can then concentrate on providing for their family within their means and capability and also enjoy their own life simply being parents. The society will be much better off and many stress-related ailments will gradually be eased.

Well, it is easier said than done, but, if my views can influence a handful of people in the society then I will really think that my writing this book has not gone in vain. I believe in chain reaction in Nature which has a multiplying effect and soon this handful of people multiply in numbers to make a real difference. Wouldn't this make our society a better place for all of us and for our future generations?

Our society has structured itself into several layers of socio-economic status and to the very upper echelon the privileged few it does not really matter how the underprivileged exist. So, the crunch is that it is mostly the haves who have it and the have nots who don't and keep on struggling throughout their lives.

Please don't get me wrong; as I am not professing equality in the socioeconomic structure in its true sense. It will be too ideal for societies, and cannot function smoothly under such conditions.

All I am saying is that there should be some scope for equal opportunity and that preferential treatments should not be at the fore front of our decision-making and or, choice enforcement.

Remember the immortal words of the 3rd President of United States of America Thomas Jefferson that *'All men are created equal'*; the question is, does it still hold and applies to our progressive modern-day society?

Medical Science has provided a number of science-based benefits of yoga and meditation and its validations published in reputable journals.

My reading through some of the published research did provide me with some credible information which are articulated below.

A collaborative study between Harvard Medical School (HMS) and a psychologist at Massachusetts General Hospital's (MGH) Depression Clinical and Research Program has found good evidence in favour of meditation. Although there were some questionable pieces of evidence due to the small sample size of the test subjects, nonetheless I felt comfortable with the findings.

In another reported article 'Mindfulness meditation improves cognition' published in June of 2010, the researchers suggested that 4 days of meditation training can enhance the ability to sustain attention; benefits that have previously been reported with long-term meditators. (Conscious Cogn. 2010 Jun; 19(2):597–60.)

In a recent article (2019) in Behavioural Brain Research, it was published that a brief session of daily meditation enhances attention, memory, mood, and emotional regulation in non-experienced meditators (Behav. Brain Res. 2019 Jan 1; 356:208–220).

Another interesting reading is a publication from Monash University Melbourne 'The Health Benefits of Meditation and Being Mindful' by Dr Craig Hassed MBBS, FRACGP Senior Lecturer Monash University (Australia) Department of General Practice.

Mayo Clinic a reputable research-based organisation in America has also reviewed (in April 2020) various publications on this subject matter and backed the following health benefits achievable from practicing regular meditation. It should however, be noted that, although there are significant numbers of scientific reports and publications which support meditation as providing some of the reported health benefits, some researchers think that due to the lack of hard-core double-blind studies it may not be possible to draw positive conclusions. Yet some researchers with some degree of reservation have suggested that meditation may have some value in assisting people in the management of the following conditions such as:

- Anxiety
- Asthma
- Cancer
- Chronic pain
- Depression
- Heart disease
- High blood pressure
- Irritable bowel syndrome
- Sleep problems
- Tension headaches

The degree of benefits received may vary from person to person and could be very subjective rather than objective. Traditional medical assessments may become necessary for complex medical conditions and must not be neglected at any cost.

My own experience dictates that yoga and meditation need not be very intensive and involved procedures in the beginning, and as soon as the benefits are realised we can formulate our own routine. Especially for a young disturbed mind it can only be a good thing; so why not give it a go. Another thing I found in this regard most rewarding is to spend a little time for our own-selves sitting quietly late in the evening and gazing skywards at the universe, and realising that in the scheme of things we are so tiny and insignificant; but, if we can let go of our mind thinking of the universal vastness then, will this not give us scope to broaden our minds just as the ancient Rishis and Munis (people with wisdom) did through yoga and meditation so many millennia ago.

The upside to all this is we can also spend this quiet time to do some **Pranayama,** a modern-day version of the ancient breathing technique to cleanse our internal organs and let them breathe. Pranayama is an ancient word for an ancient technique, which has now created a lot of interest not only in the Eastern Philosophy but also in the Western practices of meditation and breathing exercises.

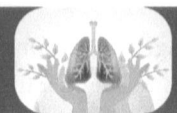

Chapter 2

PRANAYAMA AND THE CONCEPT OF 'OM' (THE PHILOSOPHY OF KEEPING WELL)

Om is considered to be the most ancient sound of the universe, linked with the primordial sound that the universe emitted at the time of its creation; a time immemorial.

– Jay Das, 2021

Origin:

Pranayama is a Sanskrit word combining 'Prana' meaning life-giving 'Breath' and 'Ayama' meaning 'Extending or Expanding'. So, Pranayama would mean extending or expanding your Prana through the life-giving breath. It is the science of life forces extension through the power of breathing; inhaling and exhaling in an organised way.

There are many scientific facts about our respiratory system; each and every cell in our body needs a supply of steady stream of oxygen for us to stay alive. In the breathing process, we inhale oxygen and exhale toxic waste majority of which constitutes carbon dioxide. Our rate of breathing is a good indicator of our heart rate and physical well-being.

A steady rate of breathing in indicates efficient use of oxygen in our body to fuel our cellular organisation, for the uptake by our brain cells for improved mental processes and for rejuvenation of our body systems and organs to perform their tasks effectively and efficiently.

In ancient Vedic times, yogis were trained in the art of meditation and pranayama; they had quite strict guidelines as to the techniques, when and where to do pranayama, how long should they do it for, etc. Now it has a bit different concept from its origin. Different yoga and pranayama studios have their own set of rules and procedures. But whatever the modern concepts are it is absolutely necessary to maintain a proper technique which has been passed on for generations as inscribed in the ancient Vedic texts.

Pranayama was developed as an ancient art or a series of breathing exercises which allows the body to breathe in oxygen in plentiful without any strenuous physical movement. The technique of inhaling and exhaling is very important, and a regular pattern needs to be maintained throughout a session. The session could be of 5–10 minutes duration for the beginners or longer if comfortable with the procedures.

Although simple in technique, the benefits gained are worthwhile. Some practitioners of pranayama are strict with their rituals and prefer the conditions to be perfect such as sitting in a lotus position and keeping the spinal contour in an upright position. In my opinion, if that can be maintained, it is good but for the beginners, it is desired that a comfortable posture and procedure may be maintained which can be improved with time and practice. For seniors is perfectly alright to be seated in a chair in an upright position, the important thing that matters is concentrating on the breathing (inhaling and exhaling) technique. So, what is the technique?

If you are a right-handed person then using the right thumb, block the right nostril and breathe in gently through your left nostril as deep as you can then block it with your ring finger and hold it in for around 5 seconds or so, just a slow mental count will do. Release the breath or exhale slowly and gently. Pause in between breathing and repeat the breathing exercise through your other nostril and so on. If you are a left-handed person, then do the opposite. Now, there is another technique of exhaling the held breath; this is a little bit more aggressive as in the exhaling procedure a forceful expulsion of held breath in smaller frequencies is required.

This allows the toxins and the carbon dioxide to be purged out of the respiratory system giving a greater chance of more oxygen to assimilate in the pulmonary region of our body. I have heard of people who are into pranayama mentioning that there is a simpler way to this technique. You breathe in as you would do in either of the two techniques as above and continually keep breathing in through one nostril blocking the other nostril and then releasing the blocked nostril, you breathe out. This frequent breathing in and breathing out while blocking one nostril or another will create turbulence thus helping the passage way to be less cluttered with mucus if you have sinus and or a stuffy nose.

However, please note that it is absolutely important that you have a professional health check to determine your suitability for performing pranayama breathing exercises and in the event of asthma or other respiratory issues exert caution and heed the medical advice.

What are the benefits of pranayama? A lot I have been told.

- It brings clarity of mind and makes our thought process more rational and sensible.
- Improves the supply and utilisation of oxygen, helps circulation and energises the body.
- Increases the lung capacity.
- Increases the metabolic rate.
- It clears the congestion in the nasal passage-way thus helps relieving sinuses and facilitating a clear flow of energy.
- It stimulates the organs of the respiratory system.
- Re-energises the nervous system and brain cells.
- Uplifts the functioning of the digestive system which in turn improves nutrient absorption, assimilation and waste elimination.

There are both, anecdotal evidence and few science-based publications which do report the benefits of pranayama and yoga. Some of the reports are cited below for your further exploration in this matter if you are interested:

Interestingly enough there are several types of pranayama as we advance through the basic breathing techniques and posture modulations. But it is more important to start at the basics and then advance to the more intricate pranayama techniques which may need professional guidance of yoga and pranayama teachers.

Slow and fast pranayama? Without stirring the pot too much let's look at simplistic formats. Slow pranayama encourages pranayama techniques using slow breathing while fast pranayama explores the benefits of breathing rapidly but steadily and expelling the held breath in more frequent, rapid bursts. All pranayama including slow and rapid types are beneficial in improving the respiratory functions in both elderly people and normal young healthy adults of both genders improving not only respiratory efficiency but also general health. Additionally, fast pranayama has additional effects on sensory-motor performance (i.e. faster auditory and visual reaction time; Ref: J Clin Diagn Res 2014 Jan; 8(1): 10–13).

Modern living and lifestyle are known to produce various physical and psychological stresses resulting in increased blood pressure and heart rate. This can lead to increased myocardial oxygen demand.

It was concluded based on a clinical study (Ref: Int J Appl Basic Med Res 2014 Jul; 4(2):67–71) that pranayama produces a relaxed state; and in this state parasympathetic activity overrides sympathetic activity. Hence, the addition of pranayama can be a useful adjunct to antihypertensive drugs for better control of hypertension in mild hypertensives.

Our body's network of parasympathetic nervous system (PSNS) primarily is entrusted to relax our body during the times of stress. It is a part of our autonomic system which is required to keep basic body functions operating. The sympathetic nerve system (SNS) network has an opposite role to the parasympathetic system activities but both systems complement each other. In a nutshell, the SNS receives signals from the brain to alert the body of imminent or impending danger or required activity while the PSNS carries out those messages and completes those activities; for example, if the light is too bright the SNS may send signals to the PSNS to fully or partially close your eyes as there may be a danger to the eyes from excess light and the PSNS complies with required activity.

In simple terms, pranayama may be viewed as an additional tool in providing relief in mild stress-related symptoms.

Further reading references:
- Pranayama Benefits for Physical and Emotional Health (www.healthline.com).
- Benefits of pranayama (www.fitsri.com).
- Exploring the Therapeutic Benefits of Pranayama (Int J Yoga. 2020 May–Aug; 13(2): 99–110).
- What Is Pranayama?—WebMD (Ref: www.webmed.com; health and balance) ...And more.

One of the earliest references to Pranayama is in verse 4.29 of the Bhagwat Gita:

"Still others, who are inclined to the process of breath restraint to remain in trance, practice by offering the movement of the outgoing breath into the incoming, and the incoming breath into the outgoing, and thus at last remain in trance, stopping all breathing. Others, curtailing the eating process, offer the outgoing breath into itself as a sacrifice." (Ref: Bhagwat Gita 4.29 with commentaries of Ramanuja, Madhva, Shankara and others).

Other references have been given in old Indian texts such as Yoga Sutras of Patanjali (verses 2.49–2.53 around 200BC), Hatha Yoga (around 15th century AD), etc.

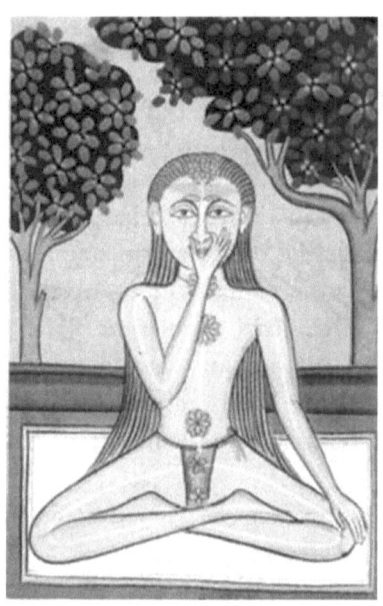

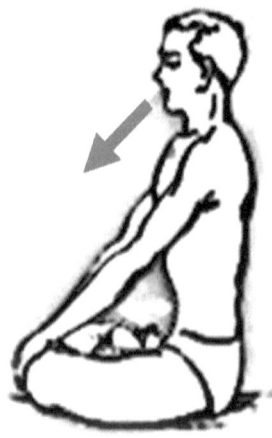
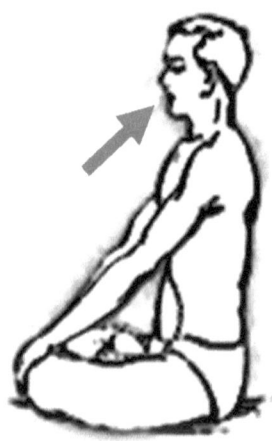

Exhaling **In haling**

Picture of an ancient yogi practicing the art of Pranayama

(Gratefully referenced: https://www.meaus.com/hatha-yoga-pradipika.htm)

The Concept of 'OM':

I often very strongly ponder on the concept and philosophy of **'OM'**. A word that has been very deeply embedded into the broader Hindu philosophy. Where did it come from and what are its origins? In my opinion, there may not be any religious connotation or implications associated with this word, and **'OM'** depicts a word or sound which holds a deeper essence a deeper inner meaning in **Life and Living,** and in all aspects of our health and wellbeing. This I will elaborate on as we navigate through the concept.

A popular view is that the sound of **'OM'** has also been linked with the primordial sound that the universe emitted at the time of its creation; a time immemorial. I do not know the validity of this theory however, my curiosity on this matter has been immense. In order to find out a bit more about the sound of **'OM'** and the universal sound emitted during the Big Bang, I came across a very potent and powerful point of view put forth by **Shiang Ying**, a Yoga teacher and Yoga therapist, in an article she wrote:

(Ref: https://shiangyingdotcom.wordpress.com/2013/08/25/om-or-aum/)

'OM or AUM? The Universe Has an Answer' (AUGUST 25, 2013; BY SHIANG YING).

Since then, I have read several articles and heard comparative sounds of collectively chanting the word 'OM' and heard simulated recordings of the sounds of the Big Bang; one such example can be heard in the following reference; (The Sound of the Big Bang, Planck Version (2013) John G. Cramer Professor of Physics University of Washington Seattle, WA 98195–1560).

It was immensely interesting to me at least, to understand the ingenuity of dedicated scientists that they could reproduce 14 billion years old residual cosmic sound frozen in time for us to hear and marvel upon. The other interesting aspect again, to me, was, the similarity of the depth in the pitch of yogis chanting **'OM'** in deep sound and the recordings of the simulated cosmic sound which sounded like a constant humming; very similar to the group chanting of the **'OM'** mantra.

Could there be any truth in that the ancient Munis, Rishis and the yogis were thinking alike only one difference is that they took spirituality into context and tweaked it with philosophy, while modern science is still searching for the absolute truth. A simple example in consideration is that modern science tells us that the universe has been expanding since the day of its creation and still expanding. While the sages of ancient times whose thoughts and theories have been recorded in writings in the great philosophical texts Vedas and Upanishads enunciate that the practices of yoga and chanting the spiritual mantra **'OM'** was a vehicle for expanding their mind and thought processes. Maintenance of these rituals continuously claimed to have not only expanded but also enlightened their universe; could this possibly be their interpretation of the physical expansion of the universe as we know it now. These great sages of the past, the Yogis, Munis and the Rishis also gave a spiritual sense and meaning to the universe as an interaction of Nature with Mankind which emitted vibes breathing life into all of their surroundings and in all the beings.

In the words of German philosopher Arthur Schopenhauer Upanishads, are the texts of the 'highest human wisdom'.

As I understand, **OM** is the original mantra (in Hindu philosophy), an embodiment of all three supreme forces of **Nature** namely **Creation (Brahma)**, **Preservation (Vishnu)** and **Destruction (Mahesh)**.

The word **'OM'** has its origins in the ancient Vedic Sanskrit; Vedas are ancient Hindu scriptures which have their roots from the earliest history of civilisation to even now and has a much deeper meaning than what it is perceived to be.

My reason for dwelling on this matter is merely to provide a philosophical outlook, a way or a sense to focus and concentrate on the job at hand so that we may be able to put some positivity in our lives, particularly in the present. Simply chanting the mantra **'OM'** may be enough to allow our mind and thoughts to be in unison to capture the essence and power of nature and help us to steady our footing in this wide world.

'OM' is where science meets philosophy.

Space scientists are in general agreement that the age of the universe is around 13–14 billion years. Human civilisation under this astronomical term is like a fleeting moment of time. Since its birth, the Universe is in a continuous phase of expansion and still continuing to expand. We as a civilisation have a long way to go.

'OM' is a Vedic Mantra which when chanted in unison emits a vibrational energy which many philosophers have compared to the pulse of the Universe since the earliest of times. Could it be that the Munis and Rishis of ancient times knew about this vibrational energy and knew of its inner healing powers?

In modern times, it has been cited that chanting of 'OM' emits sound which has been measured to be vibrating at the frequency of 432 Hz which is at a similar frequency found in all things throughout Nature.

Is this just coincidental or there is some spiritual or divine intervention? So, chanting the 'OM' mantra with reverence brings us closer to Nature and connects us to all beings around us and thus gives us the healing power from nature. In fact, it has been long known that given time our bodies do heal themselves as evident from writings in ancient texts on the uses of herbs and plant preparations.

There are hundreds of anecdotal pieces of evidence reported of the health benefits from chanting the mantra **'OM'.** Yet the scientific verifications are only few.

Why?

It is not a glamourous topic for hard core scientific community to spend their resources on; however, there are some scientific reports verifying the benefits. As a trained biochemist myself the absolute truth is yet to be found. Some of the claims made may seem to be a bit farfetched, by the disbelievers. I am sure that if some research interests are focused on this subject, then there may be some truth and possibilities.

So, what are the benefits?

I have been told that chanting **'OM'** for those who believe in it, offers several benefits; from my personal experience, first and foremost it relaxes you and gradually brings down your stress levels.

It helps you to focus on yourself and your surroundings and builds up your inner strength.

Improves your power of speech, confidence and clarity.

This is particularly significant to us senior citizens as in our advancing ages we begin to lose some of our faculties and speech impairment. At this age, we really need to be heard, and speech is an important tool that elevates our power of persuasion and mediation.

I found some interesting medical claims for which there are plausible explanations; such as by chanting **'OM'** on a regular basis and with concentration and reverence following benefits could be achieved. Cardiovascular benefits such as normalisation of blood pressure and regulation of heartbeats.

I have no doubt that meditation along with **'OM'** mantra chanting produces vibrational energy which flows through our bodies bringing them into a deep state of relaxation. It is well recognised medically that relaxation and calming of the body has a significant and measurable effect on our blood pressure and heartbeat and therefore a positive effect on the heart and its normal functions. This is assuming that there are no underlying causes which require medical intervention. There are several other health benefits that are anecdotally reported which may have some validity.

In a study entitled 'Neurohemodynamic correlates of "OM" chanting' (Ref: Int J Yoga 2011 Jan–Jun; 4(1): 3–6), it was concluded and I quote: "The neurohemodynamic correlates of 'OM' chanting indicate limbic deactivation. As similar observations have been recorded with vagus nerve stimulation treatment used in depression and epilepsy, the study findings argue for a potential role of this 'OM' chanting in clinical practice."

Strong conclusion indeed. I do not have much doubt about the validity of this study as the materials and method used in the study were relatively standard. Functional Magnetic Resonance Imaging of the OM chanting of right-handed healthy volunteers was examined in this study.

Recently, I stumbled upon an article (Mantra Medicine: the health benefits of meditation backed by science) by Suvi Mahonen, a Surfer's Paradise (Queensland, Australia) based journalist. The article has some positive arguments and I have no hesitation in recommending it as a further bedtime read.

Exploring further on this subject I found several research articles which seemed to be quite credible; one such research is summarised below a 2011 study published in Psychiatry Research lead by a team of Harvard-affiliated researchers at Massachusetts General Hospital. In this eight-week mindfulness meditation programme, researchers were able to determine measurable changes in brain regions associated with memory, sense of self, empathy, and stress.

Magnetic Resonance Images were taken of the brain structure of 16 study participants two weeks before and after they took part in the eight-week Mindfulness-Based Stress Reduction (MBSR) Program.

The conclusions were quite positive and measurable signs of improvement in the grey matter density of the brain (amygdala) which plays an important role in anxiety and stress was noticed. Interestingly enough none of these changes were seen in the control group, indicating that they had not resulted merely from the passage of time.

Chanting the **'OM'** mantra the proper way requires some efforts; it is considered to be a primordial sound which has been practiced by mankind over several thousands of years. During chanting one must control breathing by taking a deep breath hold for a few seconds then exhale. The inhaling and the exhaling part have some scientific validation as it involves a cleansing action of the lungs thus increasing oxygenation of the blood resulting in enhanced tissue oxygenation and nutritional fortification. Purified blood has more capacity to carry oxygen and nutrients to all tissues in the body thus promoting a healing and detoxification process.

This increases the body's power of self-healing and increases immunity. Besides the breathing aspect **'OM'** has a specific mantra chant involving a deep vibrational sound through the vocal cord and the paranasal sinuses which are hollow cavities around the temple zone and the nose. The vibrations produced during intense chanting clears the airways connected to our sinuses draining the excess mucus and other trapped debris through the nose.

Now, chanting **'OM'** is also thought to strengthen the muscles supporting the spinal cord hence improving the posture. How it does I am not sure but the deep-pitched vibrational sound of the chant could have some influence on the abdomen muscle. The abdomen muscle and the back muscle which forms part of the core muscle are responsible for keeping our body firm and assist in keeping our body's upright posture stable and balanced.

Scientific journals are scattered with publications, some have merit worth further exploring and many more are just linked to anecdotal observations. I urge the readers to judge for themselves and decide if they are benefited from such practices. Sometimes it is very hard to give scientific credence to empirical and anecdotal pieces of evidence but nonetheless these pieces of evidence deep down have some meaning and value which should not be discarded.

Swami Vivekananda explains "Om represents the whole phenomena of sound production. As such, it must be the natural symbol, the matrix of all the various sounds. It denotes the whole range and possibility of all the words that can be made." Or, simply it is one sound which is the fundamental sound of all humankind.

Meditation and chanting a mantra give a new meaning to self-realisation. It trains your mind and increases your power of concentration and lessens your stress level, negative thoughts and prepares you to soldier on in life. It is always a good sense to control your feelings and emotions, meditation helps you to do that and prepares you to be aware of your surroundings. However, it is a lot easier said than done; it takes a lot of self-discipline, practice and commitment, but the end result is rewarding... good health, a relaxed mental state and an overall positive outlook in life which we all aspire for and many can only dream of.

Our Planet Earth, from pole to pole (North Pole to South Pole) is energised due to the Earth's magnetic field. Although we do not feel the effect of such magnetism, it is important to realise that as the human body is made up of many atoms and elements it is not unusual that electronic vibrations emanating from our body also have a certain vibrational frequency.

Any imbalance in our vibrational energy may cause a significant concern to our health and well-being.

Deep breathing exercises, e.g., Pranayama, yoga and meditation have the power to improve our vibrational energy and unblock our chakras for the smooth flow of energy.

The human body is a living energy field and every change in our discipline e.g., mood, health conditions, anxiety, depression lack of sleep all have a cumulative effect on this energy field which can cause a disruption in the smooth energy flow essential for our simple harmonic balance. This disruption may also cause an imbalance in our homeostasis; although this has not yet been scientifically validated.

Our Energy Chakras:

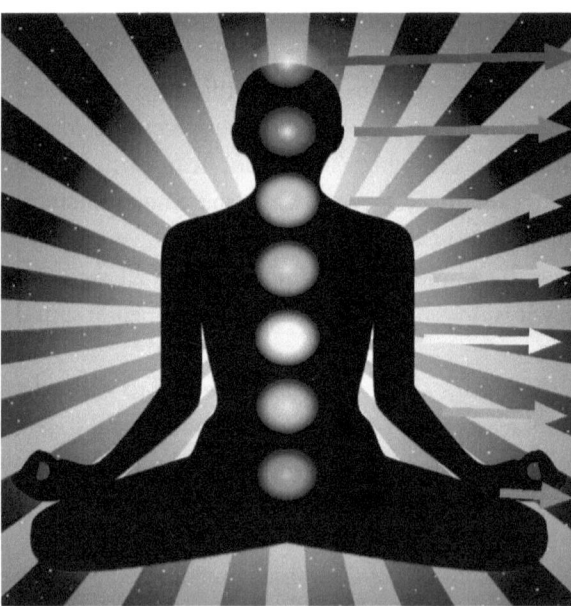

1. Crown
2. Third Eye
3. Throat
4. Heart
5. Solar Plexus
6. Sacral
7. Root

According to ancient Vedic wisdom our body has seven energy points which are called Chakras. The new age philosophy and current knowledge define these chakras as energy centres which control specific parts of our nervous system associated with specific organs.

Chakras are energy centres which when balanced, facilitate the flow of unhindered energy through our body, creating harmony and calmness and contributing to our general health and well-being.

The concept of Chakras is ancient and comes from the old Sanskrit texts.

'The Vedas' originated around 1500 BC some say even more ancient. Each of these Chakras has a fixed location and the energy flow is specific to that particular area of the body and the organs contained.

Chakras literally mean wheel or round shape and therefore can efficiently channel the energy flow. Each chakra has an energy centre called the nucleus or 'Prana' in Sanskrit, a source of pure energy ready and available for the healing power from the healer or our healthy self (**Heal-thy-self**).

As an organic body, our power of self-healing comes from this central energy which is the 'Prana' meaning life.

These Chakras start at the base of the spine to the top of the head. Each Chakra is related to the endocrine system which allows us to experience physical or emotional symptoms relating to each energy centre.

Out of balance Chakras can negatively impact our physical and mental health and interfere with our spiritual and emotional stability. Balancing the Chakras also gives us a peaceful closure of long-standing emotional hurt and paves the way to a healthy and happy life. At least, this is the belief from the ancient Hindu scriptures 'The Vedas' and also from the yogic philosophies of the past.

It must be said that balancing your Chakras and maintaining them is not an easy task as they are not tangible entities. On our planet Earth, every object has an energy component and a directional flow. This energy is a small part which is radiated from the Sun to the Earth and travels as electromagnetic waves through Earth's atmosphere.

As I have mentioned with respect to Earth's energy, every object on Earth has its share in the form of potential energy which is a stored energy in all objects and kinetic energy which is the energy generated when the stationary object begins to move. So, the stationary objects do not generate the kinetic energy but we do due to our continual movements.

I think in the derivation of ancient concepts of Chakras, the modern concepts of potential and kinetic energies are a perfect fit giving rise to the seven Chakra energy points located in the seven strategic sections of our body.

Therefore, I believe that locating the Chakras is not a difficult task and we all should be able to do that, however, balancing is not as easy as it may seem.

In a very simple and un-intrusive way, if we consider the seven locations of the chakra, we may even be able to pinpoint the blocked Chakra by looking out for any recurring health issues or any discomfort in a particular Chakra area, which may then symbolise a blockage.

For example, if you notice that your self-esteem has been low in the recent days or you lack in decision making or you have lost your fighting spirits then your Chakra number 3, **The Solar Plexus** may be out of balance. This may also be evident from the discomfort or pain felt in the stomach-navel region of your body.

The Chart below reflects some of the issues felt in relation to the Chakra blockages.

Balancing Chakras and restoring their harmonious energy flow is more involved and requires proper training and practice. Everyday stress and lifestyle processes may just be sufficient in draining energy from Chakras and therefore Chakra balancing may also need everyday maintenance.

Simple practices such as:

Yoga and meditation.

Breathing exercises (as in yogic Pranayama)

Improved diet and nutrition and the use of supplements to invigorate your body systems (e.g., digestive, nervous, circulatory, etc.) may offer some benefits.

The effectiveness of your unblocked balanced Chakras will show up as your improved attitude to life. You should feel better, relaxed, and experience high energy levels and increased vitality.

Working on your steadiness and posture will also help, remember an unblocked Chakra should allow un-hindered flow of energy through the body for its stability.

There are many different techniques and all may have many benefits to offer us. Some of us may find a particular technique suitable and compatible with our physique and constitution and get significant benefits; stick with the system you can relate to and draw out all the goodness from it to nurture your body and mind.

For seniors, I believe the breathing techniques are more appropriate and allow the techniques of pranayama and meditation in one sitting.

How?

I prefer to practice the pranayama in the quietness of the evenings. Being of senior age myself I cannot compose myself into a lotus or a cross-legged posture or even sitting on my heels and balancing the body to an upright straight posture, so, I opt for an easy solution sitting on a firm high back chair. You could do the same if you feel that you are not up to the special pranayama postures. Be mindful of your breathing techniques and do not overdo; these exercises are meant to be practiced smoothly and consistently and on a regular basis if you are serious about it.

In any form of exercise not involving weights and equipment, it is necessary to adhere to some basics concerning with physical status and environmental issues, some of these are outlined below.

It is also important that your sessions are distraction free.

Some yoga and pranayama teachers require the exercises to be done on an empty stomach, but I feel it may not be a critical requirement so long as you don't feel bloated and heavy. A lighter body will help with your breathing techniques.

Choose an area which is well-ventilated.

Select a comfortable position, and position yourself such that your body neck and posture are in an upright and firm configuration.

Relax your body keeping your shoulders in a horizontal position without stooping.

Your spine along with your head and neck should be firm and straight.

Keep your eyes closed to build your concentration levels up.

Do the exercises regularly and dress comfortably so breathing will not affect your tightness and efforts.

Crown Chakra
Head, brain and associated areas. Responsible for our emotional state, knowledge, conscience, etc.

Third Eye Chakra
Eyes, forehead, sinus areas. Mainly concerned with our awareness and Sensitivity issues.

Throat Chakra
Throat, thyroid and upper respiratory area. Expression of thought, creativity and to express ourselves.

Heart Chakra
It is mainly involved with the region of the heart, circulation and upper part of the body such as arms shoulders, etc. It guides our love, close relationships, stability and balance.

Solar Plexus Chakra
It is located in the abdomen area just above the navel. It influences our digestive organs, spinal cord, liver and also pancreas. So, apart from digestive issues it also has an effect on our self-control and esteem and helps us regain control or hold on ourselves when feeling down and low.

Sacral Chakra
Is located in the vicinity of lower abdomen and just under the navel area. It has a profound effect on our sexual feelings, reproduction and intimate relationships.

Root Chakra
Also, known as the Muladhara Chakra (the main flow) in Sanskrit, it is located in the coccyx at the base of the spine and is a manifestation of the lower part of the body, physical stability and with adrenal gland for fight or flight and the sense of community, security and emotional stability.

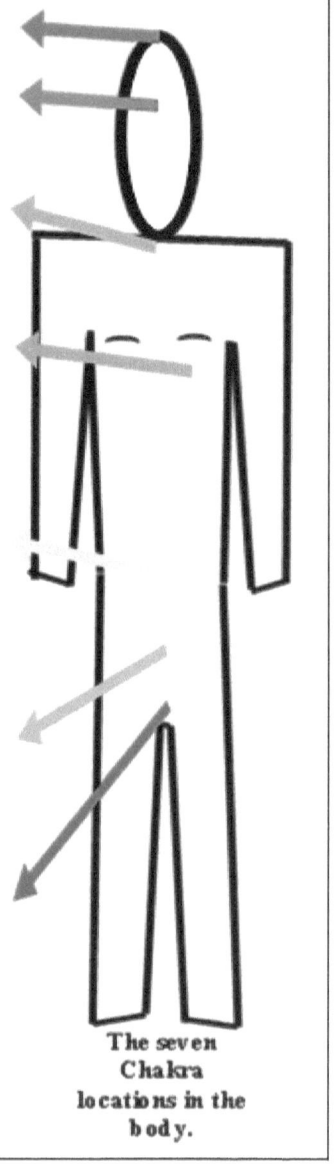

The seven Chakra locations in the body.

Although Chakras may not have any scientific basis attached to their credentials but as a mind science there are many significant evidences and interpretations attached to their meaningful existence. There are many things in life that may not be explained by science but to many of us who have had direct positive or negative experiences with those life events, a simple and plausible explanation exists in believable form; it all makes sense.

Table: Chakra Location and Fulfilment

The Root Chakra	Located at the base of the Coccyx at the tail-bone joint	The Root Chakra is the foundation of our physical body. It delivers a feeling of safety, stability and balance to our lives	An out of balance root chakra can be the main cause of in-security. Lack of confidence and the feeling of lack of purpose in life.
The Sacral Chakra	Energy point for this Chakra is located in the pelvic region below the navel	This opens up our emotions and creativity	An imbalance may cause frustrations, lack of creative energy, suffering from desires and emotional fatigue.
The Solar Plexus Chakra	Located in the Stomach region above the navel	This chakra opens up our Powerful self and brings out the warrior in us	Low self-esteem, anger, Failure to make decisions and accept challenges. Self-doubt.
The Heart Chakra	Around the Chest Cavity in the Heart region	This Chakra energy point invigorates everything to with heart; love, compassion empathy	Lack of forgiveness and hatred & jealousy for others. Fear of betrayal and rejection.
The Throat Chakra	Middle of the neck the Throat area	This chakra opens up for the smooth energy flow to develop our personality	An open throat chakra enables our free spirit to communicate and speak our feelings with truth and courage.
The Third Eye Chakra	Right between the Eye Brows	Controls our perception and our intuitions. This Chakra opens up our third dimension and the sixth senses	The third eye is the window to our inner soul and our intuition. A blocked chakra will be like working with our blind senses.
The Crown Chakra	Located right at the top of the head	The Crown Chakra is our Spiritual self and our Ego. This energises our head not heart and opens up our higher consciousness.	Crown Chakra is our connection to the universe and our own spirituality. It is the king chakra and sits right on top of our head and asserts as to who we are.

The overall wellness is largely dependent on our health condition which dictates our state of mind, attitude to life and our conduct towards others.

When our health is good and less stressful, then it is rosy all around and we ooze positivity. This is contagious and vibrates through the surroundings and people around us, and they catch it too. So, the benefits are enormous and as the saying goes "If you are smiling the whole world smiles with you." Alternatively, when you are feeling down and in the dumps, it is best to overcome it as soon as possible otherwise if you brood over it, it will get hold of you and infect others.

So, try not to spread it around as your negativity may catch on to your close associates and consequences felt widely. It is strange that bad news or bad vibes travel faster, and good news takes time to spread. It is generally weaker minds latch on to negativity quicker and are more prone to the ill effects that go with it.

Usually, weaker minds are keen to spread it around more so to get some notoriety. I am not in any shape or form condemning our weaker minds and negative consequences; we all are individuals and go through a lean period in life and also have pre-conceived ideals on how to tackle life's problems, ups and downs when these situations arise. All I am elaborating is on the well-known phrase "empty mind is a devil's playground or devil's workshop," so why not be creative and constructive helping yourselves helping others and spread the positivity around.

In the words of the famous martial artist the late and great Bruce Lee "Empty your mind be formless, shapeless like water." Unfortunately, Bruce Lee passed away too early in life.

Wellness and well-being are the central focal points within our psyche. It may be a hypothetical objective in life, or, in some, it can be a practical aspiration that defines one's character and attitude not only to one's self but also to others. As I had mentioned in the beginning wellness to me is our mind body and soul all gelled into one to shine all that is good in us.

I found a great article from the University of Colorado which caught my eyes; it captured the philosophy of wellness in depicting life's constant struggle with various dimensions.

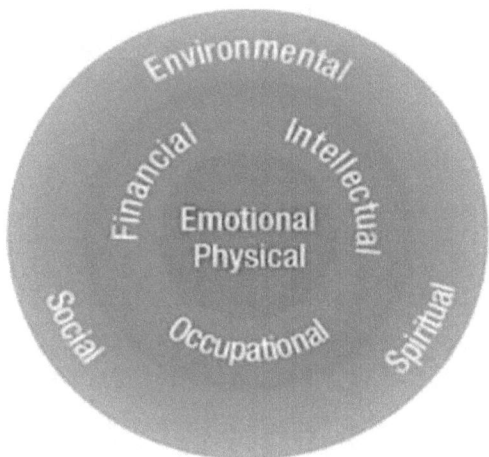

Eight Dimensions of Wellness

(Ref: Behavioural Health and Wellness Program.
Department of Psychiatry, University of Colorado Anschutz Medical Campus) bh.wellness@ucdenver.edu

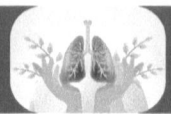

Chapter 3

PREPAREDNESS, COMMITMENT AND PLANNING (THE PHILOSOPHY OF KEEPING WELL)

Be realistic, inventive, and sincere; show empathy not sympathy.
– Jay Das, 2021

Mental Preparedness and Planning

Before proceeding and advancing to undertake a programme of any nature, there should be a thorough preparedness and planning for what lay ahead. It not only makes you aware of the journey you are about to undertake but also warns you of the pit falls along the way and constantly reminds you of your goals and objectives.

To complete this journey can be an arduous task and not recommended for all, but something of a challenge you and your conscious mind can soldier on with. You will be far more equipped if you prepare for this journey of keeping well and open to self-realisation.

Commitment is the key word.

It is a very individual thing; young children when they prepare for an exam, use different techniques, some cram the important bits from the book hoping that exam questions will be relevant to the chapters they have prepared…yes, it is a bit risky.

On the other hand, some will scan through the whole book and try to categorise similar bits of information; analyse and digest. Also, by process of memorising and regurgitating at the appropriate moment is a masterful technique. I can remember in my early teen in one of the exams papers in biology I had to respond to a question which I had never come across or at least I couldn't remember, but as I had scanned relevant bits of information it was embedded into my subconscious memory which I luckily could produce timely in an appropriate manner.

Your subconscious repository is a storage of infinite amounts of events and happenings in your life and plays a very important role allowing you to develop a myriad of skills useful in your subsequent issues if you are able to timely reproduce the relevancy.

I am merely enunciating common approaches to harnessing skills development in our progression to preparedness for a project before diving into boots and all.

It is one thing to be aware of a project the nitty-gritty of it, and, to know about your project; what it is, your commitments and how you are going to tackle it. Let alone think about what you are going to get out of it and how long you are going to commit to achieve your desired outcome.

In my view, there are 4 objectives:

Be Committed.

Strike a Balance.

Be Innovative.

Be Realistic.

Other things will fall into place such as goal setting and goal kicking. You judge your success by counting how many goals you have kicked not missed. In the relevancy of the topic we are discussing, you are the sole judge; do not allow others to judge you by counting the goals you have kicked or missed.

Your achievements are based only upon your satisfaction, answerable to none.

This is an individual quest and you are the lord or the lady of all you survey.

We have still not navigated entirely through mental preparedness and planning. We need to incorporate the practicality of all this because it is the practicality which will guide us to our destination. Our preparedness comes from mental stability and attitude. The focal point of consideration which is controlled by our mind, needs to be our goal or target. The power of the mind gives us control of the thought process, it really has a firm grip on stepwise action we need to take in our mental preparedness.

If we give it a serious thought, we will soon realise that it is simply a question of **If**, **How** and **When** of the various stages of our mental preparedness that is under consideration.

There are no **Buts** and no **Can't Do's**.

If, control our fears; are we going to succeed or fail **How,** is the processing side of it?

When, is the execution?

All these keywords must be made to work in unison and it is our duty to have full control in bringing then together to make it all happen.

Once we have addressed and understood the preparedness aspect, we need to address the planning side of things which combines **if, how and when**. How will the planning work; we will need to make some adjustments in our daily activities that we engage in and combine any free or additional time we can organise to devote it to the project so that there is a routine that we can follow and carry through. The importance of this is really our challenge. Depending of course on the level of the commitment we are prepared to make. To plan effectively allocate a time of the day that you can commit to and stick with it, unless, it is absolutely necessary for any sudden or unexpected changes that may be required to be made. Do not convert any temporary change into a permanent one unless it is absolutely necessary. Frequent changes introduce the element of uncertainty, relaxed attitude and lack of discipline. Discipline is the key to success for any project that we undertake at various stages of our lives.

Ok, so we have committed to the planning; just one thing, do not force unnecessary burden or undertake a commitment that you cannot keep, so, be relaxed and mindful about it and commit only to what will come naturally to you or you can handle.

The first step of our journey is to select a time of the day. It sounds quite a bit regimented; it does not have to be like that. But, for all projects, an early commitment is good as it shows us the pathway to adhere to, and once that commitment is realised then it may be streamlined as you go along and as you require making slight changes here and there to adapt to your particular situation and circumstances. One thing to be very mindful of is not to overdo it and control your commitment in a way that you can handle things easily.

Rewards should be appreciable and noticeable as you could find yourself not being troubled by minor ailments, aches and pains flu and cold symptoms which could have been a cause of your frequent complaints from time to time. Pill popping seems to be a common habit in many people at the slightest hint of bodily discomfort; I am not in favour of this, but in health situations which are difficult to manage I am all in favour of medical intervention. A quick evaluation by your physician or general practitioner could only be a good thing.

My choice has been that in the cases of mild symptoms of aches, pains and flu to try and weather the storm in a natural way by taking the required rest and sometimes if need be, take over-the-counter pain relievers if absolutely necessary.

Frequent use of anti-biotic medication is not uncommon and an easy way out; the consequences can be significant as this can change the bacterial mapping in our system especially in our gastrointestinal tract (GIT) eventually causing a resistance to antibiotic medication. If for some medical reason, antibiotics are necessary to be administered then make sure that certain food items such as yoghurt and other fermented cultured dairy products and soy products are also taken to repopulate your GIT system with good bacteria which may have also perished due to the effect of the antibiotic administration.

I often profess this which is nothing new, that after a certain age, our bodies lack energy and fitness. This is due to a myriad of reasons but just to elaborate on a few which are very relevant to our current subject matter, let's concentrate on the following few.

Inadequate nutrition in the diet.
Lack of exercise and physical activities.
Mental capacity and alertness:
Cognition and reflexes.
These activities within us start to slow down with age.

Also, the presence of mind and inner momentum within ourselves starts to decline. The serious question is at what age do we start to slow down and feel we are getting old? This is quite personal and varies from people to people and seniors to seniors. But if I had my way, I would probably say we are as old as we feel and as long as our mental faculties are reasonably intact and our bodies are still functional, let us carry on as a trooper and not lay down our arms. And yes, there is always room for improvement.

There have been some quite interesting studies conducted internationally; at what age a person can be regarded as a senior?

According to World Health Organisation (WHO), people in the age bracket of 60–65 years are categorised as elderly people, I like to call them seniors.

This brings globally to just under 10% of the entire population. Not bad, let's face it as time passes by, we all have to become old and time does not stand still for anyone. Remember this 10% or so is not evenly divided amongst countries of the world and seems that a decrease in population longevity is directly proportional to the increase in population above 60–65 years old and their socioeconomic status. My interest in these statistics is to verify the quality rather than the quantity of longevity and this is where the availability of good nutrition and good healthy living programmes for seniors will help immensely.

What to Do Then?

Let's look at this in light of both the growing population of seniors and the quality of life available to them.

2020 has seen a major change in lifestyle within our general population and significantly so in the senior segment. It is never easy to address complex issues of social reforms be it in the senior population group or any other age group in any society. We have almost 16% of the total population of seniors in Australia, (according to the Australian Bureau of Statistics; ABS) 2018.

(Ref: Population projections, Australia, 2017 (base)-2066. ABS cat. no. 3222.0. Canberra: ABS).

This suggests that one in every six of us is 65 years old or more age bracket. My interest in this age group of the population is relevant as I am also a member of this elite group. And therefore, I am always mindful of our situations. We have done our duty to our families and contributed to the society and just maybe it is time for us to improve our status by helping ourselves by firstly improving our physical fitness and mental alertness and then gradually work our way through improving our quality of life. Improving our fitness and alertness levels is mainly up to us and once we have done that, we will be more equipped to improve our quality and status in life; this is a societal commitment with rewarding consequences.

There are several government and private agencies entrusted with the task to uplift and improve the quality of life amongst their older citizens and it is in our best interest that we make full use of those availabilities. I am certain that many other governmental instrumentalities particularly in developing and developed nations have similar arrangements.

For your fitness and mental alertness, please read on and get proper advice regarding your health condition from your registered medical practitioner to check out if you are up to the task of making this journey with us.

Our journey starts here and is the combination of a few ingredients; mind, body and soul which are intertwined. Mind, as you will make a journey through your consciousness. Encyclopaedia Britannica describes the mind as a complex human faculty combining memory, analytical powers, emotions, sensation and perceptions and many more attributes that make our mental functions tick. I believe that the two most powerful sensations of our mind are our personality and our sub-consciousness. Medically, our neurological functions and disorders determine our mental activities and are the function of our brain.

What is Mind? It is one of the greatest mysteries of our time (Professor. Mark Solms Cape Town University).

The other two ingredients are the Body and Soul; the Soul is our essence which connects us to our cosmic being. It is the body only, which is the tangible physical entity and which is the conduit to our mind and soul. Mind and soul have no physical existence, but have a very significant spiritual role to play in our existence.

If at any stage of this journey, you feel discomfort of any kind, please stop immediately and seek medical advice.

In the past, I have been a regular guest at a local digital radio station (Radio 16 New Castle, Australia) and also have been involved for quite some time may be 6–7 years trying to promote nutritional awareness. It had been very rewarding as I interacted with the host another senior citizen to bring a 20-minute programme segment to multiple senior listeners. And I feel that, if I have been able to spread the word around to just a hand full of the listeners then I have done some positive work for the community and eventually hope this will start a chain reaction.

After waking up, start your day with a positive focus on life and affirmation; how do you want to spend your day, plan it so that there is room to reflect on without rushing and scrounging for additional time. People often rush to fit in a lot in a limited span of time and unfortunately miss out on some of the important activities.

Set your priorities right and tick them off one by one.

Start your day with a positive note and end your day with a sense of achievement.

Our sleep and wake-up cycle called the **Circadian Rhythm** is a natural process or cycle which is affected by the natural darkness and light. In the sleep cycle, the brain signals the Pineal gland a small gland located in the epithalamus region in the central part of the brain for the production of a hormone **Melatonin,** and in the wake-up cycle the production of the hormone **Cortisol** is activated by the adrenal gland; these are also activated by the darkness and natural light.

Why did I mention this; often we forget about the lethargy factor in the sleep and wake-up cycle which has a significant effect on our activity level between the time of waking up and starting an active day.

For those who lead a busy life, their set of priorities is a lot more involved than for someone like me who is a semi-retired senior and accepts life as it comes; as in, been there done that attitude.

So, what can we do in the morning, the period between waking up and starting your next activity? More importantly, being present at your job starts fresh and full of vitality.

Shaking up the lethargy and breaking up the circadian rhythm can certainly be daunting for many of us. Before **morning-itis** may set in and get a hold of our psyche a few simple things can be practiced to give us a boost from our state of inertia to a get-up-and-go mode.

If you are, a grab a cup of coffee and go kind of a person then just slow down for a moment or two and spend around 10–15 minutes for a light breathing and free hand exercise; this will do you good and stabilise your cortisol level. Have some breakfast and then by all means grab a cup of coffee on your way out, this will help your cognition and alertness levels. Some nutritionists say that drinking coffee on an empty stomach is harmful, so be mindful of this.

So, we have broken the circadian rhythm what next?

For those who have a bit more relaxed lifestyle, it would be good if we could maintain a regular walking pattern of 20–30 minutes to achieve 2000–3000 steps or more for younger sets of legs; it does not have to be vigorous just according to your age and stamina, you control the paces.

Some people prefer meditation, breathing and free hand exercises, yoga or other modalities Tai Chi and others. All will possibly lead to similar end results.

During these walks I suggest, however, to practice controlling your mind and thought waves as we all know the mind wonders at a million miles an hour. Control of mind under these idyllic situations can harness a lot of positive thoughts. A soothing and comforting thought full of positivity can work wonders for our health and well-being. People have problems in life, some have more than others and at times problems can be very challenging and often seem to try us out, but one thing to remember life cannot be without a problem or problems. It will be too ideal and monotonous. As long as we try to steer our thought processes in the right direction, we can hopefully alleviate life's worries and tribulations.

Our routine would consist of a relaxing walk as suggested earlier, and upon conclusion sitting down and reflect on yesterday (the past), casually sort out plans for today (the present) and think about tomorrow (the future). Yesterday is gone never to return yet it is a powerful teacher to learn from and improvise for the future. Yesterday is gone so do not dwell on it. Learn from it and apply lessons learnt to make your present and future, even better. Your tomorrows will always be uncertain and planning will help.

For those who can afford to have some lazy time, I feel it is the best time of the day to contemplate so many aspects of both the past and present. Contemplation encourages all of us to rationally think and generate ideas which leads us to the meaning of our very existence. We are here at this moment of time for a purpose; some are destined to do great things and some to lead a peaceful and quiet life, we all have a purpose and a meaning.

I did not know, but I realised soon enough that contemplation is also a form of self-realisation. It questions your own actions in life good or bad and can have a profound effect on those who you have interacted with in the past, currently interacting with, and will interact in the future.

Now we know what is contemplation, so what to do and how to put it to use in our real life?

As in preparing for meditation, you need to choose a peaceful time of the day and a quiet little spot. Nothing unusual be relaxed and comfortable.

Think about issues that are bugging you, and what you can do to get rid of this nagging feeling.

Think about some good time you have had in your life as a child or as a youngster or even recently and overlap it with your negativity and the annoying nagging feelings, just like dowsing a fire with water until it is completely extinguished.

Your actions (Karma) define you! Sow the seed of good karma and picture in your mind the seed you have sown growing into a large shady tree offering shade and comfort to so many weary travellers.

Muster strengths to face challenges; everyone has to go through difficult patches from time to time, your situation may be more or less challenging. You have to deal with them and find solutions; always realise that there may be someone who is worse off than you are.

I would be happy and consider myself blessed if I can do at least one good deed in a day; and contemplate how I can contribute to improving the wellness of the community and my fellow beings.

Different people have different views on life, let us not be judgemental but be open in accepting and reciprocating. Contemplation deepens bonding with our own spirituality and affirms our position on this planet.

Staying healthy as we discussed earlier requires commitment and planning. I sincerely hope all those who are reading this book and liking the thoughts are already thinking of taking the first step in mental preparedness and planning.

The success of any project depends on the acronym **RISE**; Realism, Inventive, Sincerity and Empathy. We all need to rise to the occasion and build upon these 4 pillars which are the basic support structure for all our successes, health and happiness. To be a realist, failures are temporary blocks in our path to success and activate our sense of inventiveness to achieve success.

Remember the story of the Scottish king **Robert the Bruce**; legend has it that King Robert Bruce after losing a battle, during one of his hideouts was observing a spider climbing and spinning its web but each time it tried it fell and each time it rose up again and tried and tried till successful. This gave King Robert Bruce the sincerity in his commitment which led him to his eventual victory.

So, yes be committed and if you are sincere, you will never look back; **RISE** Above all odds and make it happen.

Be Realistic; know yourself and what you are capable of. Realise all your potentials and go for maximum output, and make it for the best. Remember never to over commit or under commit yourself; know your strengths and weaknesses do only what your mind and body can handle because mind and body are both very powerful entities and must work in harmony.

Be Inventive; hunt for new ways to make your progress and programme enjoyable and interesting, it is nothing worse than harbouring negative thoughts arising out of the monotony and repetitive steps or processes and most of all fear of losing. Be mentally prepared for the road ahead, and make it as smooth a ride for you and your fellow passengers. There will be occasional bumps along the way but wear it out with a smile.

Be Sincere; in your dealings, give people the feeling of honesty and mate-ship. **Show Empathy**; not sympathy by sharing other's lows, by being constructive and practical which will give them strength and courage to convert the lows to the highs. Do not sympathise as this may further deepen their lows.

In your planning, make sure to detail all of your relevant activities or moves, importantly the time you have allocated for the project, and ensure that efficient time management is achieved. Shorter time allocated if used efficiently can be more effective and leave you with time to spare for your other activities.

I know we as human beings are individuals. We all have differing views and opinions when doing some work or making plans and so I fully appreciate that every individual reading this book will have differing views on preparedness and planning. If the goal is same, different pathways do not matter. I hope I am merely providing a vehicle to get you started and perhaps offering some points to think about and draw up your own plans to suit your own individual situation without too much of a disruption to your own daily routine.

Your Daily Routine Set Up

Are you now ready to set up your daily routine?

All you need is an allocation of half an hour time in the morning and in the evening to set your plans in motion. Always remember you are the controller and you are setting up your own plan and at your own pace. We are using walking as our basic tool and it is by choice our main menu of activity. It is an easy and simple task, so choose a route or a walking course, and make it as cluster-free as possible and with minimum obstacles. It can be indoors, outdoors or a combination of both in order to introduce an element of variety.

Both types of venues or courses have their own advantages and can offer pleasant experiences. Walking outdoors offers you both fresh air and sunshine. Plenty of oxygen to breathe in and exhale the stale carbon dioxide and invigorate your blood supply with oxygenated air. Inhaling fresh oxygen-rich air and exhaling stale air will cause revitalisation of your blood circulation and enrichment of organ tissues with nutrients that are circulating in your bloodstream ready to be deposited. It will also increase your lung capacity and lung health. Your lung health is as important as your heart health.

For your heart to work properly as a pump, it will need to be able to pump stale, oxygen-depleted air carried by your veins into the right chamber of your heart and then pump it into the lungs for oxygenation. The co-ordination between the lungs and the heart has to be a precise clockwork operation; the lungs must be healthy with adequate lung capacity to hold oxygen available for the heart. This life-giving oxygen supply is very crucial for the sustenance of our life and our tissues and organs to breathe. It also determines how healthy we are; any deviation could be a trigger point for medical intervention.

Respiratory and pulmonary disorders are caused by the inefficient working of the lungs.

The other aspect of outdoor walks is the availability of all important vitamin D when exposed to sunlight, our skin has the capability to biosynthesise vitamin D. Sun's ultraviolet radiations react with skin cells containing cholesterol forming the important vitamin D. This biosynthesis is little bit more complex but the end result is that we enjoy getting the important vitamin D from the sunshine and therefore vitamin D is often called the sunshine vitamin.

How much vitamin D do we get from exposure to sunlight, how much time we need to spend outdoors are questions that need to be answered as we also know that too much exposure is not a good thing as there are many ill effects of the excess sunshine on our general health and wellbeing.

In general, people with different skin colour will need different exposure levels. Additional melanin in dark-skinned people have that extra bit of protective factor from Sun's damaging ultraviolet rays and therefore can enjoy longer exposure to sunshine without getting sunburn. On the other hand, fair-skinned people, due to the lack of melanin in their skin are likely to get a harsher exposure and start getting sunburns much more quickly.

Sadly, the dangerous side of enjoying sunshine is sunburn causing the risk of skin cancer and melanoma which if not diagnosed and treated in the earliest phase can often lead to death.

Although it is true, that natural exposure to sunshine is a great way to absorb vitamin D through our skin. Normally a half an hour exposure is adequate, but the level of exposure should be carefully monitored depending on one's skin colour. A pale to fair-skinned person should no longer expose more than 10–20 minutes after which the skin may start to sunburn which should be avoided at all costs. An olive to darker-skinned person may enjoy a longer exposure.

It has been reported that a fair-skinned person if adequately exposed for 10–20 minutes under an intense to bright sunshine conditions will produce enough vitamin D for daily requirements.

It is very important, irrespective of your skin colour, proper sun protective measures are taken when exposed or enjoying the sunshine. It is always preferable to apply sun protective barrier cream for additional protection. So, it is quite clear that even though outdoor walks are pleasant and interactive with Nature there are risks that we all must respect and take adequate precautions.

Preparedness, Commitment and Planning (the Philosophy of Keeping Well)

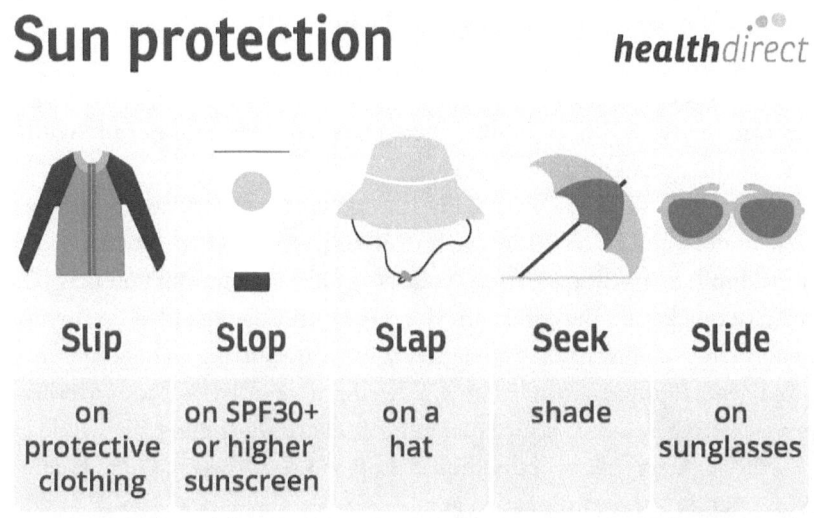

(Gratefully referenced from www.healthdirect.gov.au/sunburn)

The reference is an important reading and offers good information for exposure to sun and sunburn protection. It is a must-read from Australian Government health advice on Sunburn and Sun protection.

The environment also has a large part to play. Pollution, smog, atmospheric density, e.g., humidity, seasonal pollens in the air can be negative factors that we have to contend with. Again, adequate protection such as general-purpose masks can be helpful but they are not sophisticated enough to filter fine pollutant particles and pollens. People with respiratory disorders must seek professional guidance and take some basic protection if required.

People who smoke and or suffer from asthma must always be mindful of the environmental conditions and refrain themselves from taking outdoor walks on a moderate to high polluted days. It can cause more harm than good.

Your indoor alternatives under such conditions are a much safer bet. Your indoor course will allow you to escape the effects of the weather and offer protection from Nature's elements e.g., rain, heat and strong winds in addition to the pollutants.

Planning can be an interesting venture; it is exciting to roughly know how many steps you are taking on a daily basis and equate it to distances. To simply get an idea approximately gauge the course distance you want to walk, and then count the steps to complete it. By doing so, you will know approximate how many rounds you will need to do or how many laps you may need to complete before reaching your target.

Roughly 3000 steps twice daily is a medium to good target for a senior citizen under the age of 70 years; but of course, you must not exceed your comfort limit. Struggling to exceed your target in the hope that you may benefit or achieve quicker results will cause you more harm than good. Also, by timing the steps taken can introduce consistency in your routine. Depending on your age and general physical condition you can do more or less without overheating or over-exerting yourself; again, remember you are controlling the whole game and at the slightest feeling of discomfort stop and rest. To keep going even when you are tired is not recommended at all.

Start with a small target then improve on it. Set a goal, twice a day will be adequate and simple walks are good enough. Just so as you get the feeling of satisfaction and build confidence and a commitment that you are going to stick around and see it through. There will be plenty of scope to improvise and build on your strength and to set newer goals and targets. Records are meant to be broken and as human beings we improve on our weaknesses and thrive on our successes.

If you are in a weight management regime then it may be ok too, only that you could be required to do a bit more involved routine which will assist you to burn excess calories to slim down and build up strength. Under a weight loss programme there are several other aspects of the management that you need to be aware of and follow. You must consult with your trainer or experts in this field. All we are trying to impress upon is to set in motion a plan of action to follow and hopefully generate enough motivation to maintain reasonably good health and general well-being.

Our journey will have lots of advantages if we have an open mind and willingness to support ourselves. In due course, if we can keep it up, we will find there is an enlightenment in the attitude and outlook, which can only bring positivity in our quest for wellness, and life will have a deeper meaning of enjoyment and appreciation.

Weight management programmes can be more rigorous with strenuous exercise routine and a strict dietary plan to maintain; no milk and milk products if you are allergic to lactose, no chocolate, no sweets no ice-cream as all these condiments can load you up with unwanted calories. In some people, these food products not only cause an allergic trigger but may also have a fattening effect if you do not make an effort to trim it down. It is also important to remember that as soon as you go off these weight management programmes and deviate from the strict dietary guidelines you may find that the extra weight that you had lost is starting to come back on.

In actual sense, weight management plans are quite involved, more rigorous and requires a strict discipline. Any fluctuation and irregularity in the execution of the specific plan which may have been tailor-made can lead to an unnecessary delay in achieving your goal.

On the other hand, a simple commitment to keeping up your target of achieving a well-balanced lifestyle leading to general health and well-being can be non-regimented and so much easier to follow.

To keep up with weight management programmes you will need to be more disciplined and must be under regular supervision and a controlled gym environment. It is not for everyone. However, having said that, from my past experiences in people with whom I have consulted, a careful consideration must be given and a strong personal commitment is required.

Failure to commitment and discipline can manifest in mood changes, irritability and other irregularities which may result in some health issues and complications; such as inconsistencies in sleep patterns, anxiety, etc. It is a completely different ball game. People who train in gyms to achieve their goals and ambitions are highly motivated people. Simple distractions are no match for their commitment to their training regimen and quest for their chosen aspirations.

Making a commitment is easy but breaking them is even easier.

My comments should by no means be a deterrent. Rather I am all in favour; however, be fully aware of the involvements, see what lies ahead. Once you have done your homework and had proper guidance and orientation, if you still feel that this is for you then don't look back.

Our journey has no complications if you do not overdo, and take things light and easy. The motto is easy does it.

Now, as you think about setting up your daily routine, think about the time and effort available to you or you can allocate for this activity. I do not want people to go out of their way to create time for the activities because all you will be doing is to steal your valuable time from one activity to progress the other. This is not how our motivation works so allow only the time you can spare for this and do it in a relaxed and enjoyable way and work your own routine and style; own it and control your ownership.

If you so choose, you can break down your segments into 4 blocks of 5–10 minutes each if this works for you, otherwise modify the programme according to your requirement.

Block 1. Any time after you wake up before or after breakfast. This will break the lethargy and circadian rhythm and push you into a new and positive frame of mind. Maybe not straight away but given time you will enjoy the freshness and soon find yourself in a habituated regular pattern.

Block 2. Before lunch break or half an hour after lunch. This cycle will assist you to start the digestive juices and prepare your system for a smooth transition from food intake to digestion.

Block 3. After you have a cuppa in the afternoon (afternoon tea); this only needs to be a short stint just to break the monotony from your routine.

Block 4. After dinner; this is important as dinner can be quite heavy and filling, and you should not go to bed with a full tummy as this can cause mild respiratory problems and feeling of suffocation and occasional acid reflux in some people with a weaker digestive system. And believe me this is not uncommon as I know and had this unpleasant experience myself. Also, with light exercises such as simple yoga posture and a few minutes of meditation after dinner or even walking around your dinner table or dining hall may provide you with the all-important relaxation and bolster your digestive system for a good night's sleep.

Some people can be a bit complacent or can be a bit lazy and become couch potatoes and go to bed with a full stomach. This may sometimes cause slight to moderate discomfort leading to an unpleasant and intermittent sleep pattern. A good night's rest can do a world of good to all of us especially a relaxed and refreshed morning after. If the start of the day is good, then hopefully the rest of the day will follow suit.

The disadvantage of going to bed with food sitting in the stomach is that it will start slowly to break down into carbohydrates, fats, etc. and as the body is at rest, metabolisms are slow with less insulin available in the bloodstream to completely burn off the excess glucose circulating in the blood which may eventually be deposited in organ tissues (can be anywhere) resulting in weight gain.

Glucose is the end fragment from carbohydrates which is the fuel needed by our body. And since our diets consist of 50% or more carbohydrates it is important that a consistent supply of insulin from our pancreatic gland is maintained and available. So, a light activity in block 4 (above) is really helpful to our physical digestive system fitness. This should also help us with a pleasant night's sleep and a fresh start to the day when we wake up the next morning feeling relaxed and ready to take on the world.

I also think that breakfast is important, the very meaning of the word implies that we break the long fasting which could be up to 10–12 hours, a long time in between any food intake. Again, should this happen your body is starving for nutrition to provide the energy we need to sustain activities and to keep the body systems going.

Our next step is to monitor our progress and evaluate it on a monthly basis. For this, there will be some simple record keeping required. Make it less complicated and less involved, then it will be simple to follow and meaningful.

Check your weight on a simple bathroom scale which is reasonably accurate and has a proper display.

It may be a good idea to calibrate your scale periodically using a standard weight, this will prevent any discrepancies in your weight measurements. You may also need to note down your tummy circumference using a simple tape measure and any additional parameters that you may wish to record as a general control point. For example, a simple description of your physiological profile such as your breathing patterns, your digestive issues and any allergies. Note down these measured parameters before you start the journey preferably with time and date so you can compare as you build up your database. It may also serve as a valuable experience if you monitor your psychological profile such as how you feel about the programme, are you comfortable, are you making any progress and any other little details that you care to observe.

This reminds me of a funny joke I used to tell my students at the College of Somatic Studies in the late 80s and early 90s during Urinalysis Class. I used to tell them about the importance of observation and how important it is to be observant with this story. In one of the medical schools in London the teacher while explaining the same topic asked the students to produce their urine samples for testing and he then asked one of his students to hand over the jar of the specimen to him and said to them, "now all of you pay attention and observe me carefully."

He then looked at the specimen jars and started commenting on the physical attributes of the specimen sample like the colour, texture, odour, etc., and suddenly opened the lid of the jar and dipped his index finger and licked his ring finger and asked his students to do the same with their specimen sample. Lo and behold all students dipped their index finger and licked the same and drew up funny faces and disgusting gesture. At the sight of this, the teacher burst into laughter and said in a loud voice, "Me lads, all of you failed to observe me, I dipped my index finger and licked my ring finger."

The students realised their mistake but no harm done as they tasted their own specimen samples.

I have known of some people who have also recorded their blood pressure, pulse rate and also a brief description of their energy levels. If you do not have any facility to measure these parameters in-house by yourself, then please get someone you know who can do it for you. This way you will be able to create a profile to understand which direction you are heading to. Many pharmacies or drug stores offer a free periodic blood pressure check service which you can avail from time to time and record.

These days it is a craze to run long distances, endurance running. I have even seen elderly people in their 60s and above running quite briskly and then panting their way to rest. I ask is that of any help.

I can appreciate they may be on a cardio exercise routine; as it has been stated by many experts and also reported in several journals and articles that running is good for the heart. Yes, it may be so but surely your age and fitness levels are of prime consideration.

Heavy exercise leads to over-exertion of the heart unless conducted properly, and seniors are well advices to proceed with caution and under professional supervision. This is why our journey is so attractive and can be suitable for all; remember the motto, easy does it.

I prefer to keep control on myself and do what I am comfortable with. And for seniors, I will recommend to set your journey yourself and do what you are comfortable with.

Now that we have prepared ourselves and set up a daily routine, we are well set into our journey. Along the way, all we need to do is to monitor our progress.

As I have mentioned earlier, start with simple walks. After the comfort period which may be a week or a month after the start, if it feels comfortable add some simple free hand exercises. Nothing too complicated and then graduate to a more involved lightweight workouts, it helps. As we advance in age our muscles undergo significant wear and tear and loss in muscle tactile properties and to bring our muscles to a required strength some lightweight exercises do help.

It will not bring back the youth but certainly tone you enough to get by with dignity and confidence. A pictorial guide in chapter 9 may be of some help; follow it and see where it leads you to. Again, it is important to note down your parameters at the end of each stage and, or, when you make any changes no matter how simple or trivial it is. This will keep a log of any noticeable effect on your wellness positive or negative and will allow you to make any adjustment that you may see fit. This will also assist your primary health assessor to review your history should it be needed.

Another important point to consider in this overall package is to improve your gait, particularly as we advance in age, because of the looseness in our muscle structure and spinal curvature we tend to stoop a little from the upright stance. If it is not due to any spinal complications which needs medical intervention or Chiropractic manipulation or adjustments then simple upright exercises could be of some value. As mentioned, chapter 9 provides some easy and simple to do posture developing exercises shown for you, keeping in mind that these are not too complicated and can be easily practiced.

A very simple routine that I have found beneficial and works for me is movements up and down the stairs. Climbing up and down the stairs provides that all important circulation and activates the pump action of our heart; a mild version of cardio-exercises. Circulation in the legs and the lower part of the torso, e.g., the waist, strengthens the muscles in that part of our body to carry our body weight.

Some people carry too much weight in the upper part of the body causing a buckling effect which destabilises the legs. You do not need to overdo and depending on your body constitution and weight distribution a 5-minute climbing exercise should be enough. Your body is the best judge and will soon let you know if you are overdoing it.

I have also found it helpful in the event of unavailability of stair cases to just simply climb up and down any elevated structure that may be handy and readily accessible. This will help to build calf muscles and the feet alignments such that the body weight can be evenly distributed during workouts and other load-bearing actions on the feet. There are several muscles in our foot which control and support mobility and strength.

In our advancing age, the flexibility and elasticity of the connective tissues and cartilage which is holding the vertebrae becomes lose and weakened; also, the synovial fluids which act like a lubricant starts to dry up causing friction between bones and other joints. The best way to improve this situation is through diet and mild forms of exercise. Green leafy vegetables, omega-3 fatty acid-rich foods and supplements such as fish oils, glucosamine, and chondroitin are all good for regular intakes. If the intermittent lumber pains and discomfort persists, then medical intervention is essential.

Risks and Hazards of Daily Living

As our planet Earth revolves around the life-giving star the Sun in our solar system we encounter days and nights. 24 hours signals the completion of a full daily cycle. This 24-hour cycle is further broken down into 2 twelve hourly day and night segments. A day cycle and a night cycle, this rhythm or pattern has been permanently etched into our planet's psyche since its formation. The only difference is the duration of day light and night darkness.

In summer time when our planet is tilted on its axis closer to the sun, we experience summer and Sun's direct heat-causing rays. In summer months, we also experience longer daylight hours while the opposite is true in winter where we experience shorter duration of day light and longer nights filled with darkness. This has a profound effect on our mental and physical health.

Imagine living close to the arctic regions where winters can be long with only a few hours of sunlight and in a few remote places the situation can be even more drastic with long months without any sunlight.

If there was a census for the preference of daylight over the night darkness, I would imagine that there would be an overwhelming yes for daylight. The Sun has a very strong psychological and physiological effect on human beings throughout our very evolution into modern human beings. In the sunlight, we are inspired by the beauty of the Nature, and when night falls the gloom and doom of darkness takes over; except in the brightness of the moonlit night. "**Let there be light!**"

Hippocrates, father of ancient medicine, also linked health with availability of daylight during different times of the year and believed that changes in the season had something to do with it. There are many examples of Hippocrates's ancient views; and in modern time the so-called winter blues, feeling of lethargy, doom and gloom are all real. According to Dr Norman Rosenthal of Georgetown University (USA) winter blues are a part of the physical and psychological condition called Seasonal Affective Disorder aptly abbreviated as SAD.

In actual effect, this came about when a group of people were forced to spend more time indoors than outdoors due to seasonal and weather conditions e.g., lack of sunshine etc. suffered from feelings of sadness, helplessness and hopelessness and other negative psychological effects.

As we progress further, as a highly evolved society, and our humanity has continuous interaction with technology and modern lifestyle of working and playing indoors under bright artificial lights, could it then be, that, our future generation will suffer from an advanced form of SAD all year round? Some of the science fiction and sci-fi film depictions of recent times, makes me feel that we are already bracing for the changes.

This reminds me of Jules Vern, a 19th century French author who wrote classic fictions such as 'Twenty Thousand Leagues Under the Sea', 'Around the World in 80 Days' and who can forget his classic 'From Earth to the Moon' and my favourite 'Journey to the Centre of the Earth'. These were only imaginative stories then, and the author may have coped a few verses of sarcastic remarks for being ahead of his time in the imagination department. His stories, and in fact these were stories when he wrote them were way ahead of its time and still to this day remains favourites among many of us.

Imagine, space explorations started only in the late 1950s when Russian (then USSR) launched their first artificial satellite Sputnik to successfully orbit the Earth. This was the beginning of the space race between the Americans and the Russians and in 1961 Russian Cosmonaut Lt. Uri Gagarin became the first man to shoot out through Earth's atmosphere and orbit the Earth and safely back again. What an experience would that have been to Gagarin and what a view of our blue planet we call home he must have had, the third rock from our Sun.

It was a remarkable feat, but the highlight of space race was achieved when American Astronaut Neil Armstrong and Buzz Aldrin actually landed on the Moon on 20 July 1969, which until then to many older generations was revered as a heavenly body. Neil Armstrong was credited to be the first person on the moon but by no means was Aldrin's contribution any less. Also, not to forget the expert control of the navigation skills of Michael Collins the command module pilot without whom this would not have been possible.

Imagine, Jules Vern writing about space journeys around 1865, more than 100 years ago when space travel was unimaginable and ridiculed and so it was very appropriate and befitting that Commander Neil Armstrong of Apollo 11 made a reference to Jules Vern's book during a TV broadcast on July 23 upon their return from Moon to Earth.

I was merely digressing from the main subject to contemplate on the events or thoughts of some pioneer's so many years ago especially now, when these events have become a reality for all human kind to marvel upon.

Hence there is no reason why Dr Norman Rosenthal views on SAD cannot be a reality years into the future from now when science and technology may become the norms of our daily life.

Living our lives normally under present day conditions is fraught with risks not only from the nature and our environment but also from foods and drinks we take for our daily sustenance and also from chemicals, pollution and contaminations we have to live and cope with.

Does this mean 'Living is a Health Hazard'?

Not quite, we do have protective measures and it is up to all of us to think about our futures, our and our fellow human being's health and wellbeing and to do the right things which are helpful in our quest for health and wellness for us and our planet.

Vitamins, minerals, amino acids and very many macro and micro nutrients from our diet are needed to keep us functioning as a fine-tuned unit, both physically and mentally. Proteins from both animal and vegetable sources are also important components of our diet.

Research into nutritional biochemistry has clearly demonstrated that significant portions of our population are marginally vitamin and mineral deficient depending on a number of lifestyle and environmental factors such as age, dietary consideration, stress levels, smoking habits, drug and alcohol abuse, pollution, physical activities, use of oral contraception, metabolic insufficiencies e.g., digestive problems etc.

Nature has blessed us with all we need to sustain life. Since the dawn of civilisation human beings have been heavily dependent on Nature: our forbearers, as hunters and gatherers, sustained life by living on Nature's bounty. Since then, through our development and progress, humans have continued to rely on Nature for many aspects of our lives. Today many useful commodities from our energy needs to lifesaving drugs extracted from herbs are all derived from Nature.

The oldest surviving civilisation on earth, the Australian Aborigines who have been known to inhabit the Australian continent for over the past 60,000 years have survived on the available flora and fauna and made good use of the land and the natural environment for their health and well-being.

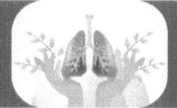

Chapter 4

FOOD CATEGORIES AND DIET

Good food and good nutrition equate to healthy-self. Healthy-self equates to Heal-thy-self.
— Jay Das, 2021

Healthy foods and healthy diet to me have separate meaning; unless you have healthy foods, you cannot have healthy diet. If you are starting from scratch, then keep these following points in mind, sure it is a challenge but accept it with a degree of humour and wit.

Don't be overwhelmed, keep it simple; these pointers may assist you keeping in mind that every body's needs are not similar.

- Fresh is best for all produce.
- Do not get sucked into bulk buys to save a few dollars. Often the excess goes to waste causing you a loss; so, stick with your needs not wants are and buy in portions that you are likely to use up in a short period of time.
- Buy loose produce rather than prepacked items, particularly fruits and vegetables so you can feel the freshness and blemish free quality of the items you are buying.
- Meat products are best fresh from the butcher.
- Pre-packaged items use plastic and other non-biodegradable materials and ends up in the land fill and causes environmental hazard.

We all are, due to the time and budget constrains have hunted for the cheaper options and there is nothing wrong with it, just a bit of due diligence would not hurt and go a long way to securing our general well-being. Healthy diet consists of healthy foods to start with then built on it with additional requirements for grains, nuts seeds fats and oils and dairy products. A wholesome combination which can be changed occasionally to introduce a bit of variety to keep the interest in our food intake alive and wanting. In April 2020, WHO published a document with key facts about healthy diet. A healthy diet helps to protect against malnutrition in all its forms, as well as non-communicable diseases (NCDs), including such as diabetes, heart disease, stroke and cancer.

Unhealthy diet and lack of physical activity are leading global risks to health. Healthy dietary practices start early in life-breastfeeding for infants fosters healthy growth and improves cognitive development, and may have longer term health benefits such as reducing the risk of becoming overweight or obese and developing NCDs later in life.

Energy intake (calories) should be in balance with energy expenditure. To avoid unhealthy weight gain, total fat should not exceed 30% of total energy intake. Intake of saturated fats should be less than 10% of total energy intake, and intake of trans-fats less than 1% of total energy intake. Try to make a transition in fat consumption away from saturated fats and trans-fats to unsaturated fats, and towards the goal of eliminating industrially-produced trans-fats altogether.

Saturated and trans-fats are becoming to be known as unhealthy fats and too much of these in our diets can elevate the levels of LDLs in our blood which can over time clog our blood vessels and cause severe cardio-vascular issues. We need to be aware of various types of fats that are commercially introduced in our diets and also in our home cooking unwittingly due to the choices of ingredients we make. Commonly we can find four types of fats or fatty ingredients in our diets.

Monounsaturated fats.
Polyunsaturated fats.
Saturated fats and trans-fats.

Of these saturated fats and trans-fats are unhealthy and should be replaced by mono and poly unsaturated fats as soon as possible.

Mono and Poly unsaturated fats contain omega-3-fatty acids and can improve to lower the cholesterol status of our body by lowering the low-density lipoproteins (LDL) and help improve heart function.

Certain facts about the omega-3-fatty acids that we all should know are following:

These lower the concentration of LDLs and triglycerides in the blood.

Reduce high blood pressure in people who have consistently high BP reading.

Reduces Plaque formation (fatty acid deposits) which hardens the arteries.

All these actions and more help heart functions and reduces heart diseases. So, how can we introduce more of the mono and poly unsaturated fats in our diets and which of the cooking ingredients contain lots of these good fats? Mono and poly unsaturated fats, are rich in food ingredients like sunflower and safflower oils, avocadoes, several nuts such as peanuts, wall nuts, pine nuts sesame and flaxseeds. Pea nuts are also a good source and so is pumpkin seeds. Olive oil can be used in cooking procedures where not a lot of heat is required e.g., salads and dressings.

Regular inclusion of oil rich fish in diet can be very beneficial. Fish protein is easily digestible and contains a significant portion of omega-3-fatty acids. For people who are interested in looking at alternatives in their food substitutions, there are several simple swaps that can be considered in their diets. Although list can be exhaustive, simple common-sense and suitable alternatives may be tried at first then put in practice on a regular basis. Full cream milk, butter, yoghurt, cheeses etc. are high in saturated fats and these can be substituted for low fat alternatives although may not be as tasty but certainly a healthy alternative. Peanut butter can be used as alternative to straight-out dairy butter.

Use leaner cuts of meat and increase the use of white meat e.g., chicken, pork and other poultry meats and where possible de-skin and trim the excess fats around the cuts of meat you are using. Binge eating can also be a cause of overweight and additional intake of carbohydrates so avoid it as much as possible; easy swap to binge snacking is nuts and seeds in moderate intakes and provides much needed polyunsaturated fats.

Limiting the intake of free sugars to less than 10% of total energy intake is part of a healthy diet. A further reduction to less than 5% of total energy intake is suggested for additional health benefits. But remember cutting down to zero may not be a good thing and cause energy issues. All carbohydrates e.g., sugars provide glucose for our cells to burn into energy.

Keeping salt intake to less than 5 g per day (equivalent to sodium intake of less than 2 g per day) helps to prevent hypertension, and reduces the risk of heart disease and stroke in the adult population.

World Health Organisation (WHO) Member States have agreed to reduce the global population's intake of salt by 30% by 2025; they have also agreed to halt the rise in diabetes and obesity in adults and adolescents as well as in childhood obesity by 2025.

(Ref: Healthy diet—WHO | World Health Organisation https://www.who.int › Newsroom › Fact sheets › Detail)

Good food intake is the key to good nutrition and to become nutritionally aware in our daily intake regime is a step in the right direction for the management and continuity for good health and our overall wellness. Especially now a days when the variety of foods available to us are overwhelming with tempting choices.

There are many reasons why we eat food; there are social reasons for feasts, BBQ gatherings when we enjoy our food mixed with pleasure of good company and the necessity to fill our belly to satisfy the hunger. Then there are fundamental reasons, our body needs nutrients for survival and sustenance to perform tasks both from within and externally to keep us alive. By within, I mean our cells which are the primary composite of our body and good nutrition is the fuel that keeps our body cells alive and functioning.

Lack of adequate nutrition for our cells and deprivation of essential nutrients can lead to cell death and ending up in sickness and diseases. Some people eat foods sometime a lot of it for pleasure, and in the process accumulate unwanted nasties which our body has to overwork to get rid of. Sometimes these wastes or nasties are too much to get rid of and accumulate within our body developing obesity leading to several debilitating diseases and uncomfortable life style.

Externally, if our body cells are working efficiently due to the availability of good nutrients then we have more energy and power to overcome feelings of tiredness, fatigue and stress. So, it is important to make the right choices of what we put into our mouths and give our body's a fighting chance to improve our health, general wellbeing and mental strength to lead a happy and healthy life.

Let's keep a simple saying in mind "let's eat the food and not the other way around; not let the food eat us."

The topic of food and nutrition is relatively simple because we can have a control over it when it comes to self-application; we just need to develop awareness and also a sense to differentiate what is the right choice and what may not be the right choice. Making a good and simple choice with lots of common sense and awareness information at hand, will go a long way. Before we consider different food categories, I believe that a common understanding of food and good storage is very important.

As a general common-sense approach to food storage, it should be stored in good clean hygienically verified storage area. In controlled commercial storage areas, control comes from regular monitoring of the control parameters. In domestic or household storage conditions, a visual inspection of the storage areas or containers on a regular basis are quite appropriate. For instance, tell-tale signs of moisture, fungal growth, vermin droppings and general lack of tidiness can be enough to determine unsuitability of the storage area.

Early detection could allow you to take precautions and preventive measures and often saves you money and wastages.

Food Contamination and Factors Affecting Quality of Food:

Nutrition in foods largely depend on soil and climatic conditions the produce are grown in; but it is equally important for their storage in the right environment and climate control warehouses. Specially designed and purpose-built bulk storage areas provided must be monitor continuously for their storage to preserve their nutritional goodness.

Once the produce has been distributed down the supply chain it becomes the responsibility of the distributors and the retailers alike to store the produce appropriately to prolong their use by date to give the end user a proper time frame from purchase to consumption. Once the produce is sold it becomes the end user's responsibility to store the purchased produce adequately to improve the nutritional value until consumed.

Food contamination and spoilage before consumption is a big issue and a cause for major concerns. Storage and food handling both at the producers end and for the end user must be critically evaluated to get best out of the food products available for us to consume. Climatic changes including prolonged dry spells can cause low crop yields in some crop growing cycle.

The reverse cycle when there are excessive rains and flood can create a complete washout and crop damage. A conducive growing cycle when there is a balance of the availability of water and sunshine, a bumper crop yield is harvested which can often create storage issues. These bumper seasons become important factor for the farmers and growers as insurance and safety net for any lean times ahead.

From the raw produce point of view, animal derived food source such as meats, poultry, fish, crustacean, milk and eggs etc. require different sets of storage conditions. Some can be stored for prolonged periods of time while others are more perishable and therefore may need to be consumed within a short span of time. In most developed countries, food storage has a very strict guidelines and managed by various government agencies and therefore storage conditions are regularly monitored with strict testing and quality control guidelines and an expiry dating or a use by date is imprinted on the packaging of the consumables.

Other commodities which are less prone to decomposition or decay due to their dry physical characteristics, the storage condition may not be as strict as the raw animal derived produces. These are basically grains, seeds, nuts etc., items that are required to be stored in a dry climate-controlled condition with main emphasis to cleanliness and protection from vermin and insects. The microbiological stress in the storage of most types of primary food products are overwhelming but less in the dry storage of grains seeds nuts etc.

There is yet another type of food supply that needs some mention is fruits and vegetables which are also required to be stored with appropriate monitoring requirements. Again, as with every other category of food storage the requirements are different. Although they are stored under a specific climate control, further protection is required from insects that initiate rotting process.

(Further reading ref: Storing food safely—Food Standards Australia New Zealand www.foodstandards.gov.au › standards)

In general household storage of consumable foods, due to a much smaller operation than commercial enterprises become more manageable. However, as the household storages are beyond the control of various government agencies the management is up to us how we handle and store primary produce. Most of us store foods, be it raw produce or cooked food in the household fridge/freezer with the most common setting at 3–5 degree Celsius for fridge and much lower temperature setting around minus 15–20 degree Celsius for freezer section.

High risk food items which are animal derived must be stored in the freezer if they are not scheduled to be consumed within 24 hours of purchase. Milk, eggs, cheeses and other frequently consumed items such as bacons, salamis and other delicacies may be stored in the fridge up to its expiry or use by date. If storage instructions are imprinted on the packaging, then that must be followed at all times.

Consumers often store meats, poultry, fish etc. which are high risk produce in the fridge and use as and when needed for consumption. Sometime the stored high-risk produce goes beyond the expiry date (in the fridge or the freezer section), but I have been told that you may store several meats, poultry and fish items more than 3 months if the packaged items are in frozen condition when purchased. But please check the storage conditions labelled on the consumable goods and if in doubt confirm with the manufacturer.

These days, consumer laws dictates that there must be a storage condition and use by date clearly imprinted on each consumable items for the consumer's awareness.

Defrosting of food is also an important procedure.

Some experts believe in thawing frozen food in the refrigerator by relocating frozen food overnight into the fridge section, or, defrosting in a microwave immediately prior to cooking. But not thawing in the open area for prolonged period which increases the risk of microbiological contamination. Only a specific portion required for immediate consumption should be thawed. Any surplus portion may be consumed immediately within 48 hours provided it has been well preserved in storage fit for consumption. Never leave a thawed-out portion of food item specially derived from animal origin unattended in the fridge or at room temperature as it can go bad and unfit for consumption. Always discard such items.

Often it becomes necessary for economic reasons to buy in bulk and store for longer duration of time and consume on needs basis. In doing so, it is important to check and monitor your storage unit for its performance and also for its efficiency.

Risk minimisation should be practiced as best as possible:

- Washing hands as frequently as possible, essentially before food preparation.
- Wash utensils, wipe-down food surfaces such as bench, table counter tops and chopping boards prior to prepping particularly immediately before serving and eating.
- Store the perishable foods particularly the raw foods with a high risk of contamination in the fridge or freezer promptly and at the earliest opportunity. Don't leave them lying around.
- Segregate the raw uncooked food from cooked ready to eat foods when storing in temperature-controlled storage units e.g., fridge/freezer and make sure that the cooked food is heated uniformly at temperatures required prior to eating to obtain maximum kill of any residual harmful organisms.
- When cooking, make sure that a temperature of 65–75 degree Celsius is maintained throughout the cooking process.

Once the storage side of things are taken care of satisfactorily it is important to know the factors which can be detrimental to the quality of stored foods. Commercially there are several monitoring steps which determines the quality of the food for its suitability for human consumption, e.g., microbiological contaminants are of major concern. There are many micro-organisms which can invade stored foods and contaminate them to the point of no return. And these can be easily monitored by conducting specific tests.

Some of these contaminants pose a real threat to our general health and wellbeing and in these situations, there are no other alternative than to destroy the contaminated items; except, where the spoilage is not to the extent which may require total destruction of the contaminated food. Under these noncritical situations, the contaminated food item can be salvages by applying an appropriate dosing of gamma irradiation. However, high risk foods such as raw meats fish poultry etc. may not be irradiated.

In many countries, feed stocks for domesticated animal also undergo a similar strict control, such as Australia, New Zealand. Canada etc.

Food poisoning is a result of bacterial, viral and parasitic contamination of food products which can happen at any time during commercial growing to harvesting followed through to processing, storage and to the point of end use before consumption.

Therefore, it is of serious consequence that storage conditions and a strict protocol for microbiological monitoring are maintained at a very high level with environmental monitoring on a regular basis. Some of the most common symptoms of food poisoning can show up within a few hours of consuming contaminated foods. There can also be a delayed onset of reaction depending on your immunity level and body constitution and may last for few hours or could prolong for a few days depending on the severity of the symptoms.

If early signs of any of these symptoms appear, it is necessary for an urgent and immediate medical intervention:

- Elevated temperatures, fever and sweating.
- Nausea and vomiting.
- Diarrhoea, dysentery with a loose motion with appearance of blood.
- Abdominal pain, cramps and bloating with flatulence.
- In more severe cases, for example food poisoning caused by Botulism which is caused by *Clostridium botulinum* more serious side effects are noticed; for example:
- Blurred vision and unclear speech.
- Muscle weakness.
- Dry mouth and swallowing difficulties.
- And in more serious cases paralysis of the body.

Food poisoning is a common infection that affects millions of people in and around the world with most people complaining of vomiting, diarrhoea, and abdominal pain with mild to strong cramps.

Most cases of mild form of food poisoning are temporary and relieved quickly with plenty of hydration and rest. Probiotics may also help. However, it is always advisable that you seek medical attention at the earliest signs of pain and discomfort so that the bacteria causing the discomfort can be identified and a course of treatment initiated to control the infection. If left untreated, problem can escalate and serious symptoms can prolong the agony and suffering.

Maintenance of personal and environmental hygiene is critical. Care must be taken in the preparation and handling of ready to eat, partly cooked cold meats, salads and raw fruits and vegetables, as, harmful bacteria can be easily transferred from one exposed surface to the other before entering into our body through the mouth. Because these foods aren't heat treated or cooked, residual harmful bacteria and parasitic organisms are still likely to cause food poisoning when eaten.

Table below may assist in the understanding of possible contaminants, onset of symptoms and transmission of several harmful organisms. This is a general information taken from Mayo Clinic for educational purposes.

Chart: Food poisoning—Symptoms and Causes, Mayo Clinic (https://www.mayoclinic.org › syc-20356230)

Contaminant	Onset of symptoms	Foods affected and means of transmission
Campylobacter	2 to 5 days	Meat and poultry. Contamination occurs during processing if meat products come in contact with faeces. Other sources include unpasteurised milk and contaminated water.
Clostridium botulinum	12 to 72 hours	Home-canned foods with low acidity, improperly canned commercial foods, smoked or salted fish, and potatoes baked in aluminium foil, and other foods kept at warm temperatures for too long.
Clostridium perfringens	8 to 16 hours	Meats, stews and gravies. Commonly spread when serving dishes don't keep food hot enough or food is chilled too slowly.
Escherichia coli (E. coli)	1 to 8 days	Beef contaminated with faeces during slaughter. Spread mainly by undercooked ground beef. Other sources include unpasteurised milk and apple cider, alfalfa sprouts, and contaminated water.
Giardia lamblia	1 to 2 weeks	Raw, ready-to-eat produce and contaminated water. Can be spread by an infected food handler.
Hepatitis A	28 days	Raw, ready-to-eat produce and shellfish from contaminated water. Can be spread by an infected food handler.
Listeria	9 to 48 hours	Hot dogs, luncheon meats, unpasteurised milk and cheeses, and unwashed raw produce. Can be spread through contaminated soil and water.

Noroviruses (Norwalk-like viruses)	12 to 48 hours	Raw, ready-to-eat produce and shellfish from contaminated water. Can be spread by an infected food handler.
Rotavirus	1 to 3 days	Raw, ready-to-eat produce. Can be spread by an infected food handler.
Salmonella	1 to 3 days	Raw or contaminated meat, poultry, milk, or egg yolks. Survives inadequate cooking. Can be spread by knives, cutting surfaces or an infected food handler.
Shigella	24 to 48 hours	Seafood and raw, ready-to-eat produce. Can be spread by an infected food handler.
Staphylococcus aureus	1 to 6 hours	Meats and prepared salads, cream sauces, and cream-filled pastries. Can be spread by hand contact, coughing and sneezing.
Vibrio vulnificus	1 to 7 days	Raw oysters and raw or undercooked mussels, clams, and whole scallops. Can be spread through contaminated seawater.

People Who Are at High Risk of Getting Infected:

First and foremost, we all are at risk. But effort should be made to stop using contaminated food as early as possible. Visually, spoiled foods which have obvious signs of deterioration such as appearance, odour and changes in colour and texture, should not be consumed.

Following group of people are perceived to be in the high-risk category.

Senior Citizens; who are vulnerable due to their advancing age and may not have access to fresh food and rely heavily on ready to eat foods. With advancing age due to gradual decline in immunity, there is a high risk of getting infected quicker than younger adults who have a stronger immunity to fight infection from food borne common organisms.

People on low social-economic existence; this group of people due to the inadequate dietary and nutritional availability and perhaps a lower level of personal and environmental hygiene maintenance, are at high risk.

This is also because of their overall circumstances their immunity may be quite low.

People with chronic disease and debilitating health conditions; are also at risk. Chronic diseases such as diabetes, cardiovascular issues, radiation treatment for cancer, chronic liver impairment etc. require constant medication which does drain on their physiological immune response and therefore, when infected with pathogens leading to food poisoning, they succumb to infection readily.

Pregnancy is also a vulnerable period for infection in women who due to their condition are restricted from taking medications such as antibiotics to kill the bacteria causing food poisoning. Under these situations they are well advised to take natural course of action such as keeping well hydrated, taking natural yoghurts which naturally have good bacteria. Medical advice is a must under these circumstances for a smooth transition for their and the baby's health.

Food poisoning is not uncommon and I call it as one of the examples of 'Living with Health Hazard'.

In a progressive society we live in, majority of our spare time is spent in leisure activities can to create a festive mood at every opportunity available. And this leads to lots of eating and drinking to release the so-called stress of modern-day societal existence. Foods eaten during these leisure occasions in Australia and New Zealand are B-B-Q's and convenient finger foods including eating straight from the fridge/freezer foods such as salads cold meat delicacies and also cooked prawns Sushi another popular Japanese dish utilising fresh raw fish.

Barbeques are a very common socialising pastime in western culture and the common denominator is lots of foods and drinks and basically enjoy the social gatherings and each other's company; after all we are a social animal.

Sometime meats and fishes on a BBQ hot plate can be under done, raw to medium raw or very rare. This can really be a cause of the food poisoning.

Cooking our food prior to consumption is very important as inadequate cooking is a very common cause for food poisoning.

It is generally recognised that most bacteria causing food poisoning are effectively killed at around 65–75 degree Celsius which is lower than the temperature at which water starts to boil (100 degree Celsius), and hot boiling water can always be used as a powerful steriliser for utensils, cooking surfaces etc.

It is not just the cooking temperature only that we should be concerned about but also cross-contamination from other sources particularly food handling from utensils used and also personal hygiene.

A course of appropriate anti-biotic as prescribed by your general practitioner should do the trick, unless there is a more complicated and sinister underlying issue which may need a proper medical intervention and investigation.

Viruses and Parasites are just as bad if not more and pack a really nasty punch when it comes to food poisoning. Viruses are much smaller than bacteria and the fundamental difference between the two are that bacteria are living organisms which can breed without a host organism to live and thrive on. In contrast, a virus is not a living organism and must have a host to multiply and multiply they do most profusely.

Norovirus, Rotavirus are common examples which are also very active in food poisoning. They are excreted in large numbers in human or animal excrements and find their way into our food chain by way of insufficient personal hygiene, unhygienic storage and handling procedures and conditions around food. Oysters and other crustacean farming can be at risk of infection from contaminated sewage, inadequate procedures around animal slaughter houses and chicken processing plants. This is a common source and can lead to contamination which can then enter into our food supply chain.

Hepatitis A and E are other common examples of viruses lurking in the environment to pounce at us without any notice and cause serious health problems particularly in liver diseases.

Similar mode of contamination route can lead to infection or inoculation of raw foods in farming and or processing plants, such as worms living inside of human and animal bodies which harbour parasites. Classic examples are *Giardia lamblia* and *Cryptosporidium parvum*. Parasites can also find their way through to our food systems particularly vegetation through contaminated soils and use of contaminated fertilisers.

One of the most common and intensely studied yeast like isolate from clinical material is *Candida albicans* (*C. albicans*) and is a pathogenic yeast which is commonly found in our gastro-intestinal tract and is primarily the cause of 'Thrush' a common infection that affects both men and women. These yeast infections occur when the population of fungal organisms exceeds 40–60%. They can also infect various parts of our bodies especially the moist and warm areas such as the mouth, skin folds and reproductive organs. It is also the cause of nappy rash in infants.

The natural immunity of healthy persons to Candida infection probably is generated early in life possibly at birth when the alimentary canal (digestive system) becomes inoculated with *C. albicans* which in time over populates the whole of gastrointestinal tract. Oral thrush is caused by the over growth of *C. albicans* in the mouth area; although it is not abnormal for small amounts of *C. albicans* to live in the mouth area without causing any notable infection or discomfort.

However, when our body's immune system is compromised and the balance shifts from good bacteria such as the *Lactobacillus acidophilus* and *Bifidobacterium* then *C. albicans* can take over and cause harm by growing out of control. Oral thrush can be contagious and passed on from one person to another with a weaker immune response.

Oral thrush can be controlled by helping the good bacteria to over colonise and squeeze out and supress the colonisation of the *C. albicans* and also by going on a course of antifungal medication. Often washing our mouths and gargling several times a day with slightly warm saline water can provide relief.

COVID-19 has taught us several valuable lessons as to safeguarding ourselves by improving our personal hygiene; and by applying these and a few more common sensible hygienic practices with respect to cooking, storing and handling procedures we can help minimise the risk of infection leading to food poisoning.

There are no set rules to preventing food poisoning, it can happen to anyone at any time. Common sense rule applies and if in doubt follow your instincts.

Before we look into various food categories, we must explore the three fundamental nutrients that our body needs on a regular basis. It may sound strange but our very survival depends on this trio. It is true to say that without these three nutrients, our body will not be able to survive; the trio of our requirements are **water**, **sugar** and **salt**. It is also important to note that excess intake of these can have adverse effects and therefore a common-sense approach to intake and in-moderation rule applies.

Water

Let's start with **water** as water is the common factor which links us to our very existence. Our adult body is composed of more than 60% water this value is even more in newborn babies and children and therefore any significant loss in our daily water intake can have a very serious implication for our health and well-being. The minimum daily required quantity of our water intake should be up to around 2 litres. Some experts have even said intake of water must not be less than that of average expulsion of water from the body.

Water can be viewed as an essential nutrient because our body cannot produce more than our daily requirement. Each little fragment within our body, from a body cell to all our organs contains water and requires replenishing on a daily basis. Lack of water intake will lead to cellular dehydration which will cause a serious disruption in the intra and extra-cellular fluid balance through the osmotic pressure mechanism.

Table below provides an approximate value of water content in our body organs (www.medicalnewstoday.com)

Body part	Water percentage
Brain	80–85%
Kidneys	80–85%
Heart	75–80%
Lungs	75–80%
Muscles	70–75%
Liver	70–75%
Skin	70–75%
Blood	50%
Bones	20–25%
Teeth	8–10%

What is the main physiological function of water and how much should we drink every day? Answers can vary depending on your constitution, e.g., your build, height, daily activities and all sorts of different physiological issues such as your rate of metabolism; and for women, pregnancy and breastfeeding where the requirement may increase. But generally, 2 litres/day for adults should be an accepted level. My simple view is that the fluid excreted (e.g., urinary output and sweat factor) should be replenished.

Table of daily recommended water intake
(www.medicalnewstoday.com)

Age	Recommended fluid intake (millilitres per day)
0–6 months	**700**
6–12 months	800
1–2 years	1,300
4–8 years	1,700
9–13 years (males)	2,400
9–13 years (females)	2,100
14–18 years (males)	3,300
14–18 years (females)	2,300

Adult male	3,700
Adult female	2,700
During pregnancy	3,000
While breastfeeding	3,800

Water is essential to life and living for every living being that exists on our planet. The simplest tangible example is, if you grow a plant in a pot and deprive it of water then the end result will be it dies off a slow death; may be a painful death, who knows if we had the means to find that out, what we would have known. So, apart from the gift of life water contributes to many other essentials in our daily lives:

- Water has many important physiological functions.
- It has an important role in our digestive processes.
- It provides the first step in breaking down the food eaten by mixing with the saliva to initiate the digestive processes by converting the food into bolus (a ball of wet food mass) and preparing for further digestion in our Gastro Intestinal Tract (GIT).
- Water also helps the absorption of the vitamins, amino acids, minerals and several other micro-nutrients available from our foods.
- Without the availability of adequate water content our digestive systems would not function optimally.
- It helps in eliminating toxins from our body from sweat, urine and faeces.
- It is very important to keep our skins hydrated and moist to prevent cracking and penetration of infection from external sources.
- It keeps our body temperature regulated.
- It can be a helpful nutrient in our weight management programmes to keep us full for a longer period of time.
- It also assists greatly in transporting and delivering nutrients to our cells.
- It is also a medium and vehicle for keeping the integrity of our cellular structure by balancing the osmotic pressure between the intra- and extra-cellular fluids.

A daily intake of sufficient water is important for the integrity and maintenance of our good health. Water has many other physiological functions some of which we have discussed above; virtually most of our physiological processes are driven by water, important ones are the manufacture of hormones and neurotransmitters (and many other important bio-chemicals).

Protection of our organs and tissue by keeping them hydrated and also safeguarding the integrity of the mucus membranes surrounding certain organs (e.g., the heart, the pericardium).

Transporting oxygen to all parts of the body.

Lubricating joints by keeping the synovial fluids intact, etc., and many more.

Just digressing, chemically water is an in-organic molecule consisting of 2 hydrogen atoms bonded to an oxygen atom.

Due to its unique chemical structure, water has many unique features and properties. First and foremost, even though its chemical formula is H_2O, water is $(H_2O)x$ meaning that liquid water is a connection of infinite numbers of water or (H_2O) molecules bonded together with hydrogen bonding.

The angle of the bonding between the oxygen atoms and hydrogen atoms is at around 104.5 degrees. Diagrammatically, it looks somewhat like this.

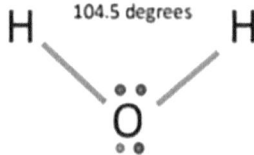

Structure of Water Molecules in Liquid Water

It is also important to note that about 75% of planet earth's surface is covered with water; it is the all life-giving elixir which all living organisms on this planet must have in order to survive.

40–50% of human blood is plasma (also, serum component) which is the watery component of blood. Both blood plasma and blood serum contain in excess of 90% water and the rest is other solid and semi-solid materials such as electrolytic elements e.g., sodium, potassium, calcium, magnesium, chlorides, bicarbonates and others. Plasma also serves as a medium for the transportation of nutrients to the tissues.

Both blood-Plasma and serum are important test tools for indicating the condition of our health and general well-being. A short table is compiled for various test parameters and related health conditions (diagnosis by clinicians).

Some Popular Test Parameters Indicative of Health Status

Test Parameters	Deficiency/Excess	Health Status
Glucose	Excess	Diabetes Mellitus, Hyperglycaemia
Proteins (Specific)	High levels or deficiencies	Indication of several health complications
Prostrate Specific Antigens (PSA)	High	Possibility of prostate cancer
Blood Urea Nitrogen (BUN)	Build-up of Urea and Nitrogen	Kidney function impairment
Creatinine	Higher levels	Kidney function impairment
Cholesterol and Triglycerides	Higher levels	Risk of high blood pressure and stroke and heart attack
Electrolytes	In-imbalance	Signs of dehydration
Vitamins and minerals	Deficiencies such as iron, B12, etc.	Specific anaemia
Various Enzymes	ALT alanine aminotransferase ALP alkaline phosphatase AST aspartate transaminase	Liver function test
Multiple cancer markers	CEA (carcinoembryonic antigen) LDH Lactic dehydrogenase PSA (Prostate Specific antigens)	These specific enzymes and antigens are indicative of the proliferation of cancer cells.

(In no cases, just one test parameter can lead to a specific diagnosis).

Liquid Water:

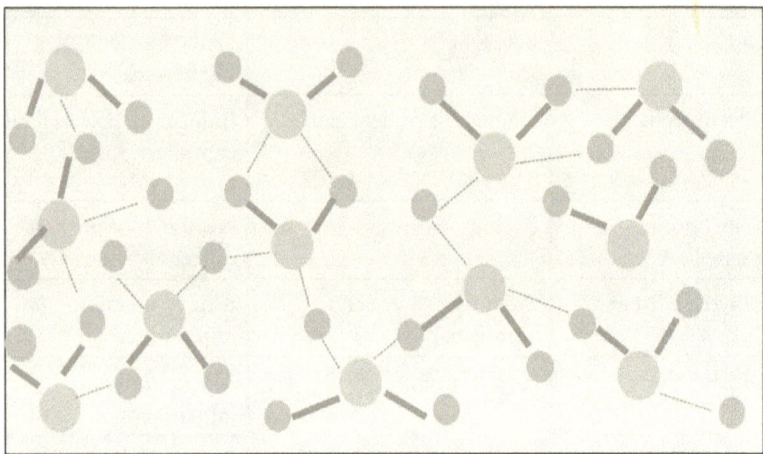

- Oxygen atom
- Hydrogen atom
- —— Solid lines denotes Oxygen Hydrogen (Covalent Bonding)
- ------ Broken line denotes Oxygen Hydrogen (Hydrogen Bonding)

Oxygen atom is bound with two hydrogen atoms by covalent bond to form one water molecule (solid black lines). While each H_2O molecule is further bound to another H_2O molecule by a hydrogen bond (broken blue lines) and this chain of hydrogen bonding of water molecules forms liquid water. Since the hydrogen bond is a weak bond, liquid water tends to evaporate.

Food Categories and Diet

Water Utility in Human Body

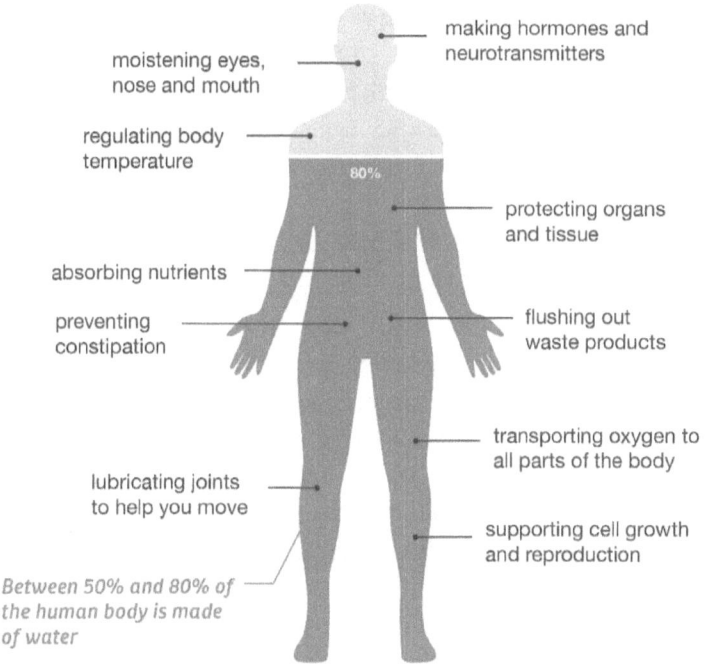

(This diagram is gratefully referenced to www.healthdirect.gov.au)

Dehydration is a common symptom in young children who have a fast body metabolic rate, higher elimination from the body, a higher sweating rate due to higher activity profile and an inadequate water intake. It is likely to happen more in a warmer temperature zone than a milder, much cooler climatic areas. Strenuous activities such as gym workouts, athletic training and performances, or just simply heavy outdoor work, e.g., gardening are also serious causes of fluid loss from our body and if not replenished adequately can become a cause of concern. Nausea, vomiting and diarrhoea are also common causes of dehydration.

Older adults physiologically may gradually lose some of their sense of thirst.

A good rule of thumb is to drink fluids throughout the day. Don't ignore when you are thirsty, drink water to quench your thirst. One of the symptoms of dehydration is the feeling of being thirsty. **Do not ignore it**.

Water Toxicity: How Much Water Is Too Much?

Water toxicity happens when there is too much or not enough water in the body. Excess water can dilute essential electrolytes in the blood, causing cells to swell, and put pressure on the brain. An electrolyte imbalance in particular a balance between the intra-cellular ion potassium+ and the extra-cellular ion Sodium+ and chlorine- can cause all sorts of physiological problems ranging from mild to serious complications. Too much water causes thinning of blood causing blood pressure to increase (hypertension).

On the other hand, dehydration can affect blood pressure; with serious consequences requiring medical intervention.

Although drinking too much water is difficult without causing discomfort, there have been cases of water poisoning in people who drank a lot of water in a very short space of time. This may be during endurance sports, heat stress, and when using recreational drugs that enhance thirst.

Frequently drinking too much water can cause kidney damage leading to loss of kidney function. Importantly also drinking too much water in a short period of time can cause serious health issues as described earlier. Some of those issues need urgent medical interventions otherwise if left untreated can develop into life-threatening conditions, especially in elderly citizens and frail or infirm people.

Seniors and Water Consumption

Older people are often at high risk of dehydration due to one or many of the following reasons.

Their limited mobility, and their immediate accessibility to drinking water.

Chronic and debilitating illness.

Decline in kidney function, with advancing age.

Imbalance in hormonal status.

Use of medication causing deliberate water loss from their system such as the use of diuretics, some heart medication laxatives, etc.

Lack of feeling thirsty due to metabolic dysfunctions.

Also, the embarrassment of incontinence can cause less water consumption.

And many more.

Elderly people have similar symptoms of dehydration as the general population; the only difference is that some of the symptoms can manifest into serious illnesses. Their need for drinking water must be attended to at the earliest sign of dehydration which in addition to the populous general symptoms are as follows:

Dizziness, fainting, confusion.

Loss of elasticity and signs of skin cracking.

Exhibiting state of delirium.

Less frequent urination.

Blood pressure fluctuation.

In general, a very dry appearance with sunken eye sockets and also bad breath.

Caring for the elderly and attending to their regular water consumption needs may not be an easy task but following certain simple etiquettes may help.

Offer elderly people under your care a drink at frequent intervals.

Make the drink a bit tasty by adding some natural flavouring or natural fruit juices. This will negate the blandness of the taste of water and keep the elderly interested in drinking fluids. Offer the drink in small portions but more frequently. Due to mobility issues elderly people may not be able to move around in search of a drink of water; this is energy-consuming for them. Keep water or fruit juice in a handy location within their easy reach.

Water requirement for elderly people is just as important as the rest of the population due to its involvement in most bodily functions as described earlier. So inadequate consumption is detrimental to health and general well-being for each and every individual young and old alike.

I have been asked on a number of occasions what is the right amount of water that we need to drink per day. There is no simple answer to this. But common sense must prevail not a blind following to some comments someone may have made in the past which may have stuck with you. Let's apply logic and break it down to some valid reasoning. Water or better still our daily fluid intake should be dependent on our physical makeup; height, weight, and food intake, our urinary output throughout the day and also environmental conditions.

Let's face it, a tall and well-built person may have an increased requirement compared to a smaller thinly built person. An active person again may require a little bit more fluid intake than a less active person, and with the same logic, people with a dietary intake of more fruits and vegetables may again need less fluid intake.

So, did you follow my logic? For what it is worth here is my explanation.

A person who has a larger body surface area will tend to lose more fluid in a 24-hour period than a person with lessor surface area and therefore, their fluid intake requirement must be more. Similarly, a person who has more fruit and vegetables in their diet will perhaps require slightly less water intake as the shortfall is compensated by the extra fluids from fruits and vegetables. It is all a matter of common-sense approach keeping in mind that too much fluid intake will put an extra filtration load on the kidneys.

As a general rule of thumb for every kg of our body weight we need 25g–35g water; this on the average equates to approximately 2.1 litre water for a person of 70kg body weight. **As I say, common sense must prevail**.

Let us now look at some of the unique properties of water as it covers up to 70–75% of our planet's surface and also our body content. So, we have a lot in common.

1. Water has a high boiling point (100 degree Celsius) and a low freezing point (0°C) and therefore it takes longer to boil and slower to freeze. This property enables water to retain heat and be used in central heating in cooler climates. This also helps the aquatic life to survive in cooler climates due to water remaining mobile or flowing even though the top layer may have frozen.
2. Water is a universal solvent and over the years it will dissolve anything in its path such as minerals, nutrients from soil and rocks and also gases.
3. Water is the only liquid which exists in all three forms within the temperature range on our planet; Ice (solid form of water), liquid water (liquid form), and vapours or steam (gaseous form of water); and strangely enough the solid form is less dense than the liquid form which is again a unique water property.

Due to the presence of such a vast amount of life-giving water on our planet, Earth is the only currently known planet in our solar system let alone the entire galaxy 'The Milky Way' where survival of any life form (Animals, insects, micro-organisms, plants and vegetation, etc.) has been possible and therefore we all are unique species living on a unique planet; it therefore becomes our responsibility to preserve our existence by looking after our planet. Water not only quenches our thirst and keeps our bodies moist and hydrated it provides the atmosphere for us to live, breathe and survive.

Sugar, a Modern-Day Villain or a Myth?

Chemically known as sucrose, it is a combination of two soluble carbohydrate molecules; glucose and fructose and occurs in nature in many fruits and vegetables. The main commercial source of sugar is from sugarcane. It is a species of tall hybrid fibrous vegetation from which sugar is extracted and is a natural source of almost 80% of the world's sugar production. Other sources of sugar are sugar beet or beet sugar and to a lesser degree corn, wheat, rice, etc., which are all grain crops grown in warm temperate climate zones.

Sugar is a carbohydrate in the macronutrient food category which also includes starches and are component of most commercially prepared food items such as bread cereals cakes and confectionaries and also a component of pre-prepared and packed lunches and dinners as a taste enhancer and offers a boost to the carbohydrate content; depending of course on the amount of the additions.

It is a primary source of energy. Another use of sugar is in pharmaceuticals, especially in syrups such as in cough syrups where the sugar loading can be around 30% or more. Sugar has found large use in confectionaries and sweet beverages.

The application of sugar in these preparations can be very high. It is also fair to say that the sugar content of many fruits and vegetables are quite high too. Some people argue that available sugars from these natural sources are acceptable and termed as a better source than that is available from the processing of sugar-rich sugarcane, sugar beets and other natural sources in factories. The bottom line of these futile arguments is that the end product is identical.

Like everything there are two sides to all stories. Sugar has many positives and some extreme negatives. It is important to consider these with proper merits and perspectives. I will try to summarise some of the positives and negatives and let the readers decide for themselves.

At the onset of this discussion, let me clearly state that currently, I do not have any commercial arrangements with sugar producers nor am I a significant user of this commodity either commercially or domestically. I do use sugar in moderation and in minimum quantities and always try to stay below the WHO-recommended daily usage. So, firstly let us see what the international recommendations for daily sugar consumption are.

According to World Health Organisation (WHO) standards sugar/s a combination of both mono and disaccharides should not make up for more than 10% of the daily energy (KJ) intake to prevent the dental caries. This includes sugars from all sources such as glucose, fructose and sucrose including honey.

This quantitatively works out to be around 50g of sugar daily.

According to the Australian Bureau of Statistics for adults on a daily 8700kJ (around 2,072 calories) intake it works out to be around 55g daily and the recommendation from the American Heart Association is that this figure should not be more than 36g daily.

The important point to remember is that table sugar or sucrose is a disaccharide which when enters our digestive system breaks down into glucose and fructose the two monosaccharide components.

Taking sugar in moderation is not all negative, there are many benefits as well which if explained in simple language comes to this.

Glucose is the primary source of energy which our body needs in performing every physiological activity. Many cells convert the circulating glucose into instant energy while several other organ cells such as the liver cells, the muscle cells store the extra glucose for later on-demand use. Insulin is a hormone which is triggered by the available glucose in the bloodstream. The instant use of glucose by the cells produces a burst of energy which gives us the stamina and power required to do various physical tasks.

Sugar is one of the most common feel-good foods; by causing a burst of release of dopamine a neurotransmitter which signals the brain to activate our pleasure centres. So, it is always a good thing to have moderate portions of dietary carbohydrates, such as sugar. A low level of dopamine is linked with several psychological and physiological state of mind such as depression, psychosis and schizophrenia.

But we must control our dietary sugar intake, as too much consumption is very much detrimental to our health.

Eating too much sucrose can convert it into glucose producing all-powerful energy. But there is a limit to what the body can handle and puts extra strain on our pancreas (a gland of our endocrine system) which will be required to overwork to keep up with the demands of producing excess insulin.

Residual sucrose and glucose will crystallise out in the blood stream causing a series of health complications resulting in circulatory issues, the integrity of our blood vessels particularly capillary vessels, lack of nutrient delivery, the inadequate oxygen concentration in the blood stream and particularly diabetes and associated diseases. It is an un-denying fact that sugar and carbohydrates in general play an important role in our daily dietary requirements but it is equally important that such dietary intakes should be restricted as overconsumption can cause more harm than good. This is a classic example where self-control and a common-sense approach must be maintained.

When sugar breaks down in our gastrointestinal system, it forms one molecule of glucose and one of fructose. Glucose and fructose are both monosaccharides and simple sugars. As we know glucose is the main energy source for our body's energy needs.

So, what happens to fructose?

Simply fructose needs to be converted into glucose before it can be absorbed into the cells for converting into energy. Conversion of fructose takes place in the liver and therefore an excess fructose in the system can have an overloading effect on the liver.

Fructose is also called 'Fruit Sugar' because it is the sweet component of almost all sweet fruits and is found in a bound state with glucose. Eating fruit will also provide a significant level of sucrose for example consuming a large apple will provide your system with approximately 23g of sugar of which around 13g is fructose. In comparison, honey contains about 80% of sugars including glucose and fructose. These foods, fruits and honey are classed as natural foods and are more popular with consumers, but remember none the less they also break down into glucose and fructose the end result of it is utilisation by the cells to produce energy which requires a continual supply of insulin.

For diabetics and people suffering from other illnesses of carbohydrate metabolism, impairment can be a significant negative physiological attribute which can lead to seriousness in their health conditions in later life.

(A Sugar/Sucrose molecule)   **Glucose**   **Fructose**

German chemist Marggraf was the first to discover glucose by isolating it from raisins in 1747 and described it as *'einer Art Zücker'*; a kind of sugar.

The name Glucose was coined by Jean Dumas in 1838, from the Greek word *glycos*, meaning sugar or sweet. But it was not until the late 1880s that the great German chemist Emil Fischer who discovered its molecular structure for which he received the Nobel Prize in 1902 for chemistry.

Sugars are a general class of compounds which are naturally occurring.

For the sake of simple understanding, the basic unit of all-natural sugars is Glucose and depending on the number of glucose units a further classification of sugars can be made such as:

Monosaccharides which are sugars with single glucose units for example glucose (also known as dextrose), Fructose (fruit sugar) and Galactose (occurs in milk).

Disaccharides are sugars which have 2 glucose units linked together; examples are sucrose (table sugar) in which glucose + fructose molecules are bound together, Lactose (milk sugar) linking glucose with galactose molecule and Maltose (malt sugar) in which two glucose units are linked with each other.

Polysaccharides are long chain structures which have several glucose units attached together, an example of this is starches from various sources.

In the following section under Food Categories, you will find that carbohydrates are an important and significant part of our dietary intake which breaks down into sugar molecules which are the major components. Reading the section through would give the readers a working knowledge on sugar-related impairment such as carbohydrate metabolism and a disease state known as diabetes.

Let us quickly look at honey which is again portrayed as a good guy and more preferable than sugar itself.

What is honey…simply, honey is a natural product made by honey bees using the nectar of various flowers that the bees collect and bring to their hives. Chemically honey is primarily composed of approx. 80–85% mainly carbohydrates consisting of 38% fructose and 32% glucose and around 2% sucrose. It also contains about 10% disaccharides, 18% water and other nutrients e.g., antioxidants, amino acids, vitamins, minerals (zinc, iron, calcium), etc., in minor portions.

Although the major component of honey is sugars, it is believed that sucrose (Table sugar) and honey differ fundamentally in so far as table sugar is compounded glucose-fructose while in honey, these two ingredients are in a free unbound state. Some people may be allergic to honey and honey products with mild symptoms such as nausea, vomiting, perspiration feeling weak, etc. Serious symptoms can also show up in the form of wheezing, arrhythmias (irregular heartbeats), dizziness, fainting episodes and respiratory problems. If untreated, these allergies may become fatal in rare instances.

Although purified, honey is quite tolerable but care and caution must be applied where sensitivity and allergic reactions are noted with certain natural products e.g., bee pollen, royal jelly, bee venom, etc. Most of these are frequently used in natural therapies.

Results of research carried out on honey to determine the possibility of its therapeutic activities suggest that it may have some benefit on cardiovascular disease, cough symptoms, gastrointestinal problems, and mild neurological disorders, wound healing, etc., however, there are no standard methods for extracting pure honey from its raw state results may vary from one source to the other.

(Ref:https://www.mayoclinic.org/drugs-supplements-honey/art20363819).

The table below compares the nutritional value of honey and sucrose and suggests their nutritional similarity.

Table: Nutritional Value Comparison:
Honey and Sucrose

Parameters	Per 100g Pure Honey Ref: McCance RA and Widdowson EM (2010). The composition of foods. 6th ed. Cambridge, England: Food Standards Agency.	Per 100g granulated Sucrose (Ref: Sugars granulated. US Department of Agriculture. Food Data Central)
Energy	288cal	400cal
Fat (g)	0	0
Carbohydrate (g)	76.4	100
Glucose (g)	34.6	Approx. 50%
Fructose (g)	41.8	Approx. 50%
Protein	0.4	0
Water (g)	17.5	0 (dehydrated)
Cholesterol	0	0
Others	Very small amounts of minerals, vitamins Amino acids etc.	Almost nil in pure anhydrous granulated sucrose.

Common Table Salt, Is It Good for You or Bad?

Common salt is also as natural as it gets; chemically known as sodium chloride; it is one of the basic human tastes. It is also one of the oldest commonly applied foodstuff used over many centuries in food preparation, preservation and enhancement of taste component. It is also essential for life. Lack of salt or sodium can cause an imbalance in the osmotic pressure between the intra and extra (within and outside) cellular fluid which has an important implication on the integrity of our cell structure. The early symptoms of low blood sodium level (hyponatraemia) are:

Nausea, Vomiting Muscle Cramps, intermittent headaches, Confusion and Feeling Tiredness, etc., and could vary from person to person in terms of frequency and severity of symptoms. It can also be an age-related variance.

The following risk group may be identified for observation:

Seniors in our community, people on medications such as on diuretic and antidepressant medications, activities which cause profusely sweating e.g., highly active athletes and gym performance, people suffering from various medical conditions such as kidney problems, heart conditions and people with low sodium diet.

People who drink copious amounts of water frequently and pass urine at very frequent intervals are also at risk.

There are many other conditions as well and must have urgent medical intervention.

I found an interesting bit of information which I think is quite relevant to our topic. I do however comment that this is an excerpt from a recent publication.

(Ref: NEMO Paediatrics Salt Replacement in Cystic Fibrosis; https://www.health.qld.gov.au › paeds salt replacement reviewed April 2020). Please read the full publication for further information. It must also be known that there is a disclaimer attached to this publication so as not to misinterpret or misuse the content information. Ref: Disclaimer: www.*health.qld.gov.au*/global/disclaimer.

Salt replacement therapy for children and adolescents with Cystic Fibrosis. Why do people with Cystic Fibrosis need extra salt? All people with cystic fibrosis (CF) lose large amounts of sodium and chloride (the two compounds that makeup salt) in their sweat, especially with exercise, hot weather, fevers and infections. People with CF lose 3–4 times more salt through their sweat than those without CF. This is because it is believed that the CF sweat gland is unable to absorb salt back into the blood. This leaves large amounts of salt in their sweat. Because the level of salt in the blood does not rise, the body has no recognition of thirst. This leads to a higher risk of dehydration. To prevent dehydration, people with CF need to replace both salt and fluid. Signs and symptoms of salt depletion:

- Fatigue, irritability, headaches.
- Poor concentration.
- Salt crystals on the skin.
- Nausea, vomiting, decreased appetite.
- Muscle cramps.
- Hyponatraemia. (Low blood sodium)
- Thicker, harder to expectorate sputum.
- Thicker secretions in the bowel leading to constipation.
  (Please read the actual publication)

Salt is an ageless ingredient which has its roots of application earlier than 8000 years in human recorded history when it was considered a valuable trading commodity in ancient civilisations such as between the Egyptian, Phoenician and other ancient Mediterranean civilisations such as Greeks and early Romans.

One of the earliest natural salt harvests, is believed to have taken place around 6000 BC in and around Lake Yuncheng in China, in the province of Shanxi.

It played a pivotal role in trade and commerce as early as 5000 BC when the ancient cultures of Greece and Samaria not only used it as a part of their culinary delight and diet but importantly also in their religious celebrations. The Phoenician seafarers are thought to have learned the use of salt and brought it to their land from the ancient Greeks. Ancient Greeks are also known to have learned to harvest salt from the sea by using the evaporation technique. The early Greeks were also accredited to have learned the art of preserving meat and fish with salt.

Salt Baths have been in use since ancient times and popularised by the Romans. Even today it is said that salt baths or natural salt pools are means to relax tired bodies and also have the ability to rejuvenate the ailing body.

Salt lamps have become a popular item as it is alleged that it keeps the room or the environment fresh, dry and clean and free of certain allergies. Most people consume too much salt—on average 9–12 grams per day more than twice what has been recommended by WHO; Ref: Salt reduction fact sheet WHO (April 2020).

In essence, salt is essential for life but in moderation; the World Health Organisation (WHO) in their policy statements has always recommended to reduce the salt intake for general consumption. In countries such as Japan, parts of the USA, China and many other areas of the world the salt intake is much higher than what has been recommended by the WHO.

For example, the consumption of common table salt amongst the adult population in China (almost 10g per day) and Japan is almost double than what is recommended by the WHO limiting to less than 5g per day (2016). Sadly, enough even with warnings associated with health issues salt consumption has not shown any sign of decrease.

The National Health and Medical Research Council (NHMRC) advises that Australian adults should aim to consume no more than one teaspoon (5 grams) of salt a day. Salt consumption in Australia is showing signs of decrease; truly a positive step.

In a 2017 study by Tokyo University, it was found that there was an alarming rate of consumption of salt among adult males (11.8g/day) and females (8.9g/day) among the Japanese population. In a 2019, Japanese study published in the Journal of Clinical Hypertension a high incidence of high blood pressure was noted in Japanese population (60% male and 45% female).

This finding corroborates with the high salt intake.

Food Categories

There are many different types of foods, some are called staple foods which we table most of the time and include in our regular main meals of the day. Foods also vary culturally and have evolved from the producers in particular regions and can be highly regional.

Scientifically we can broadly classify foods into 5 different categories for our easy understanding:

Carbohydrates.
Fats and Proteins.
Fruits and Vegetables.
Cereals, Nuts and Legumes.
Dairy.

The classification above is quite comprehensive and covers almost all food types that we consume.

Some experts classify dairy products milk and cheese etc. together with fats and proteins. Oils are also classified under fats and proteins. There are some finer points of difference but for the sake of simplicity, the above classification usually works and is considered to be complete.

Carbohydrates or carbs are macronutrients which constitute a big part of our daily dietary intakes. These mainly contain 3 types of nutrients that our body uptakes.

Sugars: These general classes of compounds have been included earlier in this chapter; all food items that we eat eventually break down in our gut system to basic glucose units (mono-saccharide) and is considered to be the most basic energy-producing unit.

Starches and complex carbohydrates are a class of their own and are complex in their chemical structure and therefore known as complex carbohydrates. These are long-chain molecules with several glucose units (more than 10 units), and eventually broken down by the digestive system into smaller absorbable glucose units.

Fibres are sourced from plants and vegetables and are indigestible by humans.

They are considered as roughage as it passes through the body's elimination system (faeces) unchanged and helps our bowel movement effectively. Like sugars fibres are also a part of the carbohydrate food chain and come mainly in two forms; soluble and insoluble fibres and each has a very specific function for our digestive system.

Soluble fibres are found in fruits and vegetables, legumes and oat and barley-like grains and are soluble in water and are the gelatinous part of the food which attracts water from the gastro-intestinal tract and forms a gel which slows the stomach emptying process thus gives the feeling of fullness. Soluble fibres by binding with the excess circulating blood glucose and cholesterol, also help reduce their levels in our body.

Insoluble fibres are also sourced from plants, vegetables and fruits and are not easily broken down into our digestive system. It is the kind of roughage which adds bulk to the faeces and helps the formation of stool to pass relatively quickly by friction through the large intestine and thus eliminates the unwanted undigested foodstuff. Insoluble fibres by absorbing moisture from the bowel help moisten the faeces and give it a slippery consistency and therefore assist in regular bowel movement.

People who are constipated and find it difficult to move bowel regularly can benefit by adding cereals such as wheat bran, nuts seeds and a good portion of fibrous fruits and vegetables in their diets.

When choosing diet plans, it is very important to keep a control on your dietary intake because the quantity of carbohydrate intake can directly affect blood glucose levels.

Excess carbohydrates will break down into absorbable glucose units and enter blood stream through intestinal absorption and finally deposit into various body tissues. Therefore, any malfunction in our carbohydrate metabolism whether genetically induced or environmental could lead to some specific problems in our health and general well-being.

Carbohydrates and Diabetes

Carbohydrates form a very important part of our food chain. As we now know that these food groups break down into smaller absorbable units to produce energy for our body to utilise. Any malfunction and or impairment in our carbohydrate metabolism whether genetically induced or environmentally propagated could lead to several disease states and affect our general health and well-being in a significant way.

Hyperglycaemia is one such condition concerned with the elevation of blood glucose (or simply blood sugar) levels. Hyperglycaemia could develop as a temporary condition and usually passes away when the underlying causes are rectified. For example, gestational diabetes which often shows up during pregnancy may cause blood glucose levels to be elevated but return to pre-gestational levels after childbirth.

However, there is a more serious side to hyperglycaemia, which if not treated or intervened medically at the onset of the symptoms could manifest as serious diabetic complications.

The most common tell-tale signs are increase in the frequency of urination, feeling thirsty, hunger associated with weight loss, irritability and some behavioural anomalies and blurred vision.

These diabetic conditions are referred to as either Type 1 Diabetes which is insulin-dependent, and Type 2 Diabetes which is non-insulin dependent. Type 2 Diabetes is a chronic condition in which the Beta-cells in our pancreas gland responsible for insulin production are impaired and insulin production is less than normal.

Insulin was first discovered in 1922 by Sir Frederick G Banting, Charles H Best and JJR Macleod at the University of Toronto Canada and is a hormone produced in our pancreas which facilitates the introduction of the glucose molecule into the cells for cellular metabolism and thus keeps a control of the free, circulating glucose molecule in our blood. For their discovery, Banting and

Macleod shared the Nobel Prize in Physiology in 1923. The early symptom of diabetes is passing glucose in the urine which can be easily detected by using a commercially available diagnostic multi-stick or a simple blood test referred by a medical practitioner. Other simple symptoms are increased thirst and frequency of urination as described earlier.

Non-insulin-dependent diabetes is less complicated and may be managed with lifestyle changes such as intake of less carbohydrate foods in our diets, weight management and cutting down on smoking, alcohol, drug abuse and in general a more regulated daily lifestyle maintenance. A good quality B group vitamin complex may also help as several B-group vitamins take part in our cellular metabolism as biochemical catalysts, to make the process more efficient.

Nutritionally, several ingredients may be included in our diet to ease the glucose load of non-insulin-dependent diabetes. Consumption of fibre especially pectin helps slow down the conversion of foods into glucose and therefore slows down the rate of availability of free glucose molecules into the bloodstream thus decreasing the overloading of circulating glucose molecules.

Chromium plays an important role in easing the body's glucose intolerance.

Diabetics lose a lot of water due to the diuretic effect of some of the medication and also excessive loss of water due to sweating and passing high volume of water as urine leads to a deficit of water in the body and consequently face electrolyte imbalance. Therefore, it is important to replenish both water and electrolytes on a periodic basis.

It is important to remember that although diabetes is not an uncommon disease these days, it is also controllable with proper medication, nutritional supplements and self-discipline. Maintaining an adequate dietary regimen, medication and adhering to a certain planned lifestyle can make a world of difference in leading a normal life, or, if proper lifestyle of self-discipline is not maintained then a life of misery can be expected all throughout our life.

Now we look at the opposite side of the diabetes coin; on one side we have diabetes due to high blood glucose on the other side we have diabetes due to low blood sugar called **hypoglycaemia**. It is a disorder of carbohydrate metabolism characterised by a very low blood glucose level. It is not a disease of an infectious nature and therefore with a reasonable adjustment in lifestyle, one can have a meaningful existence. The abnormal lowering of the blood glucose level may be caused by two important reasons. One, after meals a rapid absorption of glucose may take place into the circulating blood which then is rapidly metabolised by the facilitation of an excess secretion of insulin leaving a very low amount of glucose available for transportation into various tissues of the body.

The second reason could be that due to other associated diseases such as liver impairments, there is less than normal processing of glucose for absorption into the bloodstream. Or, certain internal problems such as abnormal cell growth, tumours, etc., which consume excessive amounts of available glucose leading to a depletion of the blood glucose levels. During excessive stress, strain, heavy strenuous exercise sessions and pregnancy situations, etc., there is a heavier demand on glucose to energise the cells thus temporarily hypoglycaemic attacks characterised by slight dizzy spells are noted which can be overcome by the intake of a candy bar or a sweet drink.

Hypoglycaemia can also be drug-induced or drug-related. The confirmation of hypoglycaemia is done by testing blood glucose levels before meals (fasting) and also after meals and comparing. However, there are certain signs and symptoms that are quite characteristic. The feeling of weakness, palpitation, nervousness, etc., are all indications of hypoglycaemia. More serious symptoms can show up as headaches, abnormal sweating, feeling hungry, weakness associated with fainting and dizzy feeling, and occasional loss of memory or blankness. It is also that some advanced cases of hypoglycaemia sufferers could have an effect on the Central Nervous System (CNS) causing loss of sense and direction, loss of co-ordination and also prolonged loss of consciousness.

If these symptoms are quite frequent or very prevalent, then professional attention should be sought at the early onset of the symptoms as these symptoms can also be signs of many other disease states. Hypoglycaemic patients have a similar behavioural pattern as the patients suffering from neurological psychological disorders and restoring the blood glucose levels to normality results in quick recovery.

The disease diabetes itself is characterised by **Diabetes Mellitus** which is the cause of hormonal imbalance (insulin) and **Diabetes Insipidus** is characterised by an imbalance of a hormone Anti Diuretic Hormone (ADH) produced by the pituitary gland.

Johann Peter Frank (1794), a German physician is credited to be the first medical practitioner to distinguish diabetes mellitus and diabetes insipidus. Interested readers can further read on by referring to **Mayo Clinic website** on this subject.

Insulin: This is a protein chain or peptide hormone, a hormone which is produced in a gland known as the pancreas within our body's endocrine system and performs a number of important functions as a carrier of glucose to all the different cells in our body and its utilisation. Glucose is the fundament unit of the food we eat which the cells use to metabolise producing energy for us to live on.

Hyperglycaemia is an important symptom of a diabetic condition and can be referred to as either Type 1 Diabetes which is insulin-dependent, and Type 2 which is non-insulin dependent.

However, it is important to remember that Type 2 Diabetic patients may need insulin treatment if their dietary intake patterns fail to regulate their general health condition to a professionally set target. It is absolutely necessary that these patients adhere to a regulated weight management programme and lifestyle change to control their obesity, body mass index (BMI), and blood pressure and improve their general fitness level.

Under normal health conditions as soon as our blood sugar level rises usually after food intake, the release mechanism for insulin is triggered which signals our body cells to accept glucose and to convert it into energy. Insulin also assists in the storage of excess glucose in our fatty tissues, muscles and in the liver for later use on a need basis.

Since its discovery insulin has been at the forefront of numerous scientific research due to its lifesaving properties resulting in the understanding of human biology and medicine which resulted in several Nobel Prizes being awarded for the study and advances in insulin.

Tracing back into the history of research and development into insulin, I came across several contributions made by notable researchers of their time. The following timeline is interesting to trace the developmental pathways from its discovery to the present day.

1869: Paul Langerhans, a medical student discovers a distinct collection of cells within the pancreas. These cells were later known as the Islets of Langerhans.

1889: Oskar Minkowski and Joseph von Mering experimenting with a dog whose pancreas was removed was found to lick its urine which was tested and found to contain glucose.

1901: Eugene Opie discovers that the Islets of Langerhans produce insulin and that the destruction of these cells resulted in diabetes.

1916: Romanian professor Nicolae Paulescu developed an extract of the pancreas which was found to lower blood sugar in diabetic dogs.

1921: Dr Frederick Banting and medical student Charles Best performed experiments on the pancreas of dogs in Toronto, Canada and later that year isolated insulin.

Late December 1921, James B. Collip joined Dr Banting's research team and started work on the purification of insulin.

1922: A 14-year-old boy named Leonard Thompson with type 1 diabetes was the first person to receive the first dose of crude insulin prepared by Banting and Best. Later that year Collip was successful in purifying a small amount of insulin from a pancreatic concoction. Which was given to Leonard Thompson which miraculously prolonged his life by a further 13 years.

In May 1922, Professor John Macleod named the extract 'insulin' in a presentation lecture to the Association of American Physicians in Washington D.C.

1923: Banting and Macleod were awarded the Nobel Prize in Physiology or Medicine. Both, however, felt that Best and Collip were equally eligible and shared their prize money with their two colleagues.

1936: Danish physician Hans Christian Hagedorn discovers the action of insulin can be prolonged with the addition of protamine.

1955: Insulin is sequenced by British biochemist Frederick Sanger, and is the first protein to be fully sequenced and structure was worked out.

1958: Frederick Sanger received the 1958 Nobel Prize in Chemistry for his work on the structure of insulin.

1963: Insulin becomes the first human protein to be chemically synthesised.

1975: Ciba-Geigy (Basel, Switzerland) first synthesised insulin in the laboratory (CGP 12 831) by recombinant technology (rDNA).

1980: Insulin synthesised by rDNA technology was first tested on human volunteers in England.

Also, in 1980 the first successful Islet cell transplantation was carried out in humans by David Sutherland and John Najarian two surgeons working in Minnesota in the USA.

1982: The recombinant insulin was named human insulin to distinguish from animal insulin which was much less allergic.

1982–1996: Saw immense developments happening in insulin availability and delivery systems e.g., insulin pen delivery system (Novo Nordisk a Danish Company in **1985**), insulin pump in **1992** by Medtronic, an American medical device company which made life much easier for regular insulin users. In **1990**, first successful islet cell transplantation was carried out by Tzakis AG, and his co-workers at the University of Pittsburgh USA (*Lancet.* **336** (8712): 402–5. 1990).

In **1991,** WHO nominated November 14th as the World Diabetes Day to honour Dr Banting's birthday.

2000–2005: Large scale trial on mass islet cell transplantation was first performed in 470 type 1 diabetes patients which reduced the dependency on regular use of insulin.

There is a further interesting timeline on insulin and diabetes improvements; those who are interested may refer to:

(Ref: https://www.diabetes.co.uk/insulin/history-of-insulin.html and Diabetes UK Diabetes History—History of Diabetes Mellitus).

Throughout our history from ancient times to now many interesting facts about diabetes and insulin have been recorded.

In ancient Ebers Papyrus (1550 BC) reference had been made of a disease which we know today as diabetes.

In Ayurvedic Medicine (Early 5th and 6th century BC), a disease known as 'Honey Urine' was known, again, we refer to it today as diabetes. Early Physicians of the medieval Islamic world, including Avicenna, have also written about diabetes in their chronicles and writings.

Johann Peter Frank (1794), a German physician is credited to be the first medical practitioner to distinguish diabetes mellitus and diabetes insipidus. From its first discovery in 1921, 100 years have gone by and insulin still remains active and vigilant helping millions of people around the world enjoy a life full of hope and promises. With the passing of each day, new information is being made available to the general public via their primary health service providers. New innovations and treatments are invented and, or updated to return the lives of diabetic sufferers as close to normal as possible.

Fruits and Vegetables

Under normal conditions, fruits and vegetables are excellent sources of good nutrition. This category of foods provided a combination of macro-and micro-nutrients, e.g., carbohydrates, proteins, starches and fibres, vitamins, minerals and anti-oxidants. In other words, fresh fruits and vegetables if chosen correctly can provide wholesome nutrition.

Fruits and vegetables also provide considerable hydration for tissues and cellular structure.

In diabetes and hyperglycaemia, it is recommended to choose your fruits and vegetables sensibly as many have a high sugar content.

The tabulated data below have been sourced from the internet from various published reports; some values have been averaged out to maintain some consistency.

(Nutritional value of some popular fruits per 100g)

Values Fruits	Calories	Proteins (g)	Carbs (g)	Fibre (g)	Fats (g)	Sugar (g)	Water (%)
Apples	52	0.3	13.8	2.4	0.2	10.4	86
Pears	59	0.6	16	3.5	0.1	10	88
Grapes	69	0.7	18	1	0.15	16	81
Peaches	39	0.7	9.3	1.4	0.7	8	89
Oranges	47	1	10.5	2	0.14	8.5	62
Bananas	89	1.1	22.8	2.6	0.3	12.2	75
Nectarines	44	1.05	10.5	1.70	0.35	7.9	88
Papayas	38.8	0.65	10.0	2	0.2	8	88
Mangoes	60	0.85	15	1.6	0.36	13.6	83
Watermelons	30	0.6	7.6	0.4	0.2	6.2	91
Strawberries	32	0.7	7.7	2	0.3	4.9	91
Apricots	48.6	1.43	11.4	2.1	0.4	9	86

(Ref: data mostly extracted from www.healthline.com benefits-of the fruit; data is also collected from www.myfooddata.com)

Food Categories and Diet

(Nutritional value of some popular vegetables per 100g)

Values Fruits	Calories	Proteins (g)	Carbs (g)	Fibre (g)	Fats (g)	Sugar (g)	Water (%)
Potatoes	73.5	4.5	17.3	1.3	0	0.7	79
Broccoli	30	2.7	5.3	2	0.33	1.33	89
Carrots	37.5	1.3	9	2.6	0	6.4	88
Cauliflowers	25	2	5	2	0	2	92
Celery	13.6	0	3.63	1.8	0	1.8	95
Cucumbers	10	1	2	1	0	1	95
Green Beans	24.1	1.2	6	3.6	0	2.4	90
Leafy Lettuce	17.6	1.2	2.35	1.2	0	1.2	96
Green Cabbage	29.4	1.2	5.9	2.35	0	3.5	93
Asparagus	21.4	2.1	4.3	2.1	0	2.1	93
Radish	11.8	0	3.5	1.2	0	2.35	95
Summer Squash	20	1	4	2	0	2	95

(Ref: Data extracted from Nutrition Information for Raw Vegetables. www.fda.gov › food › food-labelling-nutrition); and 17 vegetables highest in water. www.myfooddata.com › articles › vegetables-high-)

Fats and Proteins in Our Diet

There are two main sources of fats and proteins in our diets. **Animal Source** and **Vegetable Source** or plant protein.

Animal source protein provides a much complete amino acid profile. The quality of protein is determined by the availability and content of the amino acids from the profile. However, animal protein is much harder to digest and involves additional biochemical processing such as the requirement and availability of bile to act as a surfactant for the protein component of the food to be digested.

Most of our animal-sourced dietary protein consists of fish, meats from poultry animals, meats from abattoir animals e.g., beef, sheep, pork, etc., and also eggs, milk and milk products from farms.

In general, the available protein component varies greatly from animal to animal and also from source to source; such as poultry animals provide good quality easier-to-digest protein around 30 percent. The amino acid profile from animal source protein is relatively higher than plant-based protein (See Table). Plant-based proteins are also good wholesome protein sources which are easier to digest and universally accepted by both non-vegetarians and vegetarians.

The main sources are legumes and lentils, seeds and nuts, beans fruits and vegetables, etc. The amino acid profile in plant-based proteins are somewhat less complete than the animal proteins. Amino acids are essential nutrients which our body cannot bio-synthesise and therefore need to be supplemented on a regular basis.

So, what are **amino acids**?

Amino acids are organic compounds containing carbon, hydrogen, oxygen and nitrogen and are the fundamental building blocks of both animal and plant-based proteins.

Amino acids are classified into two main types; **essential** and **non-essential**. Essential amino acids are the ones which our body cannot manufacture and therefore must be supplemented.

Amino-acids required by our Body

Essential Amino acids (9 in total)	Non-Essential Amino acids
Histidine	Alanine
Leucine	Aspartic Acid
Iso-Leucine	Asparagine

Lysine	*Arginine
Methionine	*Cysteine
Phenylalanine	*Glutamine
Threonine	Glutamic Acid
Tryptophan	*Glycine
Valine	*Ornithine
	*Proline
	*Serine
	*Tyrosine

Although Amino acids marked with asterisks (*) are non-essential amino acids which our body can manufacture, but under conditions of stress and excess fatigue body's demand increases more than the body can manufacture and therefore under these special conditions dietary or supplementary intakes are necessary. These amino acids, therefore, are often referred to as **Conditional Amino acids**.

Arginine is sometimes classified as an essential amino acid as our body can only manufacture very small amounts not enough for everyday utilisation.

Amino acid Functions: They have a myriad of roles to play in the human body; our health and general well-being are dependent on our intake of amino acids either through good nutrition and food intake rich in amino acids and, or, daily supplementation.

The main role of amino acids is as building blocks for protein. They are also essential for repairing our muscles which suffer daily wear and tear.

Amino acids also have the following important roles:

- Muscle and connective tissue growth.
- Repair of hair, skin and nails.
- Metabolism and energy-producing reactions.
- Assists in digestive processes.
- In the production and maintenance of neuro-transmitter.
- In hormone production.
- Involvement in various biochemical processes.
- Improves immunity.

Just to name a few.

If you are an active sports person and a regular participant in gym-activities, then you must take a healthy daily dose of amino acid supplements. Also, it is an important supplement to have during weight management programmes.

For seniors, with dietary considerations amino acid supplementation is a must for building up immunity and assisting with the prevention of muscle wasting.

Nuts, Cereals and Seeds in Our Diet:

Nuts, cereals and seeds form an important part of our diet and dietary requirements. This food group is packed with nutritional goodness containing fibre, protein, vitamins and minerals and healthy fats. Nuts are low in calories containing approximately 7–10 kcal/g.

Australian dietary guidelines recommend a daily intake of around 30g of nuts in adult diets.

Seeds are equally nutritious and should also be included in our diet although nuts are more popular inclusion in our diets than seeds as nuts can be consumed individually as a part of our diet while seeds are generally included in salads and cereals and in combination with nuts.

So, what is the difference between the two? Generally, speaking, seeds contain more oils, fats and fibre and their vitamin and mineral content can be significantly different. After all, seeds contain embryo which packs in an enormous amount of nutrients in a micro-space for the initial growth and sustenance of the future plant.

What about cereals? By cereals, we always imagine foods like cornflakes, porridge, brans and other collectively combined preparations either freshly cooked or taken out from commercially prepared packets at breakfast time. The ingredients of choice are oats, bran both rice and wheat, whole grains and certain legumes, e.g., beans, lentils, and chickpeas. All have good portions of fibre and other nutrients as contained in nuts and seeds.

There is a healthy choice for us to choose from and best to rotate from time to time to take in the wholesome natural goodness that these wonderful ingredients have to offer.

Before consuming seeds and nuts, legumes and grains it is very important to observe the allergy factors. All these ingredients can trigger allergic responses to a greater or lesser degree and create several health issues. Some allergic reactions can be life-threatening so check for allergies and take adequate precautions for yourselves and others in the family. Another issue of concern can be with commercially blended and packaged cereals. Always check the content list and the nutritional panel for the composition and unwanted taste enhancers such as excessive sugars and salt and artificial ingredients.

Aflatoxin in foods: Aflatoxins are a family of toxic microscopic organisms, fungal in origin *Aspergillus flavus* and *Aspergillus parasiticus* which are poisonous and very harmful to our health. It can cause violent sickness and may become life-threatening if not medically intervened at the onset of attack in allergic children. It affects children as well as adults but because the immune response system in children are not yet fully developed children can be at a greater risk. They are predominantly found in agricultural produce such as grainy crops, corn, peanuts and other nuts etc.

The major symptoms are nausea and vomiting, convulsions, abdominal pain, etc., serious and long-term exposure if unattended may cause acute liver damage, growth retardation in children and hepatocellular carcinoma which is a common type of liver cancer.

Nut Allergies: Although nuts provide enormous amounts of health benefits it is important to remember that there is a negative side to consuming nuts in the form of triggering allergic reactions in some people. But first, let's look at the positive benefits of nuts in our diet.

They are high in good fats but low in saturated fats, high content of dietary proteins and fibres but low in carbohydrates.

Nuts contain a significant content of anti-oxidants which helps to scavenge the Reactive Oxygen Toxic Species (ROTS) and free radical species which causes damage to our cell structures.

They are rich in vitamins and minerals e.g., vitamins B3, B6, B12, vitamin E, etc., and essential and trace minerals e.g., iron, copper, zinc, selenium, magnesium, potassium and calcium.

Due to their nutritional content nuts may help in alleviating many health conditions; many of these health benefits have been validated by either clinical trials or epidemiologic studies. Some of the benefits are outlined below.

Dietary inclusion of nuts, has positive benefits in weight management (Atherosclerosis 2013 Oct; 230(2):347–53, J Nutr 2016 Dec; 146 (12):25132519).

Nuts lower LDL Cholesterol and triglycerides, and promote the good HDL

Cholesterol in our system (Metabolism 2015 Nov; 64 (11):1521–9, Eur J Clin Nutr 2011 Jan; 65 (1):117–24).

Studies have suggested that nuts in diet can reduce the incidences of Stroke and Heart Attacks (J Am Coll Cardiol 2006 Oct 17; 48(8), J Nutr 2010 Jun; 140(6):1093–8).

There are many more credible publications and reported articles which have enunciated the importance of nuts in our diets.

With all this positive side to including nuts in our diets, there is a serious worrying aspect to consuming nuts.

Apart from choking hazards in children, it can trigger allergic reactions also known as **Anaphylaxis** which can attack children of any age can show up as a tingling sensation in the throat and mouth with dryness, swelling of lips, itchy skin rash with redness, runny nose, stomach cramps pain and nausea occasionally followed by vomiting. More seriously, tightness of the throat and chest, tongue can swell up, wheezing and abnormal breathing pattern followed by dizziness and eventual collapse.

Anaphylaxis allergic reaction can also attack adults due to nuts and other forms of food allergies such as certain medications, shellfish, certain food preservatives such as sulphur compounds, etc. In such allergic cases, a thorough plan of consideration must be ready should this allergic reaction strike. Adults due to their advanced immune response may weather the storm with less seriousness but for children sudden attacks should be immediately counteracted by administering adrenaline (epinephrine) via an auto-injector (EpiPen®), if available.

Table: Nutritional content of some Nuts, seeds and grains; calculated per serving of approx. 30g (Ref: USDA Agricultural Research Service https://fdc.nal.usda.gov)

Ingredients	Energy (kcal)	Fibre	Protein	Fats	Carbohydrate
Cashew nuts	155 kcal	1g	5g	12g	1g
Macadamia nuts	200	2.5g	2g	21g	2g
Almond nuts	161	3.5g	6g	14g	6g
Peanuts	176	3g	4g	17g	5g
Brazil nuts	182	2g	4g	18g	3g
Hazel nuts	213	3g	4g	17g	5g
Pine nuts	190	1g	4g	19g	4g

Pistachio nuts	160	3g	4g	13g	8g
Walnuts	185	2g	4g	18g	4g
Sesame seeds	162	3.4g	5g	14g	6.5g
Chia seeds	138	12g	4.6g	8.5g	12g
Pumpkin seeds	134	2g	6g	12g	5g
Sunflower seeds	80	1.5g	3.2g	7g	2.8g
Flax seeds	130	7g	5g	11g	8g
Hemp Seed	155	1.1g	8.8g	11g	2.6g
Buck wheat	95	1g	3.7g	1g	1g
Whole wheat	95	3g	3.7g	1g	20g
Oats	125	3g	3.5g	1.7g	19g
Barley	99	5g	3g	1g	20g
Quinoa	103	2g	4g	1.7g	18g

When considering the nutritional data reported in this chapter or elsewhere in the book, please take note that data has been compiled from various publications and has been averaged out due to considerable variation in reporting in some of those publications. Please use the data as a guide only and if you are using some or various data for constructing a calorie-conscious diet plan then it will be prudent to obtain some form of verification from a Nutritionist or a Dietician because each case will need to be validated based upon individual needs and circumstances.

Dietary Considerations

Whenever we talk and discuss or even think about diet we immediately go into an uncomfortable zone of uncertainty; does it involve a hard core routine of weight loss with restrictive eating and, or, a full-blown sequence of exercises to facilitate our weight management plan.

Relax, it has nothing to do with that and does not have to be that way. It can be a very pleasant experience and a simple life's journey to reach our destination of health and wellness. From start to finish, you are the master or mistress of your journeys. Along the way, there are a few simple rules that complement you and guide you to your destination.

With recent advancements made in human nutrition and technology to assimilate Nature, it has become necessary for all of us who use nutritional supplements as a means to improve our health and well-being to become nutritionally aware and conscientious of our surroundings in the way of food and supplementary intakes and co-ordinate with the available information. In essence, diet is what we eat to sustain our body and it is up to us to carefully prepare the foods that we are about to put in our mouth to fulfil our need for hunger. On this planet of ours, there are more than 8% of the whole population who go hungry every night before going to bed and of these hungry people many are children.

Food Selection and Choices

Everyone should make their choice of foods based on their cultural and religious beliefs. However, there must be a common sense approach and element of discipline involved for the preservation of our general health and well-being.

These are some of the essential points that should be considered when making choices.

- The daily portions of food intake should not provide less than the recommended energy requirement.
- Our diet should be a proper mix of a wide variety of food types as mentioned earlier in the chapter.
- Food should be enjoyed and not looked upon as a compulsion.
- The diet should be combined with some form of exercise and mild physical activity.
- Cultural and Religious factors.

  This plays an important part in the food choices we make as a society or a community. For example, the Muslim religion will not eat meat products which are not slaughtered by the Halal method.

  A Jewish community will only eat food which is Kosher.

  Hindus will not eat meat products derived from beef and pork and many in the Hindu community are total vegetarians only.

  I believe that people of the Catholic faith do not eat meat and meat products during Easter on religious grounds.

- Seasonal availability.

  Many in the community prefer to purchase fresh fruits and vegetables which are seasonally grown and freshly available.

- Socio-economic factors; for affordability reasons, many in the community do not have much choice.

- Physiological factors.

There are some foods which are not suited for many due to allergies and medical reasons. For example, many children in our community are allergic to certain nuts, eggs, peanut butter, etc. Many due to physiological disorders such as coeliac and irritable bowel syndrome (IBS) sufferers cannot tolerate certain grains and legumes which contain gluten.

- Psychological Factors such as depression, mood swings and guilty consciousness, obesity and emotions may occasionally contribute to our food choices. For example, hunting, game shooting, etc. may put off some people from consuming meaty food preparations. Some in the community will not drink milk due to the emotional belief that a calf may have been deprived of its mother's milk.
- Sensory Factors also are important in determining what type of food is preferable to an individual in making a choice; e.g., sight, smell, taste, touch, etc., are all important.

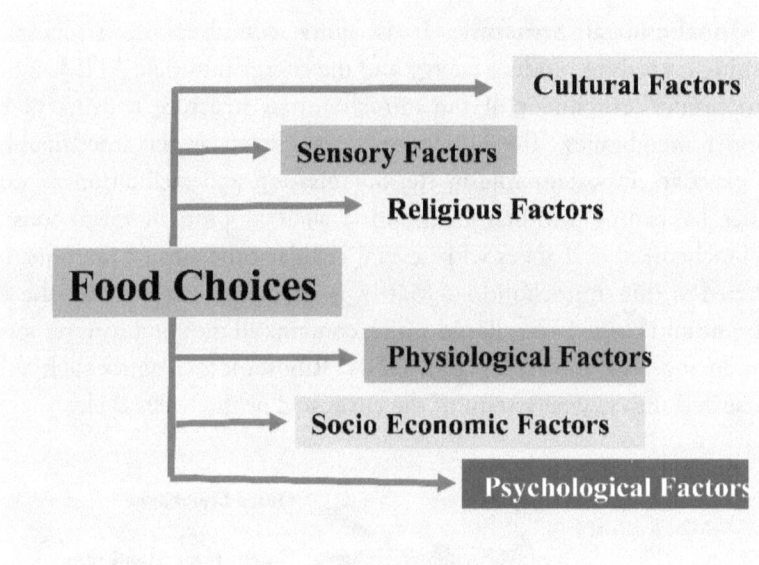

Food and Energy

All the foodstuff we eat whether it be proteins or carbohydrates, all break down into glucose molecules which then are released into our bloodstream from the stomach and intestines. The circulating glucose then enters the cells with some help from insulin.

This biochemical process takes place with the help of digestive juices containing various enzymes which are active at various stages of digestive process to complete the energy cycle (see below schematic flow diagram). The end result is the conversion of Glucose into ATP molecule. Remember, the conversion takes place deep in the core of the cell the powerhouse which we know as mitochondria.

$$\text{Glucose Molecule} \longrightarrow \text{ATP}$$

Glucose Molecule   **Energy Molecule**

Mitochondrial Structure: It is quite complex; the structure has everything it needs to produce energy and the energy molecule ATP. Just briefly the important component of the mitochondrial structure consists of outer and inner membranes. The in-between area known as the inter-membrane space plays an important role in the organisation and facilitation of various activities happening within mitochondria such as protein, metal ions, and other biochemical exchanges with several cellular processes or reactions being conducted within mitochondria. Matrix is the space enclosed by the inner membrane and has a viscous liquid which contains all the good stuff responsible for producing ATP molecules, e.g., DNA, Ribosomes, enzymes such as ATP synthase and the enzyme system of the citric acid or the Krebs cycle.

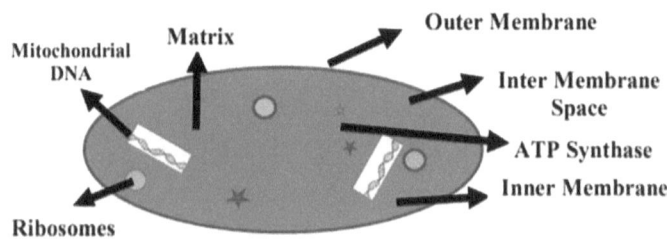

A Simplified MITOCHONDRIAL STRUCTURE

Diagram: Breakdown of Foods we eat into Glucose Molecule

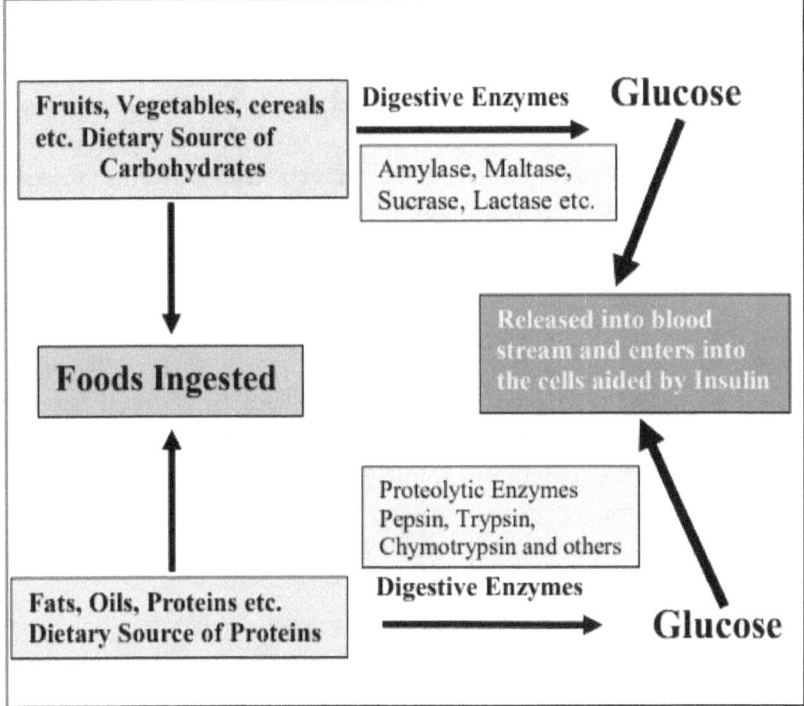

Stepwise progress can also be explained by the following flow diagram.

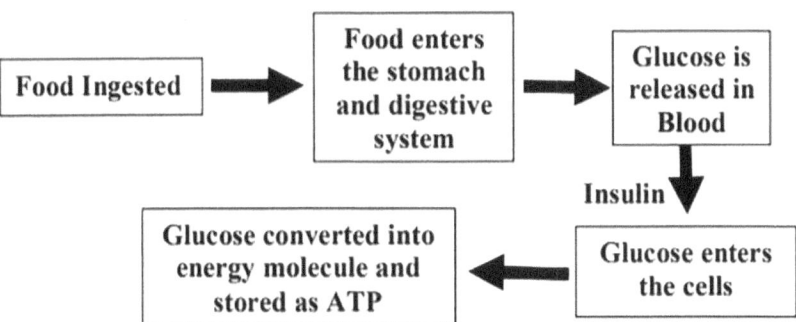

Digestion is a combination of mechanical (for instance chewing food in the mouth and grinding using teeth) and chemical processes which breaks down the ingested food into smaller fragments which are then converted into glucose units.

The majority of food breakdown happens in the mouth and the stomach. Further digestive processes occur in the intestine. Each step of the digestion process needs specific enzymes to break down the partially digested food to convert it into the final absorbable glucose units.

Carbohydrates are digested using several digestive enzymes. Each enzyme has its own specific function in the digestive system for example the enzyme Amylase is active in the mouth with the saliva and initiates the breakdown process of starchy contents of the food.

In case of proteins, fats and oils, even though the breakdown is initiated mechanically in the mouth, the actual digestion starts in the stomach where the enzyme Pepsin is active. Further down the digestive tract a series of enzymatic processes take place using specific enzymes to help further in the digestive process e.g., enzymes Trypsin, Peptidase, etc., become active. Digestion is therefore, a complex multistep process that takes place in different areas of the digestive tract to convert foods we eat into glucose to be able to be absorbed into our body cells to produce the all-important energy we need to sustain our lives.

Just to give you an idea it is a collection of organs and glands which help with our digestion process.

Digestion starts in the mouth as soon as food is taken. The mechanical action of chewing and grinding helps the initial preparation for the Amylase (an enzyme secreted from the salivary gland) to initiate the first step of digestion of carbohydrates, starches, glucose, etc.

The food in partially digested form often called bolus goes to the stomach and interacts with the stomach juices mainly hydrochloric acid and initiates a chemical breakdown. The stomach secretes an enzyme called protease which helps with protein digestion.

From there, the partially digested foods, particularly the proteins fats oils, etc., travel down to the small intestine where the bile produced in the liver and stored in the gall bladder is squirted to act as an emulsifier to help further digestion of proteins, fats oils, etc.

Our pancreas is an important organ (actually a gland) which produces a cocktail of chemicals and enzymes including a hormone, called insulin, which we all are so familiar with, and all have important functions in the digestive processes. Bicarbonates are also released in the small intestine to adjust or manipulate the pH of the environment for specific absorption of nutrients resulting from digested food.

Below is a well-defined picture of our digestive organs participating in basic digestive processes and working in unison.

Organs Involved in Digestive Juice Production
(Digestive Juices Bioninja; ib.bioninja.com.au)

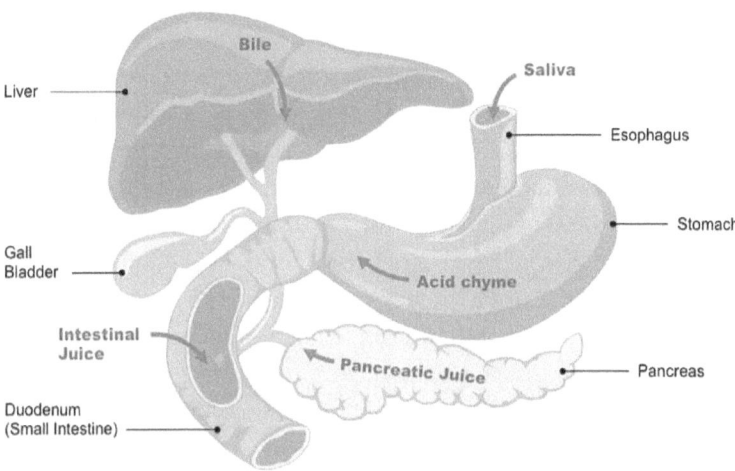

As we now have some idea as to how our food breaks down into smaller units, called glucose which is taken up by the cell with the help of insulin; the fate of the glucose is carefully orchestrated by the following processes leading to its conversion into energy.

These multi-step processes are an important part of cellular metabolism which can be explained simply as below.

The first step in the process is glycolysis which breaks down the glucose into a chemical called pyruvate and an energy unit called Adenosine Tri-phosphate (**ATP**) which is the simplest energy unit which can be directly utilised by the cells or stored for future use.

The next step is known as the pyruvate oxidation which converts the pyruvate produced from the first step into a Coenzyme A and NADH. Coenzyme A (Acetyl Coenzyme) is a very important molecule which participates in the Citric Acid Cycle for the cellular metabolism in energy-producing reactions. It was discovered by Fritz Albert Lipmann in 1946 for which he shared the Nobel Prize in Physiology/Medicine in 1953 with Hans Adolf Krebs.

The main important function of Coenzyme A is to deliver the carbon atom from its acetyl group in the molecule to enter into the citric acid cycle to produce energy by oxidative process.

NADH is Nicotinamide Adenine Dinucleotide Hydride and is an important carrier of electrons in the energy-producing process in the cells.

American biochemists Morris Friedkin and Albert L. Lehninger were the first to point out that NADH was linked to energy-producing metabolic pathways in the **Citric Acid Cycle** in the oxidative phosphorylation step resulting in the bio-synthesis of ATP. ATP is a small molecule which can be conveniently stored in the cells for further energy requirements.

Step three is perhaps the most important of all as it involves an energy-producing reaction cycle known as the citric acid cycle or more famously as the **Krebs cycle** after its discoverer Adolf Krebs. In this process, most of the energy is produced from the single glucose unit which resulted from the first step.

(Hans Adolf Krebs, discovered The Citric Acid Cycle, for which he received the Nobel Prize in Physiology/Medicine in 1953).

Krebs cycle is an overall multi-step energy-producing reaction that takes place in the mitochondria of a cell structure of all living organisms. The cycle facilitates the metabolism of glucose and other molecules to be converted into carbon dioxide and water to produce energy which can be stored in the form of ATP molecules. These metabolic reactions can only take place in the presence of oxygen.

ATP: Adenosine triphosphate is known as the energy currency in biochemical term as it is the carrier of chemical energy produced in the mitochondria of the cell as a result of the breakdown of foods we eat. All living cells require this energy to conduct numerous biochemical processes that are carried out in our cells to sustain life. ATP is continually being used up and also being produced; it is like a perpetual factory where ATP is produced and used up. Long-term storage of ATP for later utilisation is not possible and therefore our food and nutrition supply must be maintained on a regular basis.

Acetyl Co-enzyme A: is the central molecule which is the intermediate in the pathway to conversion of food into energy. Acetyl-CoA enters into the citric acid cycle as described previously and delivers the acetyl group to be oxidised in the energy-producing sequences.

Schematic Diagram of Citric Acid Cycle (Krebs cycle)

```
                    GLUCOSE
              Simplest absorbable
           energy producing unit at
              the top of our food
                       |
                  Phosphorylation
                       ↓
              Glucose-6-phosphate
                       |
                   Glycolysis
                       ↓
                   PYRUVATES
                       |
                       ↓
                                         This molecule plays a
                                         very important role in
                                         energy producing
                   Acetyl-CoA            reactions as it enters the
                                         Citric Acid Cycle
  Carbon dioxide and    |
  Water are produced    |
  As by-products        ↓
            ←      Citric Acid
                       OR
                   Krebs cycle
  Water is used up in
  Cell-hydration and
  Carbon-dioxide is expelled      Electron Transfer
  via the Expiration cycle               And
                               Oxidative Phosphorylation
                       ↓
              ATP (Energy Molecule)
```

Good Diets and Bad Diets

People often get confused with the terms Nutrition and Diet, especially beginners who all of a sudden get involved in their quest for health and general wellness.

Remember beginning has no age or barriers. From young adulthood to middle age and beyond, you can start your journey at any stage of your life. The beginning also does not have any end, it is a lifelong habit that stays with all of us to some degree. It is a practice which blends in with our lifestyle. People have often asked me what the difference between Nutrition and Diet is. Very simple,

I say! Nutrition is the Science of achieving a state of health and wellness, and diet is the vehicle or means to achieve it. Diet is more related to what you eat and nutrition tells you what to eat. It can be both positive and negative.

This is the basis of the saying "You are what you eat."

It is like a computer; if you feed the computer garbage it will spill out garbage. It is not the machine which is to blame but the operator who does the inputting. Our body is an organic matter and although, it may have the ability to mend itself in minor situations, there are some irreversible complications which require a more involved intervention. We can prepare our bodies to face such eventualities through good nutrition and diet which restores balance in our wellness factor.

A good or a healthy diet can assist you with the support you need to maintain and improve your overall health. A good diet is tailor-made for you to provide your body with essential foods containing both macro and micronutrients and other foods which will provide you with a required number of calories to sustain your daily activities.

Why tailor-made, why can't we all have similar healthy diets?

The answer is simple. We all are biochemically individuals.

According to Dr Roger Williams, we humans with our genetic similarities are enormously different in the shape and size of our internal organs. This causes different food requirements we have from each other. Not only that, ethnic heritage and genetic background also matter.

Furthermore, our food intake or variety thereof will largely depend on our metabolism and organ functionality; e.g., someone with impaired carbohydrate metabolism should be careful of their carbohydrate intake and so on. A good diet should not be too restrictive, it is all about enjoying your meal either with your family or by yourself. We all have individual choices and circumstances. Setting unrealistic goals in allocating variety and portions of your meal may take away the pleasures and enjoyment of food which may have a negative effect on your dietary consideration. The key word is, love your food, but use moderation and common-sense approach.

You will find I have used the phrase 'common-sense approach' a number of times in this book. It has a great meaning and literally has an important mentoring character.

Many foods appear to be good and tasty but please be aware they may have negative effects, e.g., allergies, bloating and digestive issues and several other effects which further on in life can manifest into more serious complications, e.g., Diabetes, Heart Complications, Skeletal Structure issues, Depression and many more.

This brings me to the modern-day fast foods. Everybody these days are busy and running around chasing a buck or two and it seems that there is no time to cook and have a proper sit-down meal. Many families are now turning to fast food and foods which are nutritionally not sound as far as food-values are concerned. Call me old fashioned but I believe that a family which eats together stays together. I will not bring back old memories as they are much too outdated for the modern generation. I do admire the new generation, as we do have a lot to learn from them. I wish they also thought likewise. But when it comes to food it is a different matter.

The modern times we live in are ever-changing in their technology and views on life. The young generation of today are the leaders and trendsetters of tomorrow. But the stigma still remains that although we have come a long way from tree-dwelling species, then hunters and gatherers and now to a more civilised modern society, the times are rapidly changing and what we think today may become obsolete tomorrow.

But the sad part of the equation is that the trendsetters of today will become obsolete to the next newer generation. The so-called fast food or the junk foods and drinks may taste good but are often nutritionally poor in their food-value content. These components of a bad diet or bad foods are high in caloric value mainly consisting of sugars and salts and a lot of it. Obviously, the primary notion of the promoters is how to make these foods tasty enough to get repeat business for the restaurants and cafes to thrive. Fast food deliveries are striving to get the prepared foods as fast as possible to their clients; it is a challenge that increases the competitiveness.

I am not entirely against fast foods I am sure they all are trying to do the right thing by them and their customers (here's hoping) using fresh produce and improved cooking techniques which are less invasive and less detrimental to the nutritional content of the food that they are supplying.

Occasional or once in a while eating of junk foods may not have much ill effect on one's health but when used and abused on a regular basis the effect can undermine the health, e.g., increase the risk of heart diseases, diabetic complications, obesity, fatty liver condition (FLC) and several other negative health problems for us to deal with for years to come.

Apart from the increased sugar and salt components in junk foods, one stark reality is that the oils and fats used in the frying process are invariably not fresh but are reused over and over again causing carcinogenicity and an increase in the trans-fats in the frying medium (the reused oils and fats) which raises the probability of cancer and increased LDL levels; the low-density lipoproteins or bad cholesterol.

Increased sugar and salt levels have their own negative health implications, e.g., increased blood sugar levels which the available insulin in our system may not be able to cope with and put an additional strain on our pancreatic functions. The end result of which can show up as type 2 diabetes in due course. Also, salt can lead to hypertension and fluctuations in blood pressure profile causing a burden on our heart.

With recent advancements made in human nutrition and technology to assimilate the abundance of natural goodness that Nature has blessed us with (as in Natural and Nature Identical raw materials), it has become easier for all of us who use nutritional supplements as an additional means to improve our health and well-being to become nutritionally aware. These good supplements are also important as they can fill in the nutritional gap left by the often-substandard dietary intake we all resort to from time to time.

Equipped with such knowledge we can now choose the supplement which has the combination of right ingredients for our supplementary needs and also check the processed foods, for preservatives and unnecessary additives which may be harmful to us, before making our purchases.

The choice now is totally with us.

In our modern-day dietary intake, there is a mix of a variety of fast foods, fried foods and frozen foods. Taste plays a big part in our choice-making. Big companies and fast-food chains are all trying to woo us with scrumptious food ads to get our attention and patronage. But at least now there are some regulatory requirements that food companies must follow to enhance consumer confidence and give them a choice. But, if you look at the immediate picture, say in the case of popular fried foods such as fish and chips, fried chicken, etc., have we ever questioned the preparatory methods such as, the prime consideration, oils that are used for frying?

What is the turnaround of the oil, how long has it been used without a changeover, what oil is being used, etc? There may be several questions hanging over the final fried preparation. But the presentation and the taste are so overwhelming that it is hard to resist, specially, when there are no real alternatives when you have to eat and run or eat on the run.

Let's look at what are the harmful causes of commercially cooked fried foods in reused cooking oil. We are lucky that in Australia vegetable oils or blended vegetable oils are used extensively. These blended oils are perhaps blends of sunflower oil, palm oil, canola oil, soybean oil and several others in various combinations and ratios. Sometimes blends are custom-made for taste enhancement unique for different commercial entities or food chains for the creation of that exclusive signature dish which projects the entity in the culinary limelight.

In many other parts of the world, fats and animal products are also used extensively. It is important to note that large fast-food chains are trying to do the right thing by putting out information about their products, its nutritional contents and calories per serve and other helpful information to give the consumers a wider choice. But it is still some of the independent producers of fast food such as local fish and chips shops or the corner chicken shops that may still have a long way to go to meet the standards and introduce consumer awareness.

I sincerely hope they are trying and, in many instances, catching up. Cooking food in overused or unchanged cooking oil is one of the sources which introduce free radicals and carcinogens (cancer producing) in the body. These free radicals or the Reactive Oxygen Toxic Species (ROTS) are the primary cause of oxidative stress and initiate many common health problems such as obesity, heart disease and diabetes.

To be fair overused cooking oil is not the only cause of free radical generation in our body but also excess smoking, abuse of drugs and alcohol and also certain environmental factors such as exposure to sun's UV radiation, exposure to chemicals, e.g., pesticides and air pollutant are also serious contributors. So, it's not a very good idea to use any oil more than once, or to heat it over its smoking point. Typically, the smoking point is a sign of oils breaking down and releasing unhealthy chemicals including free radicals which are detrimental to the taste of the foods and eating such food is injurious to our health and well-being. The lower the smoke temperature the better the oil is for cooking. The smoking point is also the temperature when smoke is released as a result of oils breaking down.

Table: Commonly used Oils and their Smoke Points

https://www.masterclass.com/articles/cooking-oils-andsmoke-points-what-to-know-and-how-to-choose	
Refined Avocado Oil	270°C
Safflower Oil	266°C
Rice Bran Oil	254°C
Refined or Light Olive Oil	240°C
Soybean Oil	232°C
Peanut Oil	232°C
Ghee or Clarified Butter	232°C
Corn Oil	232°C
Refined Coconut Oil	232°C
Sunflower Oil	232°C
Refined Sesame Oil	210°C
Vegetable Oil	204–232°C
Beef Tallow	204°C
Canola Oil	204°C
Rapeseed Oil	199°C
Unrefined or Virgin Avocado Oil	190°C
Pork Fat or Lard	188°C
Chicken Fat or Schmaltz	190°C
Duck Fat	190°C
Vegetable Shortening	182°C
Unrefined Sesame Oil	177°C
Extra Virgin or Unrefined Coconut Oil	177°C
Extra Virgin Olive Oil	163–190°C
Butter	150°C

Some Common Cooking Oils and approximate Composition

Vegetable oils	Fatty acids			Artificial antioxidants
	monounsaturated	polyunsatured	saturated	
Olive	71.3	12.7	16.0	–
Rapeseed (A)	65.2	29.3	5.5	citric acid/E vitamin
Rapeseed	65.0	29.0	5.0	–
Sunflower (A)	22.8	65.2	12.0	citric acid/E vitamin
Sunflower	23.0	65.0	12.0	–
Corn (A)	33.5	51.0	15.5	citric acid/TBHQ
Corn	34.0	50.0	16.0	–
Soybean	24.3	60.0	15.7	citric acid/TBHQ
Rice	40.8	40.1	19.1	

(A) presence of artificial antioxidants

(**Ref:** Thermo-analytical, kinetic and rheological parameters of commercial edible vegetable oils, February 2004 Journal of Thermal Analysis and Calorimetry 75(2):419–428).

The composition of cooking oil is very important. They mostly contain a mixture of monounsaturated, polyunsaturated, trans-fats and saturated fatty acids. When making a choice, the experts recommend choosing a cooking oil which is low in saturated fats and an even mix of mono and polyunsaturated fats.

Trans-fats are best avoided as they have been reported to raise blood LDL cholesterol levels and increase the risk of cardiovascular diseases. These are a result of hydrogenation and further processing of oils. Polyunsaturated fats are a good source of omega-3 fatty acids and assist in lowering cholesterol and triglycerides. Mono-unsaturated fats in the oils are also helpful in reducing the LDL (Low-density Lipoproteins often referred to as the bad cholesterol). Both Mono and polyunsaturated fats in the cooking oil are good and may assist in slowing the build-up of plaques which consist of fatty substances, cholesterol and also calcium. The two tables presented above may give some valuable choice guidelines.

What are the five most basic human tastes which we have developed as a society over many millennia?

These are **Sweetness** involving sugar, **Saltiness** involving common salt, **Bitter** taste sensation which comes from a combination of bitter components of many foods such as coffee, raw dark chocolate, some bitter vegetables and many more every day food items we consume. The other two taste sensations that are in our taste repertoire are **Sour** taste and other less common **Umami** taste.

Sour taste is associated with acidity and has a very strong influence on our taste buds and provides a tingling sensation. Umami is more of a Savoury taste and is associated with appetitive and appetisers.

No taste sensation will be complete without the pungent hot bitter taste sensation of chilli which is more prevalent in the South East Asian cooking. So, let us keep that in mind also, when we are thinking of invigorating our taste buds.

Our mind and body work in mysterious ways when many basic physiological functions are performed. What can be more basic than to eat food for our sustenance? It is now a well-established scientific fact that junk foods activate the reward system in the brain meaning that it stimulates the neurotransmitters to be released by activating dopamine. Dopamine is a feel-good chemical messenger released by the brain and produces feel-good effect like after consuming sugar, or chocolates and therefore, eating junk foods to many of us can be addictive which can be a real problem.

The modern-day pressures of life and living have diverted our thoughts and priorities such that it may not be far-off when there will be no kitchen to prepare real foods and cooking will be a lost art.

But as we develop into a multi-cultural society, the introduction of a variety of ethnic dishes e.g., (Chinese, Indian, Arabic and some Continental and from many other parts of the world) are on the rise with a good and healthy mix of meats, vegetables and salads and other combinations that are now offered for our eating pleasure.

Long gone are the nostalgic days when eating around the table for dinner and Sunday lunches and roast dinners were a pleasure part of our growing up.

Palaeolithic Diet

Palaeolithic diet literally means stone-age diet. Although we have come a long way, there are still many commonalities that we share with our cave-dwelling early ancestors.

The concept of such a diet started in the early 1970s when Dr Walter.

Voegtlin, a gastroenterologist, recommended a meat and plant-based diet. As we know now that the stone-age people were basically hunters and gatherers and foraged for foods such as tubers and roots of plants, fruits and any fleshy leaves and vegetable-like substance that they could gather and supplemented their diets with occasional hunting for meats and perhaps fishing as well.

The concept of farming and domestication of animals had not started then and as a result, there were not too many choices for cultivated plant-based produce, dairy products and perhaps poultry and eggs. It was what they gathered is what they ate. The concept and availability of nuts, grains and dairy products were completely out of their menu. However, some stone-age inhabitants were more adventurous and may have experimented with the limited availability of wild grains and perhaps nut-like substances available in their diets. Since the very early period of time, when mankind was in its very primitive stage, their diets were very basic and crude.

Although it is difficult to exactly date the periods, just to give some perspective to the ages or the time during the early human evolution and development, it was divided into several ages such as the Stone age (2.5 million years ago MYA), Bronze age (around 10,000 years ago), Iron age (around 5000 years ago), and Gold and Silver Ages (around 3500 years ago). It is very likely that there are differing references to the above quoted time line as many experts have differing views on this subject.

As societies started to take shape and our early ancestors developed tools and various life skills, they started to include a variety of foods in their diets due to the cultivation and domestication of animals.

So, based on archaeological findings and studies conducted on several ancient tribes, in particular the Hadza tribe from central Tanzania, anthropologists and several groups of scientists came to the following conclusions about Palaeolithic diet developed over generations during Stone-Ages. During the first of the Stone Age periods the **Palaeolithic Period** (around 2.5 million years or earlier) the diets mainly contained vegetation and the surrounding plant matters that were available and the game meat and fish that the pre-historic man was able to hunt and gather.

As the hunters and gatherers became more sophisticated and started using tools they started to forage for roots and tubers from underground and were able to distinguish berries, fruits and nuts and included variety in their diets. This started happening in the **Mesolithic Period** (around 100,000 years). Farming was still not developed at that stage and hunting, gathering and digging for additional food stuff was the order of the day.

Neolithic Period was a boom period for the Stone Age people when farming appeared around fifteen to twenty thousand years ago. With farming came various sophisticated food varieties with the inclusion of grains, starches and legumes. Domestication of animals started some 10,000 years later when the Neolithic societies were more societal and adjusted to communal living. This was a real boost to the quality of lifestyle improvement in our early ancestors and paved the way for modern societies to develop and thrive as we see it now.

Neolithic people were really very progressive and industrious people and introduced the wheel which greatly enhanced transportation capabilities. Also, they were able to prepare and cook their foods and had a wide application of fire. Although early humans had encountered fire long before (around 1 million years ago) probably in the form of wildfire but had seemed to have mastered the controlled use of fire not until 400,000–300,000 years ago probably at the same time learned to put raw foods on fire which gave them boost to their taste and cooked food became popular instead of raw food. In their book Challa, Bandlamudi and Uppaluri wrote at length about Palaeolithic diet and adequately summarised the findings of several anthropologists, scientists and palaeontologists that most likely the diets of Palaeolithic People consisted of the following.

Plants and vegetation—these included dugout tubers, gathered seeds, nuts, domestically grown or wild-grown grain crops such as barley, wheat, etc. Variety of fish and aquatic animals including shellfish, turtles and other smaller marine and freshwater fish and smaller animals.

A variety of insects and insect products also became a part of their dietary intake such as honey.

However, the most important inclusion was meats from domesticated animals such as goats, chicken ducks, etc., and their produce such as eggs and milk.

(Ref: Palaeolithic Diet—Stat Pearls—NCBI Bookshelf).

High Energy Diets

A high-energy diet constitutes protein and carbohydrate-enriched meal portions which deliver around 50% of the daily required intake.

The average Australian adult male weight is around 87kg while the equivalent female weight is 72kg; this is just an average, however, height and general constitution need to be taken into consideration (Australian Bureau of Statistics 2018). The corresponding figures, for adult males and females in the United States of America are around 89kg and 76kg, respectively.

These figures are average values which however depend considerably on height, general structure and the BMI (Body Mass Index which is calculated by dividing the body weight in kg by the square of height in metres). The average caloric requirement of daily energy intake is 1800–1900 kcal which converts to around 7500 KJ (Food and Agriculture Organisation, USA); while in Australia the requirement is around 8700 KJ (2000 kcal). What happens if the daily consumption exceeds these values? Not a very healthy thing to do; as these extra kcals will need to be burned off by doing extra activities or else that extra bit will be stored as fats causing obesity and other health complications.

The main reason for eating food is to convert it into calories required for our normal daily activities such as walking, working, and exercising and any other efforts that our body has to make to do something even the minimal task involving movement. Energy is the body fuel, which is like the energy and power, required to drive a motor. There are hundreds of biochemical processes happening within our body that require energy to sustain life; fuel our tiny cells to maintain and repair damages to our cellular structures due to performing everyday bio-functions; the tasks are endless.

It has been suggested that extra energy produced and stored as fat resulting from consuming as little as 24 kcal worth of extra food if not burned off can increase one kg body weight as fat over a one-year period.

High-energy diets are normally prescribed where a burst of energy is required due to a high level of physical activity. Patients who have recently undergone a traumatic stint, under medical care and are released from such care may undertake a high-energy diet for a speedy recovery and cellular reconstruction and healing; but it is absolutely important that before undertaking such dietary plan, medical appraisals and consultations are sought. High-energy diets or snacks such as bars, biscuits and drinks are also consumed by high-performance athletes in between activities. A classic example of this can be noticed during a game of tennis, contact sports and also soccer during half-time or other rest periods.

Low Energy/Weight Management Diets

Obesity and over-weight are still of great concern among the world population. According to the World Health Organisation (WHO) anyone with body-mass index (BMI) 25–30 is classified as overweight while those over 30 are obese. BMI is calculated by dividing the weight of a person by the square of the body height in kg/m². For example, if a person weighs 70 kg and is 1.7 meters tall then the BMI will be 24.2.

It is estimated that the combined percentage of overweight and obese people in the world is around 39% of adults (over 18 years) with a BMI of 25 or more. This statistic is rapidly changing and may increase to around 40% or more by the time I have completed the book.

The main causes of overweight and obesity are increase in the consumption of energy-rich diet and lack of physical activities due to lifestyle changes. The consequences of being overweight and obese are very concerning as the condition could lead to cardiovascular diseases, diabetes, and certain types of cancers such as breast, ovarian, prostate, liver, gallbladder, kidney, and colon.

And also, may cause some damage to the skeletal and muscular systems. So, what can be done?

- Enforce dietary restrictions and exercise your will power and assertiveness.
- Cut down on intakes of high-energy components from diet.
- Increase the intake of fresh fruits and vegetables and salads nuts and grains etc. which will provide adequate nutrition.
- Increase fluid intake including plenty of water.
- Low-energy dietary practices are also encouraged.

Low-energy diets can vary significantly, case by case and often is a requirement in weight management programmes. A low-energy diet consisting of 800 kcal has often been prescribed in extreme obesity; again, it is important that medical intervention and directions are adhered to. These diets are used on obese patients on a short-term basis, primarily to study the physiological changes in metabolic rates of weight reduction. A clinician will normally set up the routine for the patients.

A person on low-energy diet can feel very uncomfortable during the early stages of this dietary plan and the feeling of hunger may take over, but this phase passes quickly as the body starts breaking down the accumulated fats converting them to ketones (Ketosis) which generally are appetite suppressants. To keep body functions active, low-intensity exercises are also beneficial and of course, I tend to suggest taking a good vitamin and mineral supplement once or twice daily in between meals with plenty of just pure water.

Intake of juices can easily increase the caloric intake which is a complete no in this situation. In this type of diet, green leafy non-starchy vegetables which give you the bulk and feeling of fullness such as lettuce, cabbages, spinach, etc., and a small portion of very lean meat, a piece of omega-3 enriched fish or even egg are good. The addition of a little bit of fresh ginger as a thermogenic (heat producing) which aids in fat burning will be excellent.

Vegetarian/Vegan Diets

There are various classifications of vegetarian and vegan diets to suite individual choices for those who follow strict codes of vegetarianism and veganism. As a broad definition, a vegetarian will not eat meat, fish, poultry, crustacean (shell fish crabs, etc.) and will only eat vegetables, grains, fruits, nuts and seeds and all plant-based products and milk and milk products. The vegetarian diet has been around for more than 2500 years and is much older than the vegan diet which is relatively a modern dietary development.

According to the vegan society "Veganism is a philosophy and a way of living which seeks to exclude-as far as possible and practicable-all forms of exploitation of, and cruelty to, animals for food, clothing or any other purpose; and by extension, promotes the development and use of animal-free alternatives for the benefit of animals, humans and the environment. In dietary terms, it denotes the practice of fully dispensing off with all products derived wholly or partly from animals" from their diets and items for general use.

The Vegan Society was founded in November 1944 by Donald Watson an English animal rights advocate.

In this regard, veganism has a lot in common with the ancient Indian religion called Jainism founded by Nataputta Mahavira around 6th century BCE in Eastern India.

Jain philosophy is the oldest Indian philosophy that separates the body from the soul completely. Jain philosophy deals with reality, cosmology, and epistemology (a belief and vitalism; Ref: Wikipedia).

A vegan diet totally consists of plant-based products such as fruits, vegetables, seeds, nuts, legumes, etc., and excludes all animal-derived products. It is also that a vegan diet will exclude the vegetables of the allium family such as onions and garlic. In contrast to vegan diets, the Jain diet is stricter in so far as their dietary consideration excludes root vegetables such as potatoes and other tubers such as yams, etc.

Diabetic Diet

According to the recommendations of the American Diabetes Association and Diabetes UK, there are no strict guidelines to suggest that a particular diet is better or more helpful than any other. Inconsistency and lack of correlation in current published research reports suggest that further long-term studies are required to formulate popular guidelines which may be suitable universally. Diabetes Australia recommends following general suggestions yet making it clear that there is no single dietary plan that could be suitable for consideration. Individuals must seek medical advice before considering a diet plan.

Eat regular meals and spread them evenly throughout the day. Eat a diet lower in fat, particularly unsaturated fats.

If you take insulin or diabetes tablets, you may need to exclude carbohydrates and have smaller meals rather than large meals and where possible cut down on the binge eating habits and in-between meal snacks.

It is important to recognise that everyone's needs are different. All people with diabetes should see an Accredited Practicing Dietitian in conjunction with their diabetes team for individualised advice.

(Ref: https://www.diabetesaustralia.com.au).

The Australian Diet

The Australian diet has undergone a massive transformation from its early dietary patterns. Meat was the predominant staple as were potatoes and bread.

Milk cream and cheese were also a good part of the Australian dietary regimen. With the influx of earlier migrants mainly from Europe, the dietary mix started to change with different cultures introducing their preferences. These included pasta, a variety of cheese, vegetables, fish and poultry as the main course. Tomatoes, olive oils, red wine and some grains such as beans were a variety of mix that constituted an Italian combination. Their meals contained a very little portion of red meat on a frequent basis.

Greek migration introduced Mediterranean-style food based predominantly on a variety of fresh green salads to which a choice of meats, fish and goat cheese were added. Salads are dressed with both olives and lashings of olive oil. Modern Australian dietary pattern is a melting pot of European, Asian, Middle Eastern and Indian subcontinent dishes. Yet fast foods such as burgers, fried chicken, fish and chips and a variety of meat pies are still pretty popular with both older and younger generations. Middle-Eastern kebabs, Indian curries and rice, Asian fried rice, chicken and pork dishes are also popular as takeaway dinners. It is truly a multicultural cuisine with an ethnic flavour.

The First Nation people, the Australian Aborigines, in the heart of the Australian continent and remote parts of Australia, over many millennia have retained their unique hunter-gatherer and bush-tucker approach. However, having said that their diets in the past mainly consisted of native flora and fauna and also certain insects like witchetty grubs, bogong moths, honey ants, etc. Realistically in the past, their dietary patterns did not change from their ancestral dietary habits. This was due to the fact that they were not exposed to other cultures and possibly had no or low contact with the new migrants at the advent of Australia's migration intake and influxes.

As Australia became a melting pot of various cultures, and the assimilation of the First Nation's people the Australian Aborigines with their regular travels and re-location into all parts of Australian regional and various cities and country areas, opened up their dietary habits from hunter-gatherers to a more regularised dietary patterns. This revolutionised the Australian Diet as a whole in the last 3-4 decades.

After opening the borders to the world after the II World War, the Australian population has now become multi-cultural, which is reflected in the cuisine and culinary delights from all over the world particularly Asia; namely Chinese style and the subcontinental style of Indian and Sri Lankan dishes and also European and African tastes.

In general, now there has been a decrease in consumption of red meat, sugar, salt and flour the usual ingredients of bread and potatoes while an increase in consumption of seafood, lamb and poultry, rice and vegetables is noticeable. The introduction of oriental and Indian spices particularly turmeric, ginger, garlic and mixed spices in curries and marinating cocktails and the introduction of herbs like coriander and curry leaves are on the increase with positive health benefits.

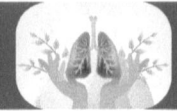

Chapter 5

BASIC HUMAN ANATOMY

The human body is the most complete and powerful piece of machinery ever built with the organs and systems laid perfectly in position for a simple harmonic motion; is it a work of science or simply divine inspiration.

– Jay Das, 2022

Our body is an organism, a cluster of chemical atoms (carbon, hydrogen, oxygen, and nitrogen) which make up cells and cellular structures; a collection of cells and cellular structure forms tissues, e.g., muscle tissues, connective tissues, nerve tissues, etc…Several tissues work their way to create organs such as heart, liver, lungs, etc. A number of organs which function together in unison is a system such as the respiratory, circulatory systems, etc., leading to an organism such as us humans. Every animal has a collection of chemical atoms at the most fundamental level or you can say a starting point, and progress to a complete organism which can function in its entirety such as us and all other animal and insect species on this planet.

(Chemical Atoms to Organisms a Sequence of Progression)

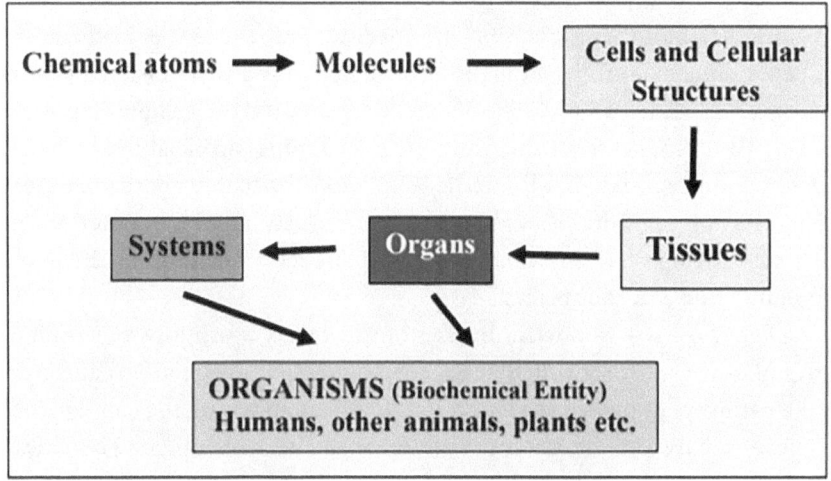

Human body is a collection of many organs of various shapes and sizes from a tiny gland to the largest external organ the skin. Just for the sake of simplification, we can say that there are 78 or so organs and all are required to perform specific functions and some systemic organs are required to work in unison. If we take the organ count further and argue about counting individual tooth as an individual organ or even try to justify multiple tissues joined and functioning together so that it could be classified as an organ, then we will have many more organs to contend with.

I have not even considered the new organs recently discovered in the counting debate. The count goes on.

There is no clear-cut nomenclature or naming system, or a preferred definition which can give us an exact count. Again, for the sake of simplification and for our understanding let us stick to the number 78, which is the general count that most anatomists agree on.

Now, the next issue is that, are all organs necessary for our survival. No, not at all. Many organs singularly or collectively have a set of specific functions which may or may not be absolutely necessary for our survival as our vital organs.

So, what are the vital organs; our **heart, lungs, kidneys, liver**, organs of our gastro intestinal system such as the **stomach**, our **brain** and also our **skin** could be classified as our vital organs without which we may not survive. Modern science is developing rapidly to keep us alive by artificial means should some of our vital organs cease to operate. Heart, liver, and lung transplantation is all a reality now with varying degrees of success and with time I am sure the success rates will improve and so will the longevity and quality of life.

Another important scientific and medical advancement is in the area of the development of artificial organs, for example, for a third degree of burn a patient can be patched up with artificial skin grafts and be well on their way to recovery. Who knows what the future holds. Cloning, artificial implants, etc., which will make today's sci-fi a reality and we will become another species of cyborgs. What a dreadful thought but it will happen only in a matter of time. But I am glad that I will not be alive to witness sci-fi mankind or the human race plundering a distant planet.

Digression is a wonderful break from so-called continuity and reality; it is an unknown territory which keeps alive our fertile imaginations and opens up the pathways to pioneering works without contemplating the consequences. Ok, now we have settled on some vital organs and we have a pretty good idea of their functions. We need a quick rundown on the vital functions these organs perform day in and day out twenty-four-seven to keep us alive.

Our human body is a uniquely devised piece of machine; finely tuned. It is an organism with trillions of cells developed over millions of years and still developing and who knows if the human race is to survive for the next million years what evolutionary changes we may have to go through. Every piece of our anatomy and its functions (Physiology) are important in some way or other even though some may believe otherwise as exemplified below. Millions of years of evolutionary changes to present-day refinements that we have undergone, it seems that quite a few of our body parts or organs that we still carry in our anatomical makeup today may not be needed anymore, yet they are there. These are vestigial body parts.

What are these vestigial body parts?

Vestigial body parts are body parts or organs, left over since our early evolution, which we do not have much use for in our modern anatomical structure or composition. I qualify by saying that during our early evolutionary origin, these vestigial organs may have had important use but as we developed into modern humans some of those body parts seem to be of no further use or of less use today.

My list is comprehensive but there are several more which I have not included.

1. Our **Appendix** features at the top of the list. It has no apparent use but can cause a lot of grief from appendicitis and the pain which follows. A group

of scientists believe that the appendix plays a limited role in the digestion of bacteria.

Questionable?

2. **Coccyx** is the left over from the tail joint that our early ancestors had. Can you think of any use now except if we had a tail, we could wag it.
3. **Tonsils** are a pair of soft tissues on either side of the uvula in the mouth. Those who have had tonsillitis and suffered the pain and inflammation would seek answers to know if these serve any meaningful purpose.

   In my opinion, it is a vestigial organ but some scientists do believe that they are the first line of defence from protection against harmful germs.

   The question still remains that in people who have their tonsils removed survive without them and do so quite convincingly.
4. **Maxillary Sinuses** are air pockets located on either side of the nose near the cheek bones. What purpose do they serve? They are connected to our nasal passages or nostrils by small channels. Their function is to drain mucus into our nostrils to keep them moist. But if blocked they can cause no end of pain and uneasy feelings. So, what is their use, if our nose is good enough to drain extra mucus?
5. **Extinct Ear Muscles (Auricularis Anterior)** we still have them and with no purpose. Our prehistoric ancestors had them pivot their ears to lock on to the direction of sound for hunting or to watch out for predators.
6. **Fabella** is a classic example of a vestigial component which was lost to us humans due to evolutionary sophistication but has now made a comeback. There have been a few scientific theories put forward for its reappearance. One such plausible reason is that this tiny bone that sits inside the tendon behind the knee has re-appeared due to the availability of good diet and nutrition to the modern humans. We are now getting bigger, stronger and heavier than our early ancestors. This additional weight has put extra strain on our knees resulting in evolution compensating for this extra need.

   According to a few experts, Fabella has contributed to some negative issues such as exertion of uneven pressure on the knees causing cartilage damage which may result in osteoarthritis. So, was it necessary to make a comeback or is it simply that we are drifting back into our prehistoric past?
7. **Wisdom Tooth** is believed to have helped our prehistoric ancestors who had to chew and grind hard and rough food whatever they could lay their hands on or shall I say their teeth on. As time passed by, we became more refined and so our shorter jaws now find it difficult to accommodate the wisdom

tooth or the extra molar. Today it is believed that less than 25% of adults have the molar tooth.

There are many more interesting vestigial organs or components that I never knew existed, which were left behind by our ancient ancestors for us to ponder upon and seriously question their usefulness.

Our human body is really a work of art and since the early times, in the renaissance period, it has been the subject of many painters' and sculptures' creations. A famous example of this is the 'Statue of David' by Michelangelo which I have been lucky to see displayed in the Academia Gallery in Florence, Italy.

It has always intrigued me; the precision, the individuality, and the harmonious way our body functions are something to behold. With around 100 trillion individual cells performing thousands upon thousands of bio-chemical processes in harmony and all they need is the right nutrition for refuelling. With so many cells, it is not surprising that large numbers perish or break down daily only to be replaced by new cells.

These cells are from various regions in the body, for example, our skin being the largest external organ produces more dead cells than anywhere else in the body. It has also been estimated that in a 24-hour period, nearly one million dead cells are lost from skin alone; there are many dead cells in other parts of the body as well which need to be disposed of.

Our body has thought of every little detail by assigning the task of removing some of the dead cells to a special type of white cells called phagocytes which munch on the dead cells and in the process produce energy which is used up to produce new white cells. What a wonderful internal recycling mechanism. Our spleen which is located in the upper left-hand side of our body behind the rib cage and just above the stomach is an important part of our body's lymphatic system. It also filters our blood and removes the wasted cells. Necrosis is the scientific word used for the process of cell death; the word has its origin from Greek word *Nekrosis* meaning the process of being dead or death.

One of the reasons cells die a premature death is due to lack of blood supply which causes nutrient deficiency and also as a result of toxin built up. Now, what happens if there is a build-up of dead cells in the body which cannot be removed from the body fast enough due to functional impairments? Accumulation of dead cells can cause several health issues which need medical intervention. If unchecked may lead to severe complications:

- They can cause inflammation.

- Cause degenerative diseases.
- Can cause hindrance to the supply chain of nutrients, including oxygen, to the good cells, thus, causing multiple tissue damages.
- Tissue damage can also lead to adverse effects on the lymphatic system, and bone tissues leading to osteoporosis and other skeletal structure-related complications.

The list is quite comprehensive, and depending on the cellular damages relating to various or specific types of cells e.g., nerve cells, can lead to any one or several nervous system, organ and tissue failures.

It can also manifest itself as a tumour growth in any part of the body where the concentration of dead cell accumulation is significant.

Some interesting facts; apart from the phagocytes which help clean up the dead cells internally; according to the American Academy of Dermatology Association (what kids should know about how skin grows), updated 2020; our skin sheds around 30,000–40,000 dead cells in an hour which is quite a significant number of cells. This equates to about a million dead cells in a day, approximately 30 million cells in a month or around 360 million cells per year which is a staggering 4kg. This is just from a normal body skin surface under normal conditions.

The arteries eventually narrow down into capillaries which are tiny with fine ends to facilitate deposition of oxygen and nutrients to the cellular structure for absorption. The capillaries are also connected to the veins and carry the toxic waste materials and flow into the larger veins which are then carried for elimination and, or, purification. Due to this extra load and the fragile nature of the capillary structure, they often suffer damage and therefore adequate nutritional supplements should be administered to preserve their integrity.

Let's Start with Our Heart

Our heart is a glorified precision pump which is a bundle of muscles. It pumps and receives blood throughout the body through an intricate network of arteries, veins and capillaries which are the part of the **Circulatory System**. Arteries carry the oxygenated blood from the heart to every cell of every tissue of every organ and the veins bring back the oxygen-starved blood to the heart which is then pumped into the lungs to be oxygenated and the process is repeated over and over again.

It is important that all of the tissue cells in our body are adequately supplied with nutrients on a constant and consistent basis otherwise nutrient and oxygen deprivation could lead to cell damage eventually leading to dead cells.

The network of blood vessels in the circulatory system carries nutrients and oxygen to the cells (via the arteries and capillaries) and removes the toxins e.g., carbon dioxide and cellular wastes via the veins.

Our heart is located slightly left on the upper side of our chest and is the focal point of our circulatory system.

Our Blood Pressure Control (BP)

When our heart pumps blood into or through the arteries, it creates pressure; so, the greater the volume and delivery of blood by the heart, the greater is the pressure build-up in the circulatory system. Blood pressure is also dependent on the peripheral resistance which is determined by the resistance offered to the flow of blood through the blood vessels.

If these blood vessels are narrower, compared to normal, the blood pressure increases. There is also an effect of the blood viscosity on pressure built up; the greater the viscosity of the blood it will offer a greater resistance to the flow resulting in greater pressure. Blood pressure is recorded by measuring two pressure numbers; the first is **Systolic Pressure** and the second is **Diastolic Pressure**.

Simply explained the systolic pressure is the pressure measured when the pressure is at the highest point and diastolic pressure is the measurement point in between heartbeats when the pressure is at the lowest point. The recording of the blood pressure is done by reporting the systolic pressure at the top followed by the diastolic pressure at the bottom.

Blood pressure can vary with age, height, weight and gender; also, your activity levels can affect your blood pressure. Your state of mind can also have a marked effect on your BP readings, for example, your readings may be normal at home but at a doctor's surgery, the pressure readings can be higher due to nervousness and tension due to uncertainty.

It is also important to note that BP increases with age due to loss of elasticity in the blood vessels. Many people these days do monitor their BP at home. It is a good idea to maintain consistency in your measurements and record keeping any inconsistency and fluctuation in the readings must be referred for medical attention.

The diagram below depicts the anatomy of the interior of our heart showing valves, arteries and veins. The white arrow shows the normal direction of blood flow **(Ref: en.wikipedia.org > wiki > Heart)**

Basic Human Anatomy

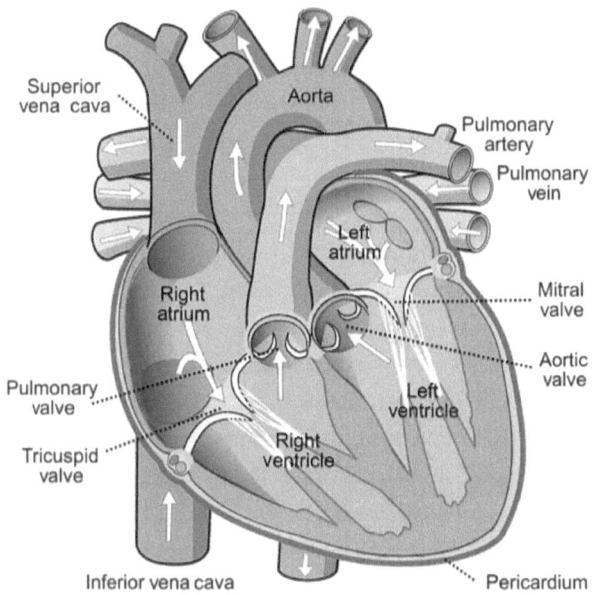

Now, here is some extracurricular; useless but interesting bit of information about our heart. It has been glorified since ancient times. Early Greek philosophers associated love and human emotions with our organ heart and this was further enhanced when Aristotle (384–322 BC) put credence to the view that the role of the heart was supreme amongst all other human organs.

Early Romans also depicted the heart with romance and love through Venus the goddess of love and her son Cupid symbolising love and heart through the powerful message of the human heart and Cupid's arrow.

Interestingly enough in the ancient city of Cyrene (modern-day Shahhat in Libya) a coin, pictured below, was found which was dated back to 510–490 BC; judge for yourself the oldest dated image of a heart shape.

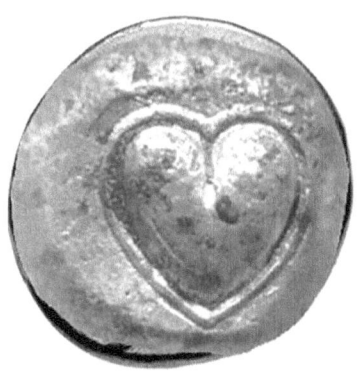

Our Lungs

Our lungs are a pair of spongy organs and form a part of the respiratory system and work together with our heart. When we breathe in (inhale), the oxygen component of the air we breathe is retained by our lungs and the carbon dioxide is expelled with the air we breathe out (exhale). The blood which is pumped from the heart's right chamber into the lungs then picks up the oxygen and the oxygenated blood is pumped back into the heart for distribution by the arteries and the capillaries to our cells. It sounds simple but the mechanism of the workings of the lung is more complex than it seems to be.

Although our lungs are described as spongy organs, it has a fine structural composition. The air that we breathe in through our nose then into our trachea which is the main airway connected to the lungs through two tubes connecting the right and left lungs. These tubes are called bronchi which are then branched out into many small and much smaller tubes which open into spaces inside the lungs called alveoli. This is where the exchange of gases takes place. Red blood cells passing through the tiny capillaries opening into alveoli exchange the carbon dioxide for oxygen which is then pumped into the heart for distribution into various parts of the body. The carbon dioxide, thus generated, is expelled from the system. So, a healthy pair of lungs will go a long way to keep our heart pumping oxygenated blood to be carried to the cells and tissues of our body.

So, what can we do to keep our lungs healthy?

Try to avoid smoking or better still give it up.

Avoid passive smoking or avoid the environment polluted with tobacco smoke.

Avoid car exhaust fumes from entering our bodies.

Avoid obesity and aim for a healthy Body Mass Index (BMI).

Do breathing exercises to increase lung capacity.

Take precautions for seasonal fluctuation, e.g., flu season, etc.

These simple activities can help strengthen our pulmonary system.

Our Lungs: Diagram (Ref: en.wikipedia.org)

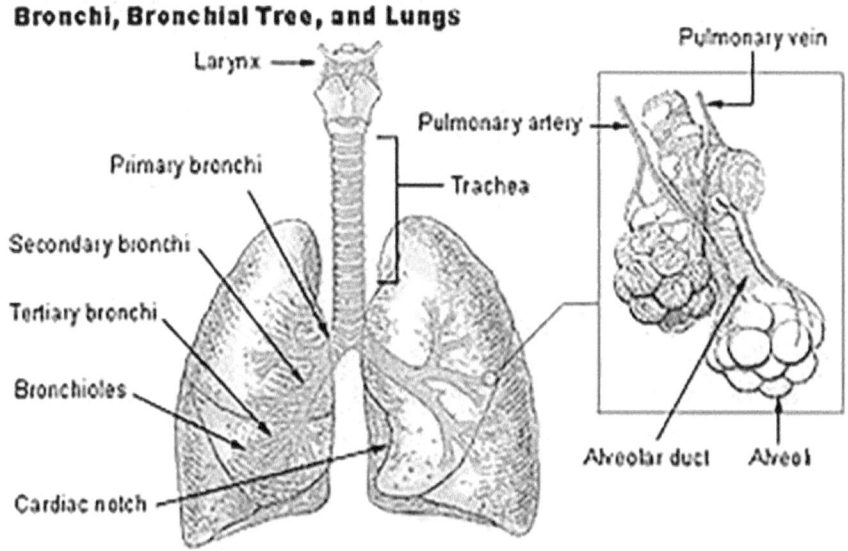

Working Diagram of our Lungs

From Anatomy and Physiology, Connexions Website (http://cnx.org/content/col11496/1.6/, Jun 19, 2013.)

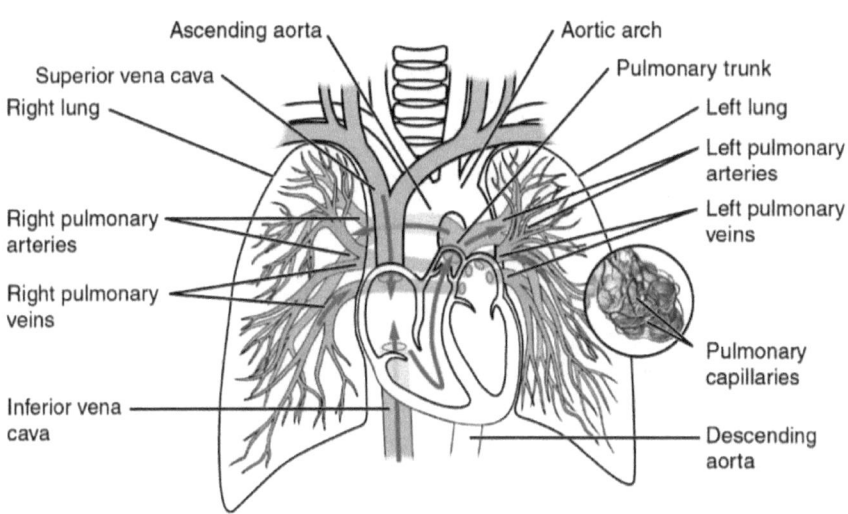

Our Liver

Our liver is the largest solid organ and perhaps the most important one for our metabolism when it comes to manufacturing various biochemicals for our body's utilisation on a regular basis. It is situated slightly right side of our chest above the stomach and tucked in behind our rib cage.

The liver has several very important functions that it carries out along with other vital organs in our body which keeps us alive and healthy.

Of the very many functions, our liver performs, a few are summarised below:

- It filters the blood from our digestive tract, before it gets to the other parts of our body.
- Our liver cleans our blood by detoxifying the circulating chemicals and preservatives which enter our body through the foods we eat and deactivates the harmful components.
- It also cleans the blood of the residual medicines and toxic compounds created from the metabolism of the drug molecules.
- It manufactures bile and stores it into our **Gall Bladder** for use in digestive processes of fats and proteins from the foods we eat especially the meat products in our diet.
- It converts excess glucose from our food intake into glycogen, which is a carbohydrate with a number of glucose units attached, and stores it for later use when the body has a requirement; glycogen is also stored in our muscles.
- Our liver manufactures proteins for blood plasma. Blood plasma is the liquid component of the blood which supports blood cells and makes up more than 50% of the blood volume in our body.
- Regulates blood clotting by manufacturing specific plasma proteins called coagulation factor without which our blood clotting mechanism will not work properly and may cause unnecessary clotting anywhere in the body that can block blood flow. This may cause a stroke or we may simply bleed to death.
- Produces cholesterol and special proteins to help carry fats through the body.
- The liver synthesises immune factors which help with our immunity by neutralising bacteria from the bloodstream and eliminating them from our body in the faeces or urine.
- It helps with iron absorption and storage and helps with haemoglobin formation using stored iron.

There are many other tasks that our liver performs 24/7 hours and days of our life.

Small mention about cholesterol; it is the primary building block of our cell membranes without it our cells will be fragile. A large portion of available cholesterol is found in our brain tissue to perform normal brain functions.

During the process of vitamin D synthesis from the sun's radiation, cholesterol from the skin is largely used otherwise the biosynthetic steps will not be complete. Cholesterol is also important for the bio-synthesis of many of our hormones and also bile salts and these are all manufactured in our liver system. Cholesterol is available to our body from two sources; dietary and from the liver where it is manufactured. Although a certain amount of cholesterol is very important for our cells and several body functions, it is important to note that too much cholesterol is detrimental and may cause serious health complications.

Lipoproteins transport cholesterol via blood to all parts of our body. There are two main types of cholesterol high-density lipoprotein (HDL cholesterol) and low-density lipoprotein (LDL-cholesterol).

The good cholesterol HDL due to its higher density expels the low LDL cholesterol from the body, especially the arteries so that it cannot travel into the heart and create the undesirable waxy or fatty deposits. The built up of excess cholesterol is called atherosclerosis and may cause many health complications such as blood pressure fluctuations, nutrient and oxygen deprivation in our cells due to lack of blood flow, stroke or heart attack.

The other fat we need to be worried about is triglycerides. This fat is also transported by the lipoproteins and in high concentrations it poses the same threat to our health as LDL-cholesterol.

There are ways to control the dietary source of cholesterol by minimising intakes of cholesterol-rich foods such as meats, oily products and dairy products which are concentrated in saturated fats.

Although cholesterol is important as mentioned earlier for several of our metabolic reactions such as vitamin D synthesis from our skin using sunlight, hormone synthesis, building and repairing cell membranes, bile production in the liver and many other vital uses, it is important to know that too much cholesterol in our body is not good for our general health and well-being. Medically, when we are assessed for cholesterol levels in our blood the individual levels of Low-Density Lipoproteins (LDL) and High-Density Lipoproteins (HDL) are assessed.

Blood is our lifeline. Lack of oxygen can seriously affect brain health and tissue starvation due to insufficient oxygen and nutrients.

HDLs are good for our health, and due to their higher density can suppress the LDLs and remove them from the arteries and other LDL-affected sites. The importance of cholesterol in our general health and well-being was recognised when the 1964 Nobel Prize was jointly awarded to Konrad Bloch and Feodor Lynen for their discoveries concerning the mechanism and regulation of cholesterol and fatty acid metabolism. But this was not all; further in 1985, two biochemists Goldstein and Brown were jointly awarded the Nobel Prize in Physiology for their discoveries concerning the regulation of cholesterol metabolism. Their discovery opened pathways for further research into Statins a group of drug molecules which are used to reduce cholesterol levels in the blood in the preventive treatment of heart attacks.

Cholesterol or cholesterol-like substance was first discovered by Poulletier de la Salle in 1769 in bile and gallstones; Poulletier's work was never published.

In 1815, Chevreul rediscovered the substance and named it 'Cholesterine'. Cholesterine was later structurally found to be a secondary alcohol consisting of four cyclic rings. The name cholesterol is derived from Greek words Chole (bile) and Stereos (solid) and being alcohol the suffix-ol was added to the name cholesterol.

Boudet in 1833 demonstrated the presence of cholesterol in blood.

Anatomy of Our Liver

A beautiful anatomical picture of our liver attached to the organs of our digestive system showing Spleen, Gall Bladder, Pancreas and Stomach (taken from John Hopkins website).

(Ref: John Hopkins Medicine https://www.hopkinsmedicine.org/**)**

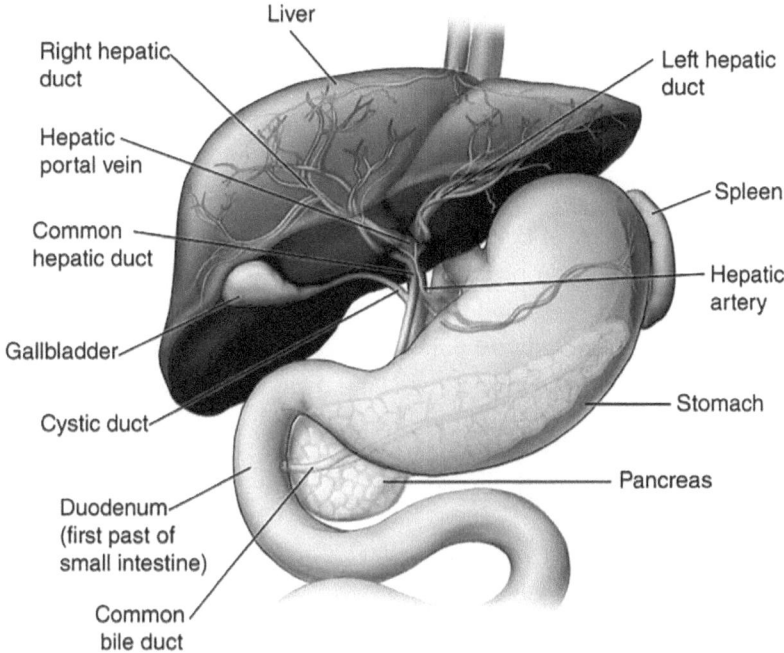

Our liver may not be a glamorous organ as our heart is, but it is the most overworked and underpaid organ which if and when given our tender loving care (TLC) will work wonders and look after our health for a very long time. Our liver is also a very forgiving organ as it can regenerate itself after a major surgery to remove the damaged portion, and interestingly enough, the regeneration mechanism ensures that the liver generates to the host weight ratio of 100% to keep the body in the state of homeostasis which is our body's way of maintaining a physiological stability within the body's constant internal environment.

In a couple of experimental studies, when animal liver (in this case a baboon) were transplanted into humans they quickly grew to the required approximate size of the host even though the baboon liver is smaller.

In another experiment, a large dog's liver was transplanted into a smaller dog and surprisingly enough the transplanted liver which was larger in size shrank to the appropriate required size for the smaller dog.

While it is impossible to live without our liver, it is possible to live with a partial liver. It is also known that some people can live with only 50–60% of their liver which can grow back to an appropriate size within months. It is the only organ of our body which can regenerate after surgery from partial removal or a partial liver transplant which cannot be done in the case of our heart, lungs, etc.

Our liver performs in excess of 500 vital functions essential to our daily life and living.

Love Your Liver

Yes indeed; The American Liver Foundation has put together a list of 25 things we can do to help our liver breathe and be healthy, and in doing so we help our self, live a happy and a healthy life.

I have slightly edited few points, however, if you want to read the full unedited version of the American Liver Foundation's publication, please log on to the reference below at the end of this list.

- Avoid taking unnecessary medications. Too many chemicals can harm the liver.
- Don't mix medications without the advice of a doctor. Mixing medications could be poisonous to your liver.
- Drink alcohol responsibly.
- Never mix alcohol with other drugs and medications.
- Be careful when using aerosol and other sprays such as paint, pesticides, insecticides and other harmful chemicals. The liver has to detoxify what you breathe in. Make sure the room is well ventilated or wear a mask.
- Get vaccinated for Hepatitis A and B and make sure your children and other family members in close contact with you are also vaccinated.
- If you get a tattoo, or any other body art make sure you only use single needles and ink pots. Do not share.
- Exercise regularly—walk a little further, climb the stairs.
- Don't share personal use items such as combs, razors, and manicure tools.
- Teach your children what a syringe looks like and to leave it alone.
- Get tested for hepatitis C.
- Use caution and common sense regarding intimate contact-hepatitis can be transmitted through blood.
- Eat a well-balanced, nutritionally adequate diet. If you enjoy foods from each of the food groups, you will probably obtain the nutrients you need.
- Keep your weight close to ideal. Medical research has established a direct correlation between obesity and the development of fatty liver disease.
- Do not smoke.
- If you have any body piercing, check that the instruments used are properly sterilised or used only once.

- Increase your intake of high-fibre foods such as fresh fruits and vegetables, whole grain breads, rice and cereals.
- At your annual physical check-up, ask your doctor to do a complete liver blood analysis and liver function tests.
- Take the right dosage of medication—too much can cause trouble.
- See your doctor for regular check-ups and share any information about health problems.
- Remember liver disease can happen to anyone—from infants to the elderly. Do your part to stay healthy.

If you want to learn more about your liver, a good starting reference will be: **(Ref: info@liverfoundation.org)**

Our Brain

It is the centre of our nervous system and controls our body's sensory activities. It receives signals from our sensory organs such as our eyes, ears and nose, etc., and passes them on to the sensory nerves attached to various muscles for relevant movements and actions. It is a very complex organ and has been likened to a supercomputer; but is it?

Our brain is an intellectual organ and drives our mind and consciousness. Anatomically our brain has three main parts **Cerebrum, Cerebellum** and the **brainstem**. Each section has its own functions.

Cerebrum: It is the largest part of our brain and has two distinct sections called the right and the left hemispheres.

The cerebrum is also known as the thinking or the conscious activity centre which is responsible for our thinking, remembering or memory, sensory feelings and interpreting various sensations like sight, hearing, touch and emotions.

Cerebellum: It is situated at the back of the brain just underneath the cerebrum and contains a number of cells which fine tune muscle movements and maintain body balance.

Brainstem: This is the bottom part of the brain and connects the cerebrum and the cerebellum to the spinal cord. It controls various autonomous functions such as breathing, blood pressure and heart rate, swallowing, etc. It also influences our sleep and wake-up cycles.

(Ref: Anatomy of the Brain | Johns Hopkins Medicine) https://www.hopkinsmedicine.org

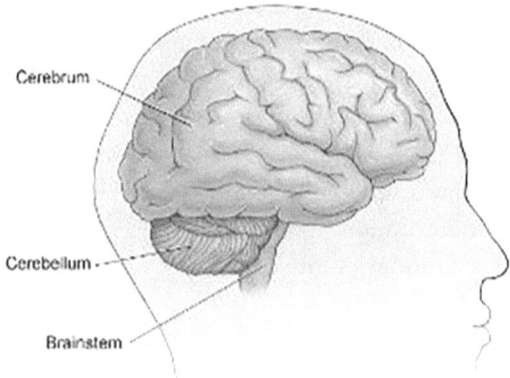

Major Parts of the Brain

Tips on How to Enhance Your Brain Function and Capacity

Simple activities like solving puzzles, reading and learning new things.

Allowing your brain to have adequate rest with peaceful sleep.

Stimulating conversations and discussions on current topics of interest. Exercises which will stimulate the flow of blood in your body and also your brain, such as mild running, treadmilling, etc.

Challenge yourself with memory games and stay alert.

A good diet and nutrition.

There have been many food items which have been suggested to help brain activity and function. Just to summarise, a few items listed below may be of benefit. It is also generally recognised that components like omega-3 fatty acids, B vitamins, and antioxidants, are known to support brain health and often referred to as brain foods. Research shows that the best brain foods are the same ones that protect your heart and blood vessels, including the following:

Green leafy vegetables: Kale, spinach, broccoli and carrots, etc., are rich in brain-healthy nutrients like vitamin K, lutein, folic acid, and beta carotene and mixed carotenoids.

Fatty fish: Fatty fish which are good sources of omega-3 fatty acids, such as Salmon, Mackerel, Gem fish, Tuna, etc., are a healthy source of good fats (unsaturated fats). There is an endless supply of these and other fish like Sardines in Australia and have been linked to lower the levels of Beta Amyloid Peptides in the brains of people with Alzheimer's disease.

Berries: Berries contain flavonoids and anthocyanin, the blue to purple pigments of blueberries, blackberries, etc. These are good antioxidants and improve circulation. Researchers at Brigham Women's Hospital found that women who consumed two or more servings of strawberries and blueberries each week delayed memory decline by up to two-and-a-half years (published in Annals of Neurology 2012). Brigham and Women's Hospital in Boston is a major teaching hospital of Harvard Medical School.

Tea and coffee: In a study published in The Journal of Nutrition (2014) researchers at Johns Hopkins University reported that taking 200mg caffeine tablets had a better effect on mental function. It may therefore seem that a cup of morning tea or coffee could offer not just a short-term boost but also some memory enhancement.

Walnuts: Nuts are healthy food and may help memory improvements. A 2015 study from UCLA linked higher walnut consumption to improved cognitive test scores. The reason given was walnuts are a rich source of alphalinolenic acid (ALA) which helps blood pressure and protects arteries, parameters good for heart and brain.

(Ref: Food linked to better brain power Harvard Health www.health.harvard.edu)

Further reading references: A Guide to Cognitive Fitness, a Special Health Report from Harvard Medical School.
11 Best Foods to Boost Your Brain and Memory—Healthline https://www.healthline.com › nutrition)

Pituitary Gland

I could not go past this chapter without referring to the Pituitary gland which is a small gland located at the base of our brain and is very small in size, yet it packs a powerful punch when it comes to our body's hormonal system. It is often called the master gland and forms a part of our endocrine system. It controls and, in many instances, regulates certain functions of the organs of our endocrine system through the process of producing various hormones required for their activities. Pituitary gland, when sensing the requirements to secrete specific hormones from different organs or glands to regulate certain body functions, it releases hormones in bursts into the bloodstream.

A healthy pituitary gland is the healthcare security system of our body, but a malfunction in the secretion has very wide negative implications and consequences for our health and well-being.

For instance, it will affect fluid retention in the body, disruption in the menstrual cycle, breastfeeding problems, over or under-active adrenal and thyroid gland responses, and an abnormal growth condition called **Gigantism** and **Dwarfism;** and many more irregular activities.

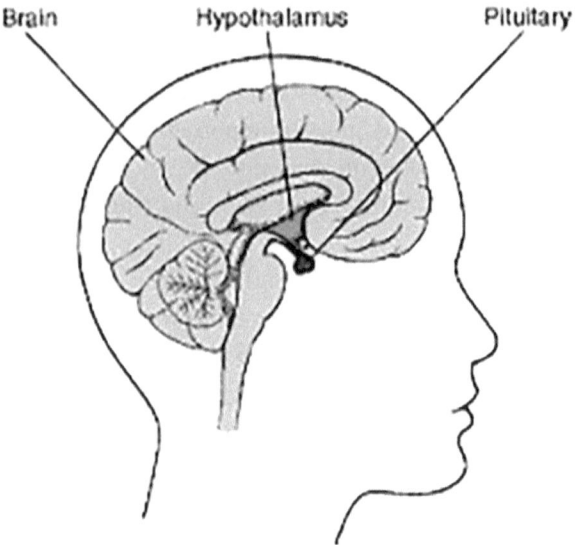

Our Pituitary Gland Hormones and Their Main Function

Adrenocorticotrophic hormone (ACTH) stimulates the adrenal gland for the production of Cortisol (for stress relief).

Thyroid-stimulating hormone (TSH) stimulates the thyroid gland for the release of TSH for thyroid gland activity.

Luteinising hormone (LH) stimulation and control of the function of ovaries in females and testes in males.

Follicle-stimulating hormone (FSH) regulates the functions of both the ovaries and testes; underactivity may cause infertility.

Prolactin (PRL) is a pituitary hormone that promotes lactation (breast milk production).

Growth hormone (GH) this hormone Somatotropin, produced by Pituitary Gland which affects growth and metabolism. Excessive secretion of growth hormone may cause Gigantism and Dwarfism.

Melanocyte-stimulating hormone (MSH) is essential for preserving the skin from harmful ultraviolet rays and also for the development of skin pigmentation.

Anti-diuretic hormone (ADH) is a pituitary hormone which regulates the water content of our body by signalling our kidneys to manage water in the kidney filtration system. It also regulates the water balance in our blood.

Oxytocin is an important hormone which is crucial in childbirth process and also regulates the male reproduction.

Our Kidneys

Our body consists of a pair of kidneys which are located on either side of the spine at the back lower end of the rib cage. These are equally important for our health and well-being as our other vital organs, e.g., heart, brain, lungs and liver are.

Kidneys are the main organ of our urinary system, which is responsible for filtering our blood and eliminating waste products such as urine, and in doing so recirculate the nutrients in the blood to be carried to the heart and then distributed in the body.

Kidneys also keep a balance between sodium and potassium concentration in blood plasma which regulates an osmotic pressure balance between the intra and inter-cellular structure. The integrity of the cellular structure depends on the osmotic pressure to be at equilibrium. Urine also contains a chemical called urea which is the by product from the digestion of meat and fats and also broken-down components of some foods including fruits and vegetables for elimination. So, what are the main functions of our kidneys?

Kidneys are the waste disposal units for our body removing harmful wastes such as toxins, drug metabolites resulting from residual drug molecules resulting from filtration of our circulating blood.

It maintains a balance between sodium and potassium and balances our body's fluid.

Kidneys also regulate the production of red blood cells which are actually manufactured in our bone marrow.

Our acid-base system is balanced by the kidneys, which also maintains our body's electrolyte balance.

Kidneys release hormones which regulate our blood pressure. Adrenal glands located on top of the kidneys produce several important hormones such as Cortisol, Androgens and Oestrogens (male and female sex hormones), Adrenaline and many others and directly release them in the bloodstream. These hormones are very important as they perform specific tasks to keep us going.

How can we safeguard our kidneys and what are the major causes of kidney damage?

There could be a number of reasons for kidney damage but the most adverse of these are hypertension (high blood pressure), diabetes, excessive drug and alcohol abuse. These affect the kidney function such as its filtration capacity. The more toxic waste the blood carries the harder the kidneys will need to work.

So, what can we do to help our kidneys?

If you are over 50, review your health profile at least once a year.

Men with enlarged prostate are at a higher risk and must review their health more frequently. Also, people suffering from cancer and degenerative diseases need regular health checks.

Women with frequent urinary tract infection (UTI) also need regular health reviews.

Early Warning Signs:

Frequently waking up at night to pass urine.

Pain, burning sensations experienced during voiding, irregularity in the urine flow, blood in the urine, very watery or concentrated dark-coloured urine may be tell-tale signs and symptoms of impaired kidney function or general urinary system problems which must immediately be medically assessed.

Several other early signs should also ring alarm bells; some of these symptoms are as follows:

Fatigue and tiredness and loss of appetite, pain in the lower back followed by abdominal pain and also a change in urine characteristics such as colour, output, appearance of froth and occasionally changes in frequency of urination.

Anatomy of the Urinary System (Ref: John Hopkins Medicine)

Front View of Urinary Tract

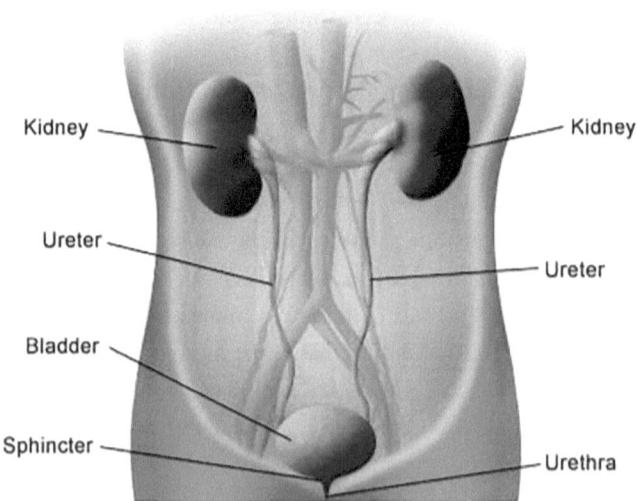

Basic Human Anatomy

Anatomy of Our Kidney (Ref: en.wikipedia.org)

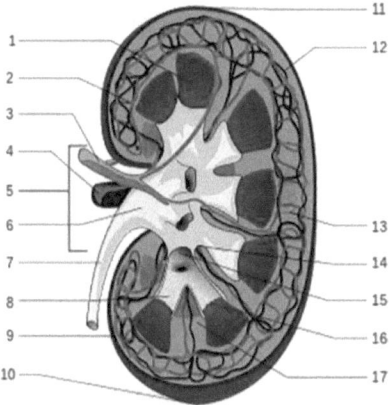

Sections of our kidney

1. Renal Pyramid	7. Ureter	13. Nephron
2. Interlobular Artery	8. Minor Calyx	14. Renal Sinus
3. Renal Artery	9. Renal Capsule	15. Major Calyx
4. Renal Vein 5. Renal Hilum Column 6. Renal Pelvis	10. Inferior Renal Capsule 11. Superior Renal Capsule	16. Renal Papilla 17. Renal Column
	12. Interlobular Vein	

Our Skin

Our skin is the second largest organ by area in our body. Not the heaviest, or the largest yet it covers the entire outer layer of our body. Only the inner area of our small intestine is much larger. The structure of our skin is quite complex It basically consists of three layers:

First the **Epidermis;** which is the outermost layer and protects our body from environmental contaminants such as infections and germs, chemicals and other effects such as heat and harmful radiation, etc.

It contains certain cells called melanocytes which produce skin pigmentation known as melanin and are responsible for the tanned skin coloration. It regulates water loss, body temperature and as the outermost covering for the body, our skin protects our organs as well. The epidermis has several layers, the topmost being the stratum corneum is not connected to any of the blood capillary vessels and therefore does not get any supply of nutrients to stay alive and active. It therefore largely consists of dead cells and is continually shedding, and is replaced by the new cells growing underneath the stratum corneum.

Underneath the Epidermis layer, there is a soft layer of skin called the **Dermis**. This dermis layer of skin is adequately connected to the blood vessels to provide the dermis cells with nutrition. This layer is highly active due to being connected with nerve cells and sweat glands. The dermis layer of the skin is much thicker than the epidermis layer and provides strength and flexibility to our skin. The primary function of the dermis layer, due to being connected with the nerve cells, is to provide the body with certain primary sensations, e.g., touch, hot and cold temperature, pressure and the feeling of pain.

It also excretes sweat from the sweat glands in hot temperature conditions and cools the body down due to evaporation. This maintains homeostasis (meaning a stable state) and regulates the body temperature even in a very hot condition.

The third layer of our skin is the deeper **Sub-cutaneous** layer which sometimes is also called **Hypodermis** layer. This layer of skin is largely made of fatty and connective tissues and is also a thick layer of skin attached to the dermis layer by collagen and fibrous material to give our skin a greater degree of elasticity. The subcutaneous skin layer has many blood vessels to maintain an adequate supply of blood for the body's storage of fats. This layer acts as the insulator and shock absorber for the body and the organs.

Layers of the Skin

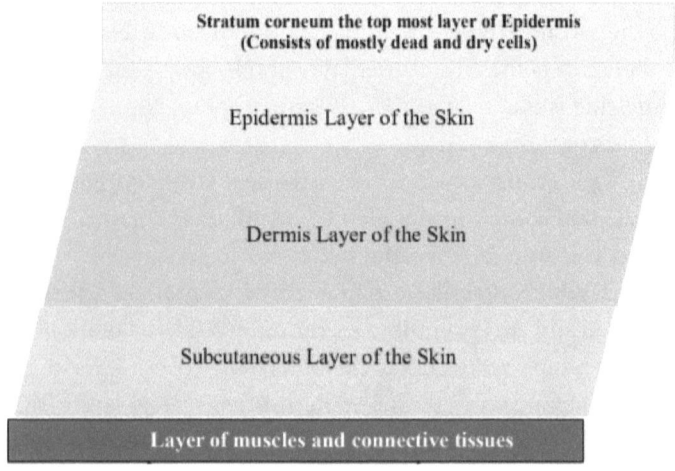

There are several systems that our body collectively defines where a group of organs and tissues work together to perform specific tasks. Let us think of a well-organised factory, and for the smooth running, it has several departments which co-ordinate with each other to fulfil the factory's objectives to make money and exercise a high degree of quality control, to make deliveries to its customers on time and also to work efficiently.

Each body system is a collection of organs and tissues performing several and or specific jobs and collectively all the systems are functioning to keep our body alive and healthy. As there are several systems in operation in our body with the involvement of many organs; let's narrow it down for the sake of simplicity, to the systems which are associated with our vital organs.

A few of the important systems which I have left out from our discussion are the **Lymphatic System, Muscular System, Reproductive System,** etc., and mentioned the more vital systems; although for a perfectly functioning organism, all systems are equally important but none the less some body systems get mentioned more often than others.

As I have mentioned before all body systems must work effectively and efficiently to keep our body alive and healthy. It is a wonder that how intricately our body parts are assembled and work in unison; there is yet a more complex and efficient machine that can ever be built. Mind you it has taken Nature millions of years to create this perfection. Highly efficient robots have been created and built but none are as humanly and conscious as us let alone spiritual.

Just a quick mention of our **endocrine system** which contains mostly glands located all over our body. These glands have the task of regulating the hormonal activities which in turn has an effect on almost all the processes in our body. Let us see which glands are a part of our endocrine system. **Pituitary gland**, is a tiny gland located at the base of our brain and controls how other glands are functioning in producing various hormones that control various processes within our body. Just like a boss who controls, commands and directs his/her staff. Read about Pituitary gland as described earlier in this chapter.

Pancreas is a very important gland which regulates the release of hormone insulin into the blood for the blood glucose to be carried into the cells for energy conversion. Pancreas, as we know from an earlier section of this chapter, is also an important organ of the digestive system producing digestive juices containing enzymes to help with digestive processes. It produces insulin.

Adrenal glands sit on the top of each of our kidneys. These produce several hormones which regulate our blood pressure and also stress levels. **Ovaries and Testes** are female and male glands which are responsible for producing hormones such as oestrogens, progesterone, etc., in women and testosterone in males which have important male and female functions. Ovaries produce hormones which play an active role in the female reproductive system, facilitate menstruation and fertility issues. Similarly, testes produce hormones which are active in male reproductive system, e.g., control of the production of sperms.

Then there are **Thyroid and Parathyroid** glands; they are located in the vicinity of each other. There are two Thyroid glands located just at the base of the neck below the Adam's apple. It is a vital gland and produces hormones which play important roles in many metabolic processes such as in our growth and development, it also controls our body temperature and fatigue levels. Parathyroid glands are tiny and there are four of them. The hormone produced by Parathyroid glands called Parathyroid Hormone (PTH) regulates calcium levels in our body and the amounts of calcium, phosphorus and magnesium in the bones and blood.

I almost forgot about the **Pineal** gland. It is a tiny gland which sits in the middle of the brain and releases the hormone melatonin which controls our sleep patterns and regulates our day and night rhythms (Circadian Rhythms). It is important to know that our body is a finely tuned machine run by several organs and systems not by just one; it is a collective effort. Lack of or insufficiency in any one organ or a system can bring about complications in our health and well-being. There are a number of other components of our body systems each of which has certain task to perform. A body system function will not be complete without the collective co-ordination of each component of a particular system.

Our Body Systems with Certain Organs, Tissues and Cells and their Main Functions

Systems	Main Organ	Other useful components of the System			Activities
Circulatory System	Heart	Blood Vessels (Arteries Veins Capillaries)	Blood (is a tissue of specialised cells)	Heart, arteries, veins, capillaries.	Carries blood throughout the body, deposits oxygen and nutrients into the cells.

System					Function
Respiratory System	Lungs	Trachea or the wind pipe	Nose and Mouth	Throat (Pharynx)	Breathing in and out; absorbing oxygen in the lungs and exhaling carbon dioxide.
Digestive System	Liver	Stomach	Gall Bladder	Intestines	Processing food and absorbing the nutrients the body needs then eliminating the waste.
Nervous System	Brain	Spinal Cord	Nerves	Sensory Organs e.g., ears, eyes, nose, etc.	Responds and activates our senses, processes and co-ordinates other organs and systems
Immune System	Thymus gland	Leukocytes (White blood cells)	Lymph nodes	Bone marrow tissues	Protection against infection and disease; most of the immune cells are made in bone marrow.
Skeletal System	Bones	Cartilage	Ligaments	Vertebral column	Offers body frame for support, protection for internal body organs, body movement.
Urinary System	Kidneys	Bladder	Ureters	Urethra	Filtration of blood, Re-absorption of nutrients, adjustment of blood pH.

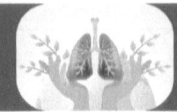

Chapter 6

VITAMINS IN OUR HEALTH AND WELLBEING

A healthy diet is a healthy beginning of good health and wellbeing; adding vitamins to your daily supplementation could mean a healthy beginning and also a healthy end.
— Jay Das, 2022

What Are Vitamins?

Vitamins are organic molecules which our body needs as a catalyst or a helper molecule to conduct numerous biochemical processes happening within our body to promote good health and vitality. We need vitamins in small quantities, a majority of which may be supplied by our diet of fresh fruits and vegetables and the 5 different kinds of food categories we have explained in an earlier chapter. Vitamins are classed as essential nutrients as our bodies cannot manufacture them or produce them in very small quantities which may not be sufficient for our body's regular needs.

Without the availability of vitamins on a daily basis for utilisation in biochemical processes, there could be an increased risk of developing mild to significant health problems. It is also important to remember that in most cases the availability of vitamins in our diets may not be enough and so we need to supplement the additional requirement through an external supplementation programme. Until today, there are 13 vitamins that are known to us which are split into two categories; water-soluble including vitamin C and fat-soluble as listed here.

Water-soluble Vitamins	Fat-soluble Vitamins
Vitamin B1 (Thiamine)	Vitamin A (Retinol)
Vitamin B2 (Riboflavin)	Vitamin D (Calciferol)
Vitamin B3 (Niacin)	Vitamin E (Tocopherol)
Vitamin B5 (Pantothenic Acid)	Vitamin K (Phylloquinone; vitamin K1 and Menaquinone Vitamin K2)
Vitamin B6 (Pyridoxine)	
Vitamin B7 (Biotin)	
Vitamin B9 (Folates or Folic Acid)	
Vitamin B12 (Cyanocobalamin)	
Vitamin C	

Vitamin K is split into K1 and K2 which are basically the two forms of the K vitamin (*Koagulation* from Danish word for coagulation) but possess two different properties both essential for our health and general well-being. Certain adjunct molecules to the vitamins such as inositol is also referred to as vitamins; and sometimes referred to as vitamin B8.

Water-Soluble Vitamins:

As the name suggests water-soluble vitamins, they dissolve in water readily and so do not stay in the body for long. Due to a higher solubility and faster clearance rate of elimination from the body, the need for the B-group vitamins in the body are more regular than the fat-soluble vitamins.

Water-soluble vitamins quickly dissolve in water and quickly to be absorbed into the tissues. These are mostly B-group vitamins and vitamin C which cannot be stored in our bodies for long and need to be replenished regularly to keep up with our daily vitamin requirement and status. It has been widely speculated by many experts that a complete diet containing the 5 food categories (as in the previous chapter) may be adequate in supplying our daily need for vitamins be it water-soluble or the fat and lipid-soluble variety. But is it really so?

As the B-group vitamins are highly water-soluble they are most likely to be leached out during food preparation, particularly at the washing and clean-up stages. There are many other factors which we will see later in the chapter that have a strong and significant effect on the availability of various water-soluble vitamins from fruits and vegetables in our diets. Adding to this we also need to consider other de-stabilising factors such as the effect on storage, heat and other environmental factors. Particularly so, at the household storage facility levels and the effect of oxidation which could lead to significant losses.

So, in addition to a diet of mixed fruits and vegetables, it is always a good idea to plan for a regular supplementation.

Fat-Soluble Vitamins

The fat-soluble vitamins on the other hand require dietary fats to help absorb these vitamins in the small intestine, from there they form micellar globules and are transported into various cells in the body. Because these fat-soluble vitamins require fats and lipids to help their assimilation they tend to stay much longer in the body and their clearance rate of elimination is poor. It is therefore not unusual to generate a large pool of reserve of these vitamins and over time build up toxicity.

Both water-soluble and fat-soluble vitamins are needed in our body for basic functions, growth and maintenance of our body's cellular structure and tissues. Vitamin deficiency in our system is caused by nutritional inadequacies resulting from a number of issues as presented in the diagram below for easy understanding. An adequate reserve of vitamins in our body helps protect us from degenerative diseases caused by free radical tissue damage and minor stress-related conditions. In several cases of minor disorders, which are vitamin dependent and, or vitamin responsive, the use of specific vitamins can assist to rectify the ailment at least temporarily until further investigation and medical interventions can be planned.

Although vitamins are needed in small quantities, a deficiency in any one or a combination of multiple vitamins can make a significant change to our health and general well-being. A large quantity of both water-soluble except Vitamin C and fat-soluble vitamins are stored in the liver.

The diagram highlights the physiological steps involved with vitamins and the availability or lack of them within our body.

Diagram: Vitamins and physiological steps in the body
(Inadequate availability and deficiency state)

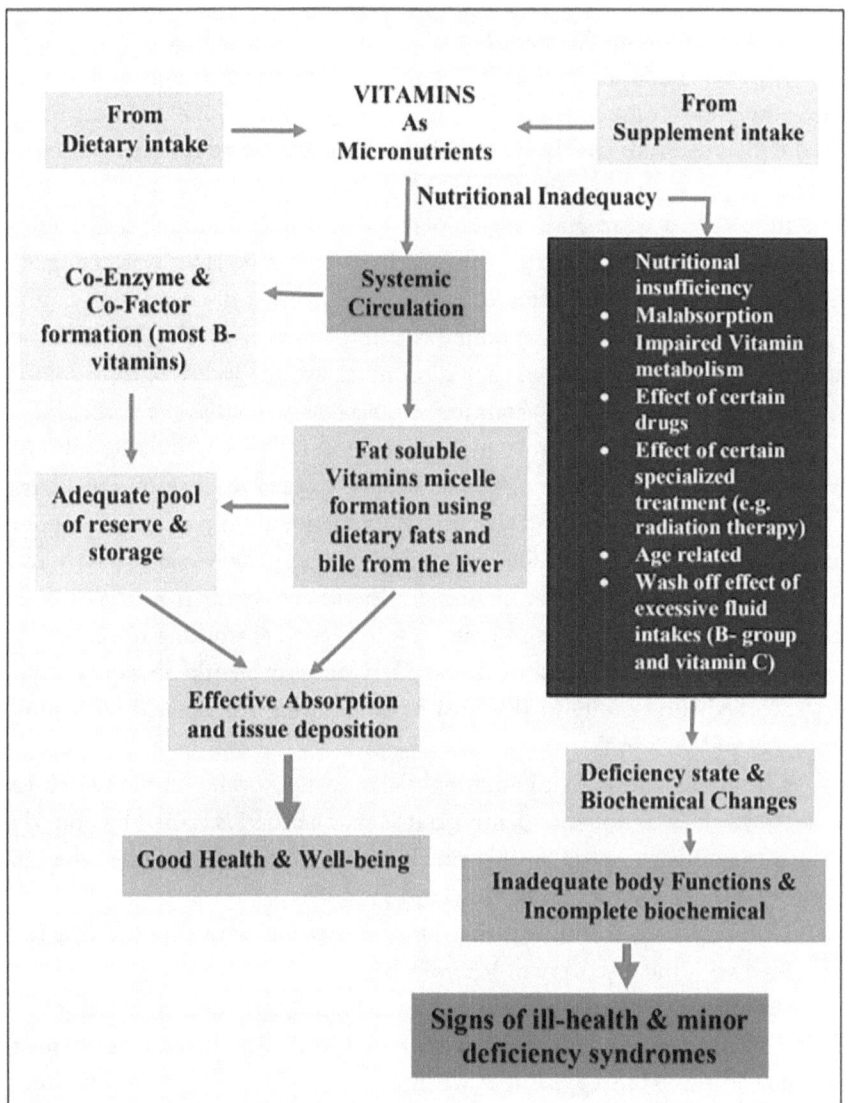

Many scientists and researchers in various fields of biochemistry and physiology have made significant contributions to the discovery and advancements of various vitamins, but only one is accredited with the title of 'The father of Vitamin Therapy'.

Casimir Funk (b. 1884–d. 1967) a Polish-born biochemist in 1911 coined the word **'Vitamine'** and suggested that there exists a group of amine-like compounds which are vital to life and are also essential to curing several diseases. Hence Casimir coined the word from Vita meaning life and Amine from his concept of amine-like compounds. Unfortunately, his concept that these amine-like compounds which are required in very small amounts to cure specific diseases were largely ignored by the scientific fraternity in those early days.

In 1912, a year after he coined the word 'Vitamine' the scientific community accepted the word which after several years later, was changed to **Vitamin** by dropping the letter 'e' as some of the latter discoveries of vitamins were demonstrated to be not of amine or nitrogenous nature, e.g., ascorbic acid (Vitamin C). The instigator of such a proposal was Sir Jack Cecil Drummond who in 1920 proposed that 'Vitamine' should be renamed as 'Vitamin'.

In 1911, in order to prove his theory Funk isolated an organic substance from rice hulls which he demonstrated to have a curative effect on Polyneuritis in birds which were fed on a diet of polished rice devoid of the compound Funk extracted from unpolished rice hulls. This organic molecule later came to be known as Vitamin B1 (Thiamine). The disease beriberi in the early 20th century was a big challenge and many researchers were working towards a cure around the world. It is acclaimed that **Dr Umetaro Suzuki** in Japan around 1910 worked successfully in this area by discovering Aberic acid with similar properties of Vitamin B1.

Christiaan Eijkman a Dutch physician while working in the Dutch East Indies (now, Java, Indonesia) demonstrated that beriberi is caused by poor diet; this led to the discovery of antineuritic vitamins for which he shared the 1929 Nobel Prize with **Sir Frederick Gowland Hopkins.**

Unfortunately, this meant that Funk missed out on being the first to be accredited with the discovery of Vitamin B1.

Riboflavin (**Vitamin B2**) was discovered much earlier in 1922; a combined effort by German biochemist **Richard Kuhn** and the Austrian biochemistry **Theodor Wagner-Jauregg**. But if we look back some credit should be due to the 1872 English chemist **Alexander Wynter Blyth** who had paved the way for vitamin B2 discovery by suggesting that the very faint fluorescent yellowish tinge in milk was a biochemical which has some nutritional quality.

Vitamin Nomenclature

The naming of vitamins is just as interesting as the biochemistry of vitamins themselves. For his tireless work in 'Vitamine therapy', Casimir Funk was nominated four times for the Nobel Prize but it was unfortunately that he missed out on each of those occasions. It is still believed by some that he should have won the coveted prize at least once, but it was not to be. The naming of vitamins is really a bit complex as it did not follow a clear logical pattern. It is believed that the first 5 vitamins A, B, C, D and E were all discovered between 1910 to say 1925 as vitamins D and E were isolated around 1922–23 and were allocated or assigned alphabetically on a first come first served basis.

Thiamine (vitamin B1) was isolated before vitamin A and should have been allocated the letter A. However, as both vitamin B1 (Thiamine) and vitamin A were isolated closely to each other and that during the isolation of vitamin A it was referred to as the factor 'A' it was designated the alphabet A.

After the discovery of vitamin A, and the naming of thiamine was achieved (as B-vitamin), vitamin D in (1922) followed immediately by vitamin E (in 1922–23) were named in accordance with the alphabetical rule. The odd one out seemed to be vitamin K (in 1929) which should have been named using letter F; but it was designated K for Koagulation by the Danish researcher **Henrik Dam** who also happened to be the discoverer of vitamin K as well.

With time, as other water-soluble vitamins similar in properties to Thiamine (vitamin B) were discovered, e.g., Riboflavin (in 1922) Niacin (in 1936), Pantothenic Acid and Biotin (in 1931), Pyridoxine (in 1934), Folic Acid (in 1941) and cobalamin (in 1926) they were assigned in addition to the letter B, a numerical order for identification. However, the order of numerical assignment was not systematic. For example, Niacin was assigned B3 while Pantothenic Acid and Biotin were assigned B5 and B7 respectively and Cobalamin was assigned B12 even though it was discovered much earlier than B3, B5 or B7.

Confused! Don't be; as the numbering in these B vitamins are not necessarily assigned in chronological order.

The Era of Vitamin Discovery

Early to middle part of the 20th century, there was a buzz of excitement. Many of the early observations made by researchers in the mid-1800s to the early part of the 1900s paved the way for new discoveries of vitamins, and, vital research into nutrition. This laid the foundation for modern nutrition. Many of the diseases as we know now or diseases prevalent in the early part of the 1800s and the 1900s were due to nutritional deficiencies in particular the unknown factors which are now proven to be due to specific vitamin deficiencies.

Scurvy, beriberi, pellagra, rickets, xerophthalmia, nutritional anaemias and many more diseases are attributed to nutritional deficiency and, or, due to a particular vitamin deficiency. I do applaud the resilience of the foresighted pioneers who experimented with what was available in the Nature, e.g., the French explorer Jacques Cartier in his first voyage in 1534 of early exploration of North America on the advice of the local Iroquois tribes of the St. Lawrence River region of Canada was able to save his crew suffering from a mysterious illness by simply boiling the needles of the spruce tree.

As we today know the mysterious illness was scurvy and the spruce tree needles offered significant levels of Vitamin C for a curative effect. There are many similar entries in the annals of history and many more scientific discoveries in various journals which have been now scientifically validated.

Professor **Paul Karrer** a Swiss Scientist, born in Moscow in 1889 extracted vitamin A from cod-liver oil and determined its composition in 1932 and worked on Vitamin B2 (riboflavin, in 1935), Vitamin E (tocopherol, in 1938) and Vitamin K (phytonadione, in 1939). He was awarded the Nobel Prize in 1937 for his outstanding work on Carotenoids, Flavin and Vitamin A.

There is another great name which springs to my mind, that of **Robert Burns Woodward**. Woodward (b. 1917–d. 1979) was an American Organic Chemist whom some say was one of the most brilliant synthetic chemists of the 20th century.

He received the Nobel Prize in 1965 for his outstanding achievements in the art of organic synthesis.

As I have been a fan of Professor Woodward let me indulge in some of his marvellous works during his career; although he received only one Nobel Prize award in 1965 many say he was deserving of a couple more.

Selected Scientific Milestones Achieved by Dr Robert Burns Woodward and co-workers.

1944 Synthesis of quinine and proposed β-lactam formula for penicillin.
1951 Synthesis of cortisone and cholesterol.
1953 Structural determination of Terramycin (an antibiotic)
1954 Determined structure and synthesis of both strychnine and Lanosterol.
1956 Determined the structure of and synthesised reserpine.
1960 Total synthesis of Chlorophyll.
1962 Total synthesis of Tetracycline (an antibiotic)

1966 Total synthesis of cephalosporin C.
1973 Total synthesis of cobyric acid and Vitamin B12
1981 Total synthesis of Erythromycin A.
And many other synthetic chemistry projects that he had part taken with distinction.

Ancient Egyptians, Babylonians, Greeks and Arabs all had the knowledge of night blindness and used animal liver for treatment and successfully cured the disease. However, there seems to be no reference that the ancients had the knowledge that night blindness is caused by the deficiency of a specific Vitamin A like compound in the diet. They only by trial and error found out that feeding animal liver had a beneficial effect. Today we know that animal liver is a concentrated source of Vitamin A. It is a classic case of cure without knowing the cause.

In modern times, the discovery of Vitamin A is the culminated effort by a number of researchers who made it easier for the next generation of research workers to reach the discovery destination. The work of French physiologist François Magendie with nutritionally deprived dogs (1816), high mortality of poorly fed, abandoned infants in Paris suffering from corneal defects and ulcers pointed to a common clinical disorder caused by nutritional deficiency. During the 1880s, Nicolai Lunin studying at the University of Dorpat in Estonia demonstrated that mice can live in good health when fed with milk. Soon after Carl A. Socin demonstrated that there was an unknown substance in egg yolk that was essential to life, and he raised the question of whether this substance was fat-like in nature.

In 1913, **Elmer McCollum** and **Marguerite Davis** claimed that butter and egg yolk contained a growth-supporting factor which they called factor A that ultimately was recognised as Vitamin A and for which they finally received credit for. So, this heralded a new era of vitamin A discovery after many years of painstaking research work.

Vitamin A was first synthesised in 1947 by two Dutch chemists, **David Adriaan van Dorp** and **Jozef Ferdinand Arens**.

Vitamin D

Vitamin D chemically known as Calciferol was thought to have been discovered by Elmer McCollum and Marguerite Davis around 1913 during their research into 'factor A' later known as vitamin A. During experimenting with cod liver oil in 1922 Elmer McCollum destroyed vitamin A in the cod liver oil by heat treatment but demonstrated that a separate anti-rachitic substance (which helps to prevent and or cures the disease rickets) was produced as a result which he named 'vitamin D'.

The 1928 unshared Nobel Prize in Chemistry went to **Adolf Otto Reinhold Windaus** a German scientist for his studies on the constitution of the sterols and their connection with vitamins; he also had worked out the synthesis of vitamin D from the plant sterol Ergosterol.

I feel that Dr Elmer McCollum was hard done by on two occasions; vitamin A and D which he had discovered. Logically he should have been awarded a Nobel Prize for his discoveries and works.

In frustration, McCollum in his book which was fairly comprehensive 'A History of Nutrition' published in 1957, again claimed that he was the discoverer of vitamins A and D and was a bit critical of several of his colleague's works including experiments conducted by F.G. Hopkins (referred above as the co-discoverer of vitamin B1).

It does seem the awards of Nobel Prizes in a few instances were fraught with injustice the two main characters in this injustice were Casimir Funk and Elmer McCollum; wouldn't you say so?

Vitamin D has so much to offer us from our health perspective; like vitamin C it is also essential to our general health and well-being the only difference being that Vitamin C cannot be synthesised in our body while vitamin D is free and can be synthesised within our body by the sun and that's why vitamin D is also called the sunshine vitamin.

The diagram offers the readers a basic understanding of the necessity of Vitamin D in our everyday life.

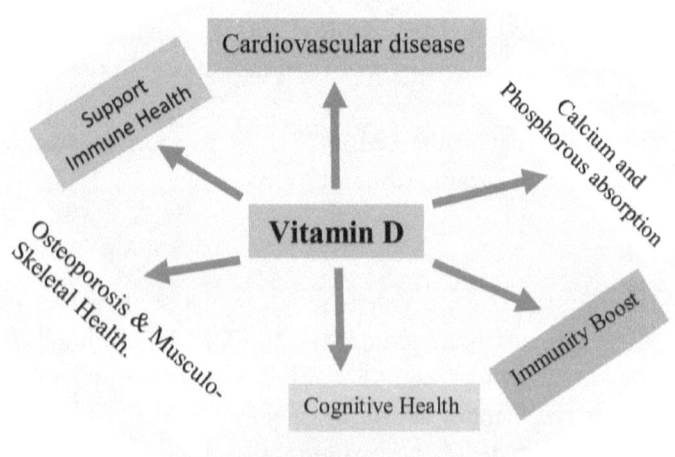

As we all know vitamin D is very important for the absorption of both calcium and phosphorous; a low vitamin D level in our system indicates an impairment in calcium absorption which results in a disruption in Parathyroid hormone (PTH). PTH is important in balancing calcium absorption in the bone tissue.

In a recent publication (Ref: Nutrients 2021, *13*(10), 3603), the authors have elegantly detailed the current understanding of Vitamin D in Chronic Diseases, Acute Respiratory Infections and All-Cause Mortality (death from any cause). For interested people, this is a worthwhile read. The second schematic diagram as represented in the above publication is also a very self-explanatory link between Vitamin D and Cardiovascular disease (CVD).

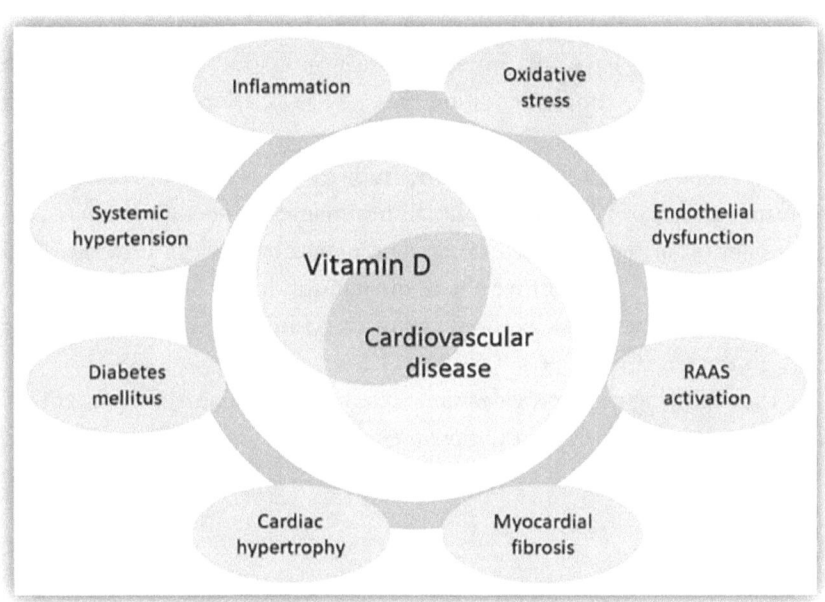

(Ref: Nutrients 2021, 13(10), 3603)

The RAAS (Renin-Angiotensin-Aldosterone System) is a complex endocrine hormone system which is involved in regulating a number of cardiovascular processes. In the early stage at the onset of heart failure when there is a drop in Blood Pressure (BP), the RAAS hormone system springs into action in a compensatory role by regulating the BP by increasing the fluid and the electrolyte absorption in the kidneys. It is also worth knowing that RAAS can be detrimental to the progression of CVD where vital medical intervention becomes necessary.

CVD is one of the leading causes of death; it is estimated that globally in 2019 around 32% of people died due to CVD of which 85% deaths were due to heart attack and stroke. Alarming numbers indeed. More than 75% of CVD deaths occur in poorer nations with low to middle-income groups.

(www.who.int/en/news-room/fact-sheets/detail/cardiovascular-diseases-cvds)

In a recent highly reputable publication (Ref: European Heart Journal 05 December 2021), the researchers concluded that Vitamin D deficiency can increase the risk of CVD. The researchers also concluded that the burden of CVD could be reduced by population-wide correction of low vitamin D status. This research was undertaken at The Australian Centre for Precision Health at the University of South Australia Cancer Research Institute Australia. In another report (JAMA Cardiol. 2019; 4 (8):765–776), the authors concluded that vitamin D may not have any protective effect on CVD; the research question was Does vitamin D supplementation have any association with cardiovascular disease risk?

Throughout medical and scientific studies there are overwhelming reports on positive effects of vitamins on human health and well-being. There could be only a handful of reports based on epidemiological and clinical studies which may not confer with the positive effects of vitamins, it should not be a deterrent against the use of vitamins as supplements as positive reports overwhelmingly outweigh the negative reports.

The following chart provides some reference to the timeline of events that led to the discovery of vitamin D now proven to be an essential nutrient for the human species.

Discovery and Time Line for Vitamin D

Timeline of events that led to the discovery and understanding of vitamin D (Unravelling the Enigma of Vitamin D)
http://www.nasonline.org/publications › beyond-discovery/ vitamin-d.pdf)
(Time-line Mid 1600s–1931)

(1) Rickets was first identified as a disease in mid-1600

(2) Sir Frederick Gowland Hopkins in Early 1906 demonstrates that certain whole untreated foods contain an unknown constituents essential to health and growth.

(3) 1906 Christiaan Eijkman and Gerrit Grijns extract the antineuritic factor from rice hulls, later shown to be vitamin B1

(4) 1918 Sir Edward Mellanby induces rickets in dogs and then cures the disease by feeding the dogs cod-liver oil.

(5) 1919 K. Huldschinsky cures children of rickets using artificially produced ultraviolet light.

(6) Early 1920s Harry Goldblatt and Katherine Soames, H. Steenbock and A. Black, and Alfred Hess and Mildred Weinstock independently discover that irradiating certain foodstuffs with ultraviolet light renders those foods antirachitic

(7) 1922 Elmer V. McCollum destroys vitamin A in cod liver oil and shows that the separate antirachitic substance remains. He calls the newly identified substance "vitamin D."

(9) 1931 F. A. Askew defines the chemical makeup of the form of vitamin D found in irradiated foods (now called ergocalciferol), derived from the precursor molecule Ergosterol.

(8) 1927 Adolf Windaus, O. Rosenheim, and T. A. Webster deduce that Ergosterol is the likely parent substance of vitamin D in food.

(Time-line, mid-1930s–2000s)

(10) 1936 Windaus deduces the chemical structure of vitamin D3 produced in the skin (now known as cholecalciferol) and identifies the structure of its parent molecule, 7-dehydrocholesterol.

(11) 1968 Hector F. DeLuca and colleagues isolate an active vitamin D metabolite and identify it as 25-hydroxyvitamin D3. They later prove that the substance is produced in the liver.

(12) 1968–1970 The existence of a second active metabolite produced from 25-hydroxyvitamin D3 is reported by Anthony W. Norman, Mark R. Haussler, and J. F. Myrtle; by E. Kodicek, D. E. M. Lawson, and P. W. Wilson; and by DeLuca and Co-workers.

(13) 1970s Researchers discover the relationship of vitamin D to the body's endocrine system and calcium regulation.

(14) 1971 Three research groups identify the chemical/molecular structure of the final active form of vitamin D as 1, 25-dihydroxyvitamin D3, which is soon reclassified as a hormone controlling calcium metabolism.

(15) 1975 Haussler confirms the discovery of a protein receptor that binds the active vitamin D metabolite to the nucleus of cells in the intestine.

(16) 1980s A Japanese research team and, independently, Michael F. Holick and co-workers show that vitamin D hormone inhibits skin cell growth. Holick and colleagues demonstrate that topical applications of the vitamin D hormone are a remarkably effective treatment of psoriasis.

(17) Mid 1980s Researchers find that vitamin D hormone seems to play a part in modulating the immune system.

(18) 1994 The U.S. Food and Drug Administration approves a vitamin D-based topical treatment for psoriasis, called Calcipotriol.

Vitamins in Our Health and Wellbeing

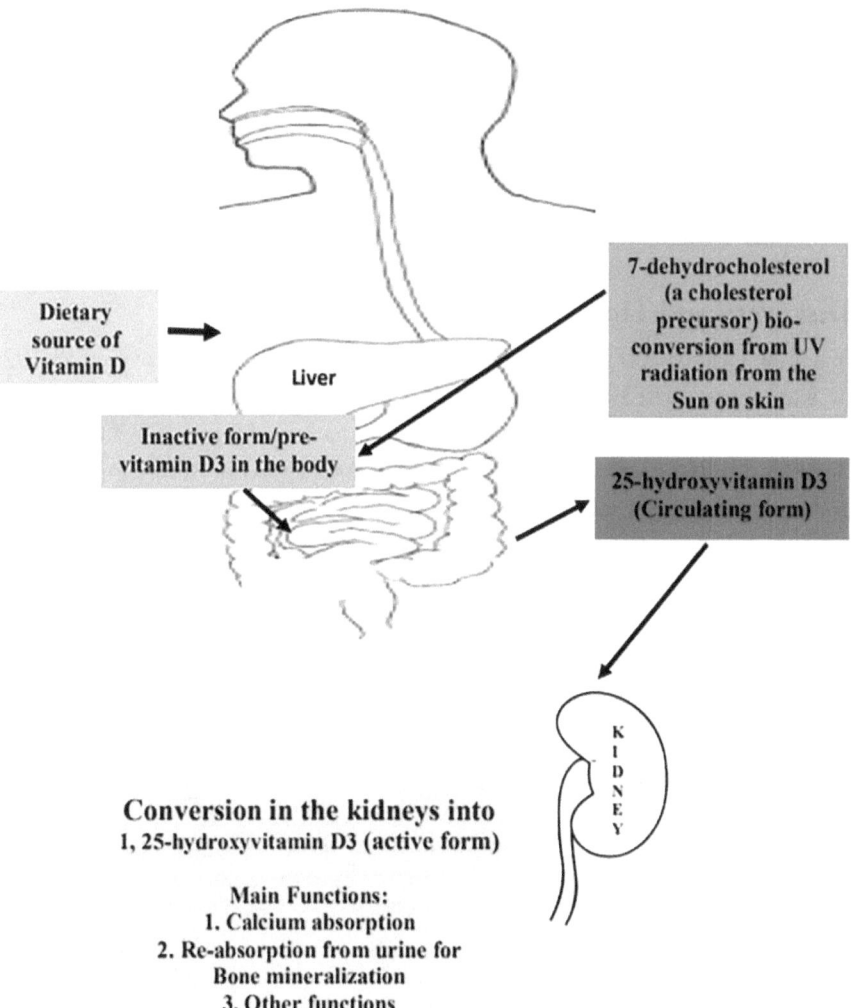

Just under one in four Australian adults (23%) had a Vitamin D deficiency, which comprised 17% with a mild deficiency, 6% with a moderate deficiency and less than 1% with a severe deficiency.

Vitamin D levels varied considerably by season, with rates of deficiency being much lower in summer (14%) and much higher in winter (36%).

In winter, rates of Vitamin D deficiency were particularly high in the Australian southeastern states of Victoria (49%), ACT (49%) and Tasmania (43%) compared with the northern states of Queensland (15%) and Northern Territory (17%). One in twenty Australian adults (5%) were taking Vitamin D supplements in 2011–12. As expected, those who took Vitamin D supplements had lower levels of Vitamin D deficiency than those who did not take supplements (7% compared with 23%).

(Ref: Australian Bureau of Statistics 2013, Australian Health Survey)

Discovery and Time Line for Vitamin E

It will be exactly 100 years (2021–22) since vitamin E was discovered in 1922 by **Katharine Scott Bishop** and **Herbert McLean Evans**.

While working in the Department of Anatomy University of California, Berkeley, Dr Bishop then working under Professor Evans an American anatomist and embryologist on the subject of the reproductive cycle of rats discovered the vital reproduction factor which was initially called the 'Factor X' was essential for a healthy pregnancy.

Vitamin E was named Tocopherol from the Greek word 'Tokos' meaning birth and 'Pherin' meaning to carry or pregnancy. This was due to the early findings that Vitamin E promoted a dietary fertility factor in rats. The word pherin was changed to pherol signifying its chemical structure as a complex alcohol molecule. Vitamin E like several other vitamins e.g., vitamin C and D has been the subject of numerous research topics and periodic reviews.

The table highlights the important and noteworthy research conducted and published on vitamin E.

> 1922—Discovery (Bishop and Evans)
> 1924—Nomenclature (B. Sure)
> 1930s—Anti-Oxidant properties of Vitamin E (Henry A. Mattill and Co-workers)
> 1936—Isolation from wheat germ oil (Evans HM, Emerson OH, Emerson GA.)
> 1938—Synthesis and Structure elucidation (Karrer and Fernholz)
> 1940s—Protective nature of vitamin E for unsaturated fatty acids in all tissues against Oxidation (Filer and co-workers)
> 1949—Serum vitamin E levels in the complication of pregnancy (Scrimshaw NS, Greer RB, Goodland RL.)
> 1950s—Beginning of interest in infant nutrition, Vitamin E and Neonates 1980 (Richard A. Ehrenkranz), and many other publications.
> 1967—Tocopherol Deficiency in Man (Binder HJ, Spiro HM.)
> 1968—Inclusion by US Food and Nutrition Board (RDA Tables)
> 1988—Vitamin E inhibits protein kinase C activity (Mahoney and Azzi)
> 2000—Gene-Regulatory Activity (GRA) of Alpha-Tocopherol (H. Fencher, A. Stoker, J. Yamauchi)
> 2005—The discovery of Antioxidant properties (Wolf G.)
> 2010—Saremi and Arora—Vitamin E and cardiovascular disease research on Vitamin E is an ongoing undertaking.
> 2010—Vitamin E and all-cause mortality (Abner EL, et.al.)
> 2018—Role of Vitamin E in Preventing and Treating Osteoarthritis-a Review of Current Evidences (Kok-Yong Chin, Soelaiman Ima-Nirwana)

Henrik Carl Peter Dam the Danish-born scientist won the Nobel Prize in 1944 in Physiology for his discovery of vitamin K. The prize was shared with Edward Adelbert Doisy for his **discovery** of the chemical nature of Vitamin K.

Dam was born in Copenhagen, Denmark in 1895. While working on coagulation experiments, Dam and his co-workers investigated the role of dietary cholesterol on Chickens and found that when animals fed on low-fat diets suffered from prolonged bleeding, but as soon as the diets were supplemented with hemp seeds the bleeding stopped. Dam and his co-workers concluded that hemp seed contained a substance which had the ability to reverse the bleeding effect. This was the start of the discovery of vitamin K in 1929.

Edward Adelbert Doisy of the University of Saint Louis also worked out the chemical structure of vitamin K which led to the understanding of the importance of this vitamin and its application in many physiological disorders e.g., the successful treatment of cases of Jaundice with prothrombin deficiency (Warner and his co-workers from the University of Iowa in 1938). An important milestone was reached in 1974 when researchers discovered the exact function of Vitamin K in the body when they isolated prothrombin, a vitamin K-dependent coagulation factor; for this reason, Vitamin K is also known as the 'Koagulations vitamin'. As was first reported in German journals.

Vitamin K is a cofactor with enzyme carboxylase which produces gamma carboxyglutamic acid, which undergoes a cycle of Oxidation and Reduction which allows the vitamin to be reused in the vitamin K cycle.

Vitamin K produces a protein which helps blood to coagulate and helps blood to clot. This prevents excessive bleeding both internally and externally. Haemophilia may be a condition defined by vitamin K deficiency both in adults and newborn children.

The mechanism of clotting is explained step by step for easy understanding; however, it must be known that each step has a complicated and involved set of procedures to manage biochemically.

Mechanism of Blood Clotting:

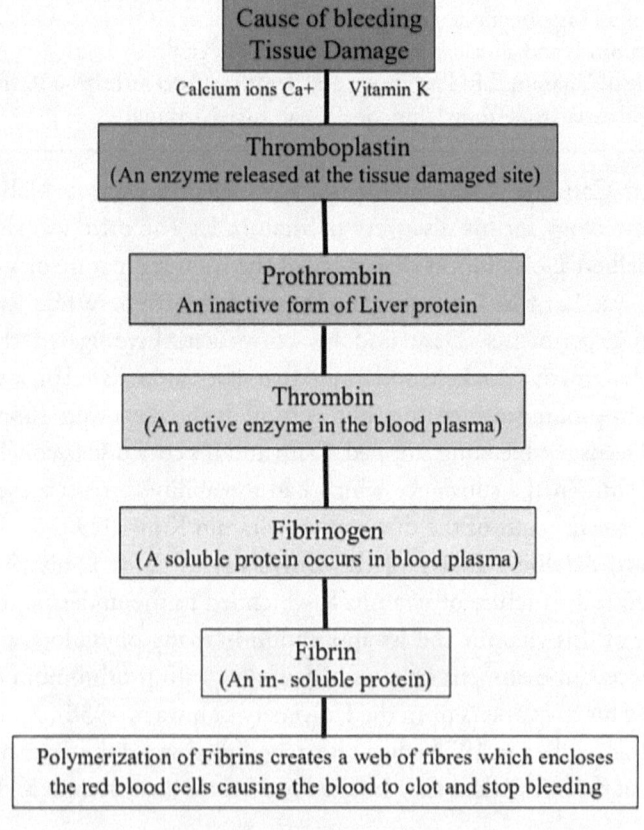

Vitamin Safety and Risk Factors

Everything in life has its own risk. Therefore, from this perspective use of vitamins has its risks too. If you use more than the prescribed dose hoping for a quick result or if you think more is better then you may sadly be mistaken. So, stick with the dose and use vitamins, minerals or any other supplements in moderation and sensibly.

Many people have a valid reason for asking the following questions.

Are Vitamin and mineral supplements safe to take?

Why do we need vitamins?

How much do we need?

Are we meeting our daily requirements?

All these questions have very basic simple answers. Information on vitamins and other health supplements has become readily available with relative accuracy and in simplistic terms if you know where to look for them. There are many research and scientific studies conducted globally in reputed research laboratories and Universities and results are published widely in journals and research citations. Most research works are now being validated and articles are reviewed before publication.

Public scrutiny is so investigative that there is no escape. Somebody is always there to take a particular research finding and analyse it diligently in search of the truth.

When I started out as a young researcher and nutritional biochemist, there was a lack of good information. A common misconception existed that vitamins and mineral supplements are possibly a waste of money and resources. Meaningful debates were of no significant value as people had preconceived ideas leaning towards the orthodox opinions that vitamins and mineral supplements alike were of not much value as far as the health benefits go. And there was a common perception that all you need, you can get from your diet if your diet consists of the required mix and portions of nutrient-rich produce be it vegetable and fruit and, or, a combination of animal proteins included.

These opinions were biased as the members of the medical fraternity just simply ignored the issue or went out of their way to discredit nutritional benefits from supplement intakes. They were early days; but now perceptions have changed and a lot more information and research validations are available for public scrutiny.

Since I was involved with the industry, I was keenly interested in taking the supplements myself and in due course got significant benefits. But the sad part of it was that several of my medical practitioner friends dismissed those beneficial results as either inconclusive or aberrations; and today, I am glad to see that many scientists and medical people be the medical researchers and medical practitioners are noticing the benefits offered by the supplements and reading the fact sheets published by renowned researchers including Nobel Laureates.

In the late 70s and early 80s, when the regulatory considerations came into effect and the required daily amounts (RDA's) in America by The Food and Nutrition Board of the National Academy of Science-National Research Council, and (RDI's) required daily intakes in Australia were published by the National Health and Medical Research Council (NH & MRC) the nutritional industry became more credible and acceptable. This was the preliminary step in the right direction upon which the fundamentals of nutritional supplements were based and further recognitions were achieved.

But still, no consideration was given to the great vitamin controversies, and, evidences that nutritional supplements do really work were largely ignored. The values for the RDA's and RDI's that were established then, still largely remain the same today. The efforts put in by many researchers in vitamins and supplements in general, and many medical and natural practitioners who worked tirelessly in dose-related trials and observations are continually updating our knowledge in these emerging subjects.

As a result of the compelling evidences compiled and published from time to time, the knowledge gained cannot be ignored anymore and the regulatory bodies are pleasingly evaluating and reviewing the RDA, RDI tables accordingly but in a cautious and conservative manner. Opinions in favour of the use of nutritional supplements, in general, have changed and several working concepts on dosages have evolved through studies in North America and other parts of the world which have laid the foundation for the introduction of the concept of ODI's (Optimum Daily Intake), TUL (Tolerable Upper Limits), etc., which have now become source points for many credible formulations of vitamin and nutritional supplements.

With the introduction of the Therapeutic Goods Administration (TGA) in Australia, Food and Drug Administration (FDA) in America and equivalent regulatory bodies in other parts of the world, the nutritional industry has now become standardised globally. This has introduced a greater credibility and confidence and promises of a better future and universal acceptability of the supplement industry and supplements in general.

It is now, more so than any time in the past 30 years that the intake of vitamins and other nutritional supplements has become an integral part of our daily ritual.

The 2017 CRN Consumer Survey on Dietary Supplements shows 76% of Americans are taking dietary supplements, up from 64% ten years ago in 2008. In Australia, over 8.3 million Australians buy vitamins, minerals and supplements as per the survey by Roy Morgan Research. (26 Apr 2019).

Having mentioned the positivity of vitamins and supplements in general, we occasionally come across a few examples of manufacturers who escape the regulatory network and self-regulatory assessments, and market products which could have been better if more care had been taken in their manufacture and quality assurances.

Sorry, I digressed from offering answers to the above-mentioned frequently asked questions. I hope that the above background material is not only informative but also prepares you for the issues involved.

Are Vitamin and mineral supplements safe to take?

Vitamins and Minerals are not drugs and if we follow the dosage levels as prescribed in the RDA, RDI. ODI and UL tables then there should not be any adverse reaction; unless the user has an inherent in-tolerance or allergic response to these. Also, make sure that you follow the dosage requirement if you are taking a supplementary product and always if in doubt consult with your health care and, or, your general medical practitioner. Do not mix supplements with prescribed medicines.

Why do we need vitamins?

As organic entities, we are made of trillions of cells, and in each of these cells numerous biochemical reactions are being processed continuously which are life-sustaining and are important for our life and well-being. Vitamins form co-enzymes and co-factors with many enzymatic systems for the maintenance and continuity of these processes, and therefore an adequate supply of these vitamins is essential. The unavailability of vitamins could disrupt the effectivity of such life-sustaining processes which can manifest as one or several diseases resulting in a weaker body.

What are these life-giving processes you may ask; these are the conversion of food into energy, growth and repair of tissues, helping to resist diseases, building and maintenance of cellular structures, etc., and many more metabolic reactions essential to basic life processes.

Our fundamental biochemical processes start in our cellular system. For the cells to perform their functions, the body needs to be in homeostasis. Which means the cellular environment must be fairly uniform or constant. The word homeostasis is a combination of two Greek words 'homeo' meaning the same and 'stasis' literally meaning standing. Combining the word has the meaning of staying the same or constant.

Human beings represent the most complex cellular organisation compared to all living beings and therefore we experience complexity of life processes which somehow, are inter-related to each other. To categorise life processes simply we need to identify the series of actions or activities which determines if we are alive or dead. Simple! Not quite. The following are the basic life processes that we need to look at:

We start with **Homeostasis** meaning the environment in which our cells can live and survive.

Energy production and utilisation; every life form must have energy to live on. Nutrients from our food get converted by our cells into energy to perform various activities for our survival.

Respiration and expiration; we need to breathe in air/oxygen for our cells tissues and organs to stay alive. We also need to exhale to breathe out the toxic air/carbon dioxide as a by-product of our breathing in.

All living beings must be capable of **re-producing** for the continuity of the species.

Movements: All living beings must be capable of moving around and being active. This allows us to experience a flight or fight response. This is a basic instinct which all living animals including us experience.

Senses: Humans have 5 sensory organs which lets us see, hear, smell, taste and touch the objects around us and therefore be aware of our surroundings.

There are a couple more basic life processes that we can characterise; e.g. **Digestion** and **Elimination**.

All of the life processes as defined above and more are benefited by vitamins.

How much vitamins do we need?

The RDA's (recommended Dietary Allowance), RDI's (recommended Dietary Intakes), and other regulatory parameters set by various governing bodies (such as Food and Drug Administration in the USA, Therapeutic Administration Australia, Medicines and Healthcare Products Regulatory Agency in UK, etc.) are reference starting point. Then build on it depending on individual circumstances. Questions then to ask of ourselves; are we getting enough nutrition from the foods we intake, are we healthy enough to qualify for the definitions of Reference Man and Woman. This is elaborated below when we embark on a discussion on the great vitamin controversy.

Also, we need to be mindful of any underlying disease condition that we may be suffering from. There are several options such as the ODI (Optimal Daily Intake), TUL (Tolerable Upper Limit) requirements also the daily values (DV) for consideration and it may be a good idea to sort out or tailor make your requirement on the advice of a health care professional. Remember vitamin intake does not accumulate in the body specially the B-group and vitamin C due to their high clearance rate from the body. Fat-soluble vitamins are not soluble in water and stay longer in the body and gets stored in the fatty tissues.

But these too over time degrade and become rancid and ineffective. Before we look at the RDA, RD, ODI and the UL values let us define these in simple terms what they are.

The RDA is the bare minimum amount of nutrients which is required to keep the population healthy. RDAs are developed generally for the American population but is also safe to be followed internationally.

The RDI's are similar data specially tabulated for the Australian population and are pretty much at par with the RDA data.

The UL (Tolerable upper limit sometimes referred to as TUL) is the maximum amount of vitamins and mineral supplements which can be taken on a daily basis without overdosing or serious side effects.

The concept of ODI is explained a bit later in the chapter.

Are we meeting our daily vitamin and mineral intake requirements?

In countries where the majority of the population is sufficiently well-off and well-nourished, it is anticipated that the intake requirements will also be adequate. But surprisingly enough in many western developed countries and Australia nutritional survey often reveals widespread deficiencies. These deficiencies may be marginal and may not be as pronounced as in much of the poorer nations where mal-nourishment is not un-common.

This is also true in countries where there is a wide gap in the socio-economic structure and purchasing supplements are way down the shopping priority list. In a recent survey carried out in 2017 in Australia by the peak research scientific organisation CSIRO, found that four out of five Australian adults were not eating enough fruit and vegetables in order to meet Australian Dietary Guidelines.

In a recent publication, it was reported that nearly 10% of Americans have a nutritional deficiency (Ref: Most common nutritional deficiencies—USA

Today https://www.usatoday.com › news › health › 2019/08/20) Although the calorie intake is more than adequate it is the mix of primary food source that is questionable; perhaps containing high portion of meats and alcohol with high carbohydrate intake in the form of sweet and after dinner desserts. Very often marginal or nutritional gaps go un-noticed and unrecognised until these subtle deficiencies manifest themselves into clinical and morphological changes resulting sometimes in nonspecific symptoms requiring medical intervention.

A marginal supply of nutrients for instance lack of vitamin C could cause wounds not to heal properly, or a skin infection due to lack of B-vitamins could enhance into an un-manageable legion which may in due time show up into something more serious and debilitating for the patient. It is therefore very important to understand marginal deficiencies which may require an early re-enforcement of nutrients to alter the nutritional balance and profile.

How to recognise the important signs of vitamin deficiency?
The most common signs to recognise are:

Brittle nails and split hair-ends; also, development of some preliminary signs of rough patches on your skin. There could be dandruffs appearing with signs of hair falling more than normal.

Additional signs of B-group vitamin deficiencies are:

Mouth ulcers, chaffed lips and signs of cracking at the corner of your mouth.

Pimple formation, sore tongue as result of vitamin B12 deficiency. Bleeding gums which become very sensitive at the time of brushing your teeth; vitamin C deficiency.

Dry eyes, and eyes turning red and also blurry vision at night are common sign of Vitamin A deficiency.

Un-usual skin legions appearing on your body could be a cause of vitamin B12 deficiency and, or, a general sign of B-complex deficiency.

Vitamin D deficiency can show up as weak and unsteady knees, joint aches and pain.

Capillary fragility can be a cause of low vitamin C in our system. Capillary fragility can be noticed by reddish coloration in the face area.

Vitamin E deficiency can manifest as muscle pain and loss of balance.

Bleeding and unusual clotting could be a sign of vitamin K deficiency. The symptoms exhibited above can also be due to several other reasons, for example, problem with balance can be due to middle ear infection. It is also considered that the examples cited are generalised symptoms of vitamin deficiencies, however, there can be several specific clinical reasons which must be investigated professionally.

Some of the more common vitamin deficiencies are summarised below. But bear in mind that the symptoms and deficiency signs are not due to a single vitamin deficiency but could be a multi-B vitamin deficiency. Several B group vitamins exhibit a similar deficiency profile. All the 8 B-group vitamins physiologically work in unison; however, the level of deficiency may dictate the physiological deficiency status. The level of deficiency varies greatly from person to person depending on age, dietary and supplementary intakes, level of physical activity and also metabolism which could have some bearing on the availability of the individual B-vitamin from foods and supplements taken.

Vitamins and Signs of Deficiencies

Vitamins	Signs of deficiencies (early signs)
Thiamine (Vitamin B1)	Tiredness and Fatigue, loss of appetite, Nervousness
Riboflavin (Vitamin B2)	Mild skin disorders, mouth ulceration, hair loss
Niacin (Vitamin B3)	Diarrhoea, vomiting and headache. Sometimes associated with constipation.
Pantothenic Acid (Vitamin B5)	Burning sensation in hands and feet, restlessness and lack of sleep.
Pyridoxine (Vitamin B6)	Confusion, depression. Weak immune system
Biotin (Vitamin B7)	Deficiencies in hair, skin and nail health, depression and fatigue.
Folic Acid (Vitamin B9)	Weakness, periodic headaches, heart palpitation, etc.
Cobalamin (Vitamin B12)	Tingling sensation in hands and feet, memory loss and depression. Anaemia.
Ascorbic Acid (Vitamin C)	Bruising easily, takes longer for wounds to heal, bleeding gums and fragile blood vessels. Iron deficient anaemia, loss of immunity.
Retinol (Vitamin A)	Dry eyes, night blindness, growth problems in children.

Calciferol (Vitamin D)	Deformity in bone structure and formation, fatigue and tiredness. Bone joints and muscle pains.
Tocopherol (Vitamin E)	Impaired lipid anti-oxidation, heart and brain health, hormonal imbalance. More serious deficiencies may cause pain in the nerve endings and other neurological conditions.
Phylloquinone (Vitamin K)	Bleeding and haemorrhaging, bone weakness, etc. In women, heavier periods causing heavy bleeding and pain.

The Great Vitamin Controversy

The National Health and Medical Research Council (NH&MRC) a peak body in Australia provides nutritional guidelines and recommendations and is involved in funding for research work into various aspects of health and nutrition and medical research. Formed in 1926 as a government agency it became an independent statutory body in 1992 and enacted as (NH&MRC Act) on 1 July 2000 within the portfolio of the Australian Government Minister for Health and Ageing.

This paved the way for setting up the Recommended Daily Intake (RDI) amounts which were based on so-called allowances for healthy **Reference Man** and **Reference Woman**. These targets were probably set around the early part of 1988 with the expectation that these will be the guidelines for manufacturers and practitioners to follow.

Definition of reference man and woman is very interesting as you will notice. The **reference man** is defined as a 25-year-old healthy individual who is free of diseases and is normally healthy. He weighs around 70 kg eats a well-balanced diet and neither gains nor loses weight. He has an ideal living condition performing 8 hours of physical work on working days and engages in active sports not of an extremely strenuous nature on each non-working day. The **reference woman** is similarly healthy, aged about 25 years and weighs 58 kg. Her lifestyle is very similar to that of the reference man and engages in general household duties and light industrial work.

What a definition; and if I recall correctly around the early part of 1988 when I had read this in one of the publications from NH&MRC it dawned on me that the objective of the RDI's is not to make unhealthy people healthy but to keep normal healthy people in the state of continued good health.

So, what about the population at large who do not fit in the category of reference man and woman; their nutritional requirement does not seem to be addressed adequately.

On the other hand, if we apply the concept of **Optimal Daily Intake** (ODI) which has been developed with the view to promote good health in individuals who do not meet the required levels of intake from their diets and those who are normally un-healthy seems to be worthy of consideration.

So, what is ODI?

Optimum Daily Intake (ODI) is a modified dietary guideline that is suggested to meet optimal nutrition, instead of the bare minimum to prevent ailments.

(Ref: Lieberman; Bruning (2007), The Real Vitamins and Minerals Book (4 ed.), Penguin Group).

The concept of the ODI has been long in discussion but seldom applied in the dietary guideline considerations (Ref: 'The Vitamin C Content of Apples', Ulster Med J, 1938; and, The Vitamin C requirement in man, estimated after prolonged studies of the plasma concentration and daily excretion of Vitamin C in 3 adults on controlled diets J Clin Invest., 1939). The table of ODI as presented gives a more meaningful interpretation of the daily requirements.

Table of ODI

(Piatkus (1999), Institute for Optimum Nutrition, ION archives)

(https://en.wikiversity.org/wiki/Optimum_Daily_Intake)

"Optimum nutrition is the medicine of tomorrow."
– Professor Linus Pauling

Vitamins	ODI
Vitamin A	7500i.u
Thiamine (Vitamin B1)	75mg
Riboflavin (Vitamin B2)	75mg
Niacin (Vitamin B3)	100mg
Pantothenic Acid (Vitamin B5)	75mg
Pyridoxine (Vitamin B6)	100mg
Cobalamin (Vitamin B12)	10mg

Folic Acid (Vitamin B9)	100mg
Biotin (Vitamin B7)	50mg
Ascorbic Acid (Vitamin C)	1000mg
Cholecalciferol (Vitamin D)	400i.u
Tocopherol (Vitamin E)	500i.u

In a recently updated version of 'Nutrient Reference Values for Australia and New Zealand Executive Summary 2006 Version 1.2 Updated September 2017' published by NH&MRC; I am really encouraged that considerable thought has been put into the report. There have been some definitions adapted which probably gives a wider choice for requirements and hence administration.

I was also pleased that there was no mention to reference man and woman.

Estimated Average Requirement (EAR)

A daily nutrient level is estimated to meet the requirements of half the healthy individuals in a particular life stage and gender group.

Recommended Dietary Intake (RDI)

The average daily dietary intake level that is sufficient to meet the nutrient requirements of nearly all (97–98 percent) healthy individuals in a particular life stage and gender group.

Adequate Intake (AI)

(Used when an RDI cannot be determined)

AI The average daily nutrient intake level based on observed or experimentally determined approximations or estimates of nutrient intake by a group (or groups) of apparently healthy people that are assumed to be adequate.

Upper Level of Intake (UL)

The highest average daily nutrient intake level is likely to pose no adverse health effects to almost all individuals in the general population. As intake increases above the UL, the potential risk of adverse effects increases.

Of the above categories, the upper level of intake (UL) interests me most.

A table (Ref: Tolerable Upper Intake Levels (UL) for Vitamins; National Institute of Health (NIH.gov) https://www.ncbi.nlm.nih.gov › NBK278991 › table › di...) may be a good reading for those who are interested in this matter.

Vitamins and Nobel Prizes

In order to add some variety and interest in the discovery of vitamins, I searched relevant areas of several literature and came up with some interesting facts as represented in the table far down below. To my surprise and joy the number of Nobel Laureates in the field of vitamins during the last century (1901–2001), have been quite significant since the awarding of Nobel Prize started in 1901 for outstanding research and scientific discoveries and for the literary and outstanding humanitarian works.

It was the vision of Alfred Nobel who left his large fortune to be awarded as prizes for outstanding research in several disciplines of subjects of human interest and enhancement of knowledge and co-operation. It is a very interesting read and those who are interested may find reading matter of interest by logging on to the following website: https://www.nobelprize.org/prizes/facts/nobel-prize-facts Alfred Nobel's life and work—NobelPrize.org www.nobelprize.org › Alfred Nobel.

The first ever Noble Prize recipient in physiology was **Emil Adolf von Behring** for his work in researching serum therapy (in 1901). He successfully discovered **Diphtheria** antitoxin thus helping to save thousands of children from death. For this, he was widely known as a 'saviour of children'.

Diphtheria, according to the Australian Department of Health website is a contagious disease, spread by an infected person's coughing, sneezing or infection through open wounds. Symptoms include a sore throat and breathing problems. It is a bacterial infection affecting the mucous membranes of our nose and throat. Diphtheria can affect people of all ages but can be prevented with vaccination. Treatment includes antibiotics and diphtheria anti-toxin.

There are many researchers who worked tirelessly in the field of biochemistry, chemistry and physiology and gave credibility to what we today know as vitamins.

Casimir Funk was an extraordinarily gifted biochemist and his name has been associated with many B-group vitamins as we know it now.

Let's look at the **vitamin B3** which is also known as Niacin, Niacinamide (and also Nicotinamide). Vitamin B3 has been strongly linked with the disease state Pellagra since the early 1900s when it became a significant health problem in America. Casimir Funk in 1912 while experimenting with brown rice hulls during his experiments to isolate Vitamin B1, also extracted Vitamin B3 and associated its curative properties with Pellagra. It was however the American biochemist **Conrad Arnold Elvehjem,** who subsequently worked out the structure of Vitamin B3 in 1937.

Vitamin B5 (Pantothenic Acid) was discovered by **Dr Roger J. Williams** during 1931–1933 while experimenting with 'Yeast growth stimulation' experiments. He was able to isolate pantothenic acid which he named after.

Greek word 'Pentos' meaning from everywhere. Pantothenic Acid and its derivatives e.g., Calcium Pantothenate (Vitamin B5) are essential vitamins required for humans and most living entities; it is also available from both plant and animal sources. One of the most important bio-function of vitamin B5 is the bio-synthesis of Coenzyme A which is essential to many biochemical reactions that sustain life.

Vitamin B6 also known as Pyridoxine was discovered by **Gyorgy** in 1934, however, its activity was unknown until Samuel Lepovsky in 1938 studied it at the Berkeley campus, University of California. The structure of vitamin B6 (Pyridoxine) was finally determined by **Folkers and Harris** in 1939. This work was done in the laboratories of Merck. Simultaneously to the work of Folkers and Harris, Kuhn in Germany was also successful in determining vitamin B6 structure.

Richard Kuhn received Nobel Prize in Chemistry in 1938 for his work on 'Carotenoids and Vitamin B6'. He was a well-known Austrian-born biochemist and died in Germany in 1967.

Biotin is often referred to as vitamin B7. It was isolated from egg yolk in 1932 by Koegl and his student Toennis and also named the isolated substance biotin. In 1936, **Dean Burke** an American biochemist also isolated biotin from egg yolk. The structure and properties of biotin were established by US and the European investigators between 1940 and 1943. The first chemical synthesis was completed by Harris and his associates at Merck Company in 1943.

Discovery of **Folic Acid** (also known as vitamin B9) and its role in human biochemical function can be largely attributed to the works of researcher **Lucy Wills** who first identified it in 1931. She found that this vitamin was needed to prevent anaemia during pregnancy. She also demonstrated that anaemia could be reversed by administering brewer's yeast. Dr Lucy was an English Haematologist who had conducted her research on pregnant women of Mumbai textile workers (Then Bombay, India) after receiving a grant from Tata Trust in 1928. Her work greatly helped in the prevention of birth defects in babies. Folic Acid was finally synthesised by Bob Stokstad in 1943 in the research laboratories of Lederle, American Cyanamid Company in Pearl River New York. Angier and his co-workers subsequently were also successful in Synthesising Folic Acid in 1945.

Folic acid received its name in 1941 when it was isolated from spinach leaves; Latin for leaf (folium).

Medical Science has now ascertained that Folic acid helps not just the mother during pregnancy but also the physiological development of the child. Millions of pregnant mothers taking Folic Acid supplements for a healthy pregnancy thank Dr Lucy Wills for this wonderful gift for which her name will live on. She died in 1964 in England.

The role of **Cobalamin** (vitamin B12) and Pernicious Anaemia has been the subject of many years of research work by several individual researchers and research institutions alike which became the subject of two separate Nobel Prize-winning works.

In the early 1900s, Pernicious Anaemia was the cause of debilitating blood disorder which killed a significant number of people.

Pernicious Anaemia is an extreme form of blood disorder caused by vitamin B12 deficiency. James Combe, a Scottish physician as early as 1822, recognised the symptoms and administered his patient's liver to combat the disease which he was quite successful at.

Although many reasons were put forward in the early stages of Vitamin B12 discovery time line, it was **George Richards Minot** and **William P. Murphy** who shared the Nobel Prize of 1934 with **George H. Whipple** for their work with Pernicious Anaemia. Dr Whipple was a pathologist at the University of Rochester USA and planned meticulously his experiments feeding dogs with pernicious anaemia liver and reversed the disease. Dr Minot and his co-worker Dr Murphy conducted their work in collaboration with Dr Whipple at Harvard University Medical School. These researchers suggested that Pernicious Anaemia was due to dietary inadequacies.

Vitamin B12 is an important factor in the revitalisation of red blood cells. Let us not however forget contributions made by William Bosworth Castle who in 1927, working directly under George Minot in Boston City Hospital (run by Harvard Medical School) paved the way for further research leading to the awarding of Nobel Prize in 1934 to Minot and Murphy.

I felt compelled to include an immortal quote by William Bosworth Castle which I feel be-fitting in this context.

"Let us never forget that Nature is the most original of all experimenters and that it is the patient's physician who is privileged to learn most directly from her sometimes cruel, but never meaningless, clinical presentations." The second Nobel Prize in this subject was awarded to the English chemist and crystallographer

Dorothy Mary Hodgkin for her work on the molecular structure of vitamin B12 which was essential to the understanding and control of pernicious anaemia.

Dr Dorothy Hodgkin was born in Cairo in 1910, Egypt and passed away in 1994 in England. She had a very distinguishing career in the scientific world and will also be remembered for her other major works such as involvement in the crystalline structures of Calciferol (vitamin D) and haemoglobin. There is another recipient completing the vitamin B12 puzzle, **Robert Burns Woodward** received the Nobel Prize in synthetic chemistry in 1965 for the synthesis of vitamin B12.

Professor Woodward was an outstanding Organic and Synthetic Chemist who is not only accredited for the complex synthesis of Vitamin B12 but also analysis and synthesis of many complex molecules, such as cholesterol, cortisone, lysergic acid (LSD), strychnine, reserpine, chlorophyll and many more and aptly hailed as one of the most disciplined minded synthetic chemists of our times.

The discovery of other vitamins is just as interesting as the B-group vitamins and again to my amazement and dismay the achievements and contributions made by a large fraternity of the scientific community are really something to behold; we are truly in awe of them.

There have been many distinguished scientists and researchers who have been recognised for their ground-breaking research works with Nobel Prize awards and many who missed out due to controversies beyond my comprehension yet nonetheless their works have enriched our life and health for which we all are indebted. The table below lists all the great scientists and researchers who have worked tirelessly for their discoveries into vitamins without which many diseases would have been rampant.

I counted 15 names as per the list below; greater than any other category since the beginning of history of awarding the Nobel Prizes in 1901. It is also important to note that a few of these names also appear elsewhere for their works and contributions to several other vitamin research. Also, some may have been awarded the Nobel Prize for their work in other field of science which somehow are linked with vitamins. For example, Dorothy Crowfoot Hodgkin won the prize in 1965 for her work on determining the crystal's structure by X-ray techniques of many complex molecules such as penicillin in 1946 and also the structure of vitamin B12 some years after, which has the most complex structure of all the other vitamins.

Let me again indulge in a bit of trivia on vitamin discoveries. There have been Nobel Prize winners (Nobel Laureates) who were awarded this coveted prize not just for one research area, but in multiple areas of vitamin discoveries.

For example, in 1937 **Paul Karrer** won the prize for synthesising vitamin E and also in the same year for establishing the chemical structure for vitamins A and B. While in the following year, Richard Kuhn had the distinction of isolating Vitamins B2 and B6 and also working out the chemical structure of vitamin B2.

From my list of Nobel Laureates who have worked on vitamins, I see that almost all the currently known vitamins have been mentioned with notable exceptions of Folic Acid (vitamin B9), Niacin (vitamin B3), Pantothenic Acid (vitamin B5) and Biotin (vitamin B7). Discoveries, extraction and isolation of each of those vitamins are quite complex and deserve credit. However, the glaring omission from the Nobel Prize list in my opinion is Folic Acid. Lucy Wills had tirelessly worked on pernicious anaemia in the 1920s and came up with the discovery that there was another 'nutritional factor' which is responsible for the curative effect of the disease. So, it wasn't just vitamin B12. This nutritional factor was then known as the 'Wills Factor' which was later around 1941 was known as the folate or the folic acid.

Nobel Laureates and their Work with Vitamins

Christiaan Eijkman	**1929**	Vitamin B1	For his discovery of the antineuritic vitamin.
Sir Frederick Gowland Hopkins	**1929**	Growth Stimulating vitamins	Discovery of essential nutrient factors—now known as vitamins.
George Hoyt Whipple*	**1934**	Vitamin B12	Discoveries concerning liver therapy in cases of anaemia.
George Richards Minot	**1934**	Vitamin B12	**(shared *)**
William Parry Murphy	**1934**	Vitamin B12	**(shared *)**
Henrik Carl Peter Dam	**1943**	Vitamin K	Discovery of Vitamin K
Adolf Otto Reinhold Windaus	**1928**	Vitamin D isolation	For the services rendered through his research into the constitution of the sterols and their connection with the vitamins.

Albert von Szent-Gyorgyi	1937	Vitamin C	For his discoveries in connection with the biological combustion processes, with special reference to vitamin C and the catalysis of fumaric acid.
Richard Kuhn	1938	Vitamin B2 and B6 and B12	For his work on carotenoids and vitamins.
Edward Adelbert Doisy	1943	Vitamin K	For his discovery of the chemical nature of vitamin K
Walter Norman Haworth (1937)	1937	Vitamin C	For his investigations on carbohydrates and vitamin C.
Paul Karrer	1937	Vitamin E and A	For his investigations on carotenoids, flavins and vitamins A and B2
Robert Burns Woodward	1965	Vitamin B12 (in 1972)	For his outstanding achievements in the art of organic synthesis
Lord (Alexander R.) Todd (1957)	1957	Vitamin B12	For his work on nucleotides and nucleotide co-enzymes.
Dorothy Crowfoot Hodgkin	1965	Vitamin B12	For her determinations by X-ray techniques of the structures of important biochemical substances

Vitamin Deficiency Is Not Rare

Many people think that they are getting plenty of vitamins from their food intake, however, it is not surprising to know that a large percentage of us could be suffering from marginal vitamin deficiency. A couple of subject matters of interest that I thought needed to be covered before going into individual vitamins and their deficiency status.

We all need a well-balanced diet but let's be honest and practical, and face the facts that it is impossible to regulate our food habits. And why should we; it is one of the last pleasures in life under our control.

Experts often comment that eating good wholesome food with a good balance and mix of all five categories of foods should be adequate in providing us with the necessary vitamins and other nutrients that our body needs on a daily basis. Yes, I say that too. But I also say that we do need some form of supplementation to fill in the gap for the lack of nutrients that our idealistic mix of foodstuff may provide. In my mind, the controversy is in the question; how much do we need and are we getting enough from our diets?

This and more will be revealed as we read further on in this chapter.

Our body's nutrient needs vary from individual to individual which largely depends on our metabolic abilities and due to our biochemical individuality. Women have different needs from men and so do senior citizens. A young active adult or children again have a different set of requirements.

It is not denying that a good mix of dietary food intake will provide adequate nutrition but will it be adequate to top up our nutritional reserves?

Vitamins in particular and other nutrients, e.g., amino acids are thermolabile or heat sensitive and are also affected by the environmental conditions such as moisture and oxidative degradation, it is therefore important to remember that food preparations and cooking can have a significant loss of these nutrients from foodstuffs we eat.

Freshly harvested raw produce may need further processing due to possible bacterial and fungal contamination which does more harm than good. So, food preparation before consumption is essential.

A review of the preparative methods and the cooking procedures to get the most nutritive value from our foods is important.

Freshly harvested vegetables straight from the paddock to the table offer significant benefits but I wonder how many of us are willing to forgo the intense cooking methods which introduces the delicacy factor thus compromising the choice between cooked and freshly procured raw foods fresh from farm to table. Also, consider the contamination factors, e.g., pesticides and herbicides, residual fertilisers, etc. Some people believe that consuming raw fruits or vegetables can be detrimental to health because many raw products contain a number of organisms which are harmful and potentially can cause serious illnesses or even death in some cases.

This is more common and applicable to regions where hygiene and storage conditions are not maintained properly. Also, during fruiting time, there could be fruit flies and other air-borne insects carrying diseases burrow into host fruit and vegetables and cause widespread infestation. Unsuspectingly, when this infected produce is eaten raw the parasitic organisms can enter into unsuspecting human hosts with a serious consequence.

Cooking not only deactivates harmful organisms but also helps improve the digestion and absorption processes. Classic examples are that in certain global regions if the drinking water is not boiled or purified prior to use then gastric infection, diarrhoea, dysentery and stomach cramps and pains may occur leading to serious complications and even death. Another example is that of raw eggs which could contain harmful organisms if they weren't cooked. An effective way of destroying harmful bacteria in raw eggs is applying heat, this way the egg protein is a lot more digestible when cooked.

As mentioned, cooking prepares food well suited for your digestion and compatible with your digestive system. Often food left uncooked or un-heated prior to consumption lends itself to bacterial contamination as discussed in a previous chapter. CDC; the Centre for Disease Control and Prevention has listed 10 hazardous food safety measures consumers should pay attention to. Sometimes due to people's belief and, or, interest in consuming raw fruit and vegetables and often animal products (e.g., unpasteurised milk, raw eggs and fish, etc., and some crustaceans) the advice given by CDC is in many cases being ignored. The likelihood of raw or un-cooked food contaminated with *Salmonella* can get into our food system and cause food poisoning with serious consequences. Also, *Botulism* toxicity as a result of contamination in raw food particularly of animal source can lead to paralysis and even death.

Ref: (https://www.cdc.gov/foodsafety/ten-dangerous-mistakes.html).

Depending on the method of cooking, there will always be a degree of loss in nutritional content. Particularly the water-soluble vitamins are thermolabile and leach out in significant quantities when water is used as the cooking medium.

Fat-soluble vitamins are also at risk of losing their potency when heat is applied such as baking and Barbecuing. Minerals in fruit and vegetables are mainly in the form of simple compounds and many are water-soluble such as calcium, magnesium, potassium, sodium, zinc, etc. As we read on further, it will become obvious that loss of nutrients is not uncommon and that storage of raw produce which were at some stage deemed as fresh lose their nutritional potency to some extent which exacerbates upon cooking or other means of heat application.

Therefore, I believe in just that extra bit of nutritional support from supplement intake will put us over the line towards a healthy being. It is from this consideration alone, let us consider the Recommended Daily Intake (RDI) as set by the **National Health and Medical Research council** (NH&MRC of Australia) and the great vitamin controversy that has been debating since the early settings of the RDI's in Australia and RDAs in America. It is the minimum target intake levels of vitamins and other nutrients that we should take to stay healthy. Now let us look at, and, question the basis upon which the NH and MRC's guidelines are set and who sets them.

As I understand the recommendations are set by the board members of the NH&MRC who also set these targets, whether there is a community consultation or some discussions with the **Complementary Medicine Association** (CMA) of Australia regarding these targets, I do not know. Perhaps, these targets were set many years ago and in light of present-day interest in the vitamins and nutritional supplements worldwide there should be some review from the appropriate authority for amendments and rectification.

It is important to review one's inherent vitamin status by evaluating dietary intake which lets us assume, is ideal; by which I mean adequate intake of fresh fruits and vegetables and proportional quantities of the other 5 food categories which are required for proper nutrition. Would we still meet the requirement; it is a question which does not have a very straightforward answer. Let me look at the issues which may influence the nutritional uptake from the dietary intake. Sounds mouthful but needs certain assurances from our dietary practices.

Let us consider the food procurement followed by the food preparative steps.

1. Organising the daily food ingredients we are about to prepare into a consumable portion.
2. Preparative work; meaning washing, cutting, trimming blanching followed by cooking which requires heat application and perhaps storage for a period of time.

Each of the steps can lead to significant losses in nutritional values. Additionally, consider the point that storage of fruits and vegetables in raw state before distribution through retail outlets can also have losses in nutritional content. Many staple produces such as potatoes, carrots several root vegetables and fruits apples, oranges, bananas and many more are held in storages for future distribution. These storages can easily be from 3 months–12 months duration before a consumer may procure them for consumption.

We will soon notice the effect of nutritional depletion as a result of storage of raw produce. Looking at some of the published information I found many interesting references on this subject matter; only a few relevant references are cited below to prove the point that nutrition depletion is inevitable from raw produces such as fruits and vegetables on storage followed by further losses in step wise progression of food preparation leading to consumption. The first example that we can look at is potatoes which is the most common vegetable consumed throughout the world.

The table below indicates the losses in vitamin C resulting from steaming and boiling processes. Other cooking procedures where higher temperatures are applied such as backing, bequing will all end up in higher losses.

Vegetables	Vitamin C content (mg/100g) in fresh produce	Vitamin C lost (%)	
		Steamed	Boiled
Potatoes	21	7	27
Celery root	5	25	51
Spinach	34	18	66
Brussel Sprouts	99	9	26
Cauliflower	74	7	35
Kohlrabi	44	26	46

Ref: Vitamin C Deficiency-Part 4: Chem Views Magazine…
https://www.chemistryviews.org › details › ezine › Vita…

In another study (The *International Journal of Scientific and Technology Research*), the effect of heat on different vegetables and the percentage of vitamin C lost at 5, 15 and 30 minutes was studied; results are presented in the table below; a constant heat of 60 degree Celsius was applied which is a fairly mild cooking temperature.

Vegetables	% loss in 5 minutes.	% loss in 15 minutes.	% loss in 30 minutes.
Pepper	11.76	35.26	64.71
Green Peas	10.59	33.33	58.28
Spinach	9.94	29.94	60
Pumpkins	12.43	37.43	62.43
Carrots	16.57	33.33	49.91

Ref: Degradation of vitamins, probiotics and other active… https://www.nutraceuticalbusinessreview.com › article page.

Dr John Marks in his book 'A Guide to the Vitamins, Their Role in Health and Disease' has also mentioned that most vegetables when stored at room temperature loose a significant portion of their nutritional content.

Green vegetables have an even greater percentage of losses.

The data presented below on the effect of vitamin C stability on the length of storage of potatoes has been taken from his above-mentioned book.

Main Crop of Potatoes	Vitamin C content mg/100g
Freshly dug	30
1–3 months storage	20
4–5 months storage	15
6–7 months storage	10
8–9 months	8

Let me now explore other avenues of cooking and storage, e.g., freezing, drying, cooking and reheating prior to consuming our food.

It will be evident from the data generated and presented that almost all processes have a negative effect on the stability of the nutrient content of the food. The harsher the process the lesser is the stability. Heat, humidity or moisture effect, light, Oxidation on prolonged exposure all have detrimental effects on the nutritional content of our foods. We have not even considered another critical aspect of food preparation and that is the washout or leaching out effect of the water-soluble nutrient. For example, peeling, cutting and washing of the raw vegetables and fruits.

Boiling of cut vegetables render themselves for a transition of the highly water-soluble vitamins B-group and vitamin C into the fluid medium due to increased exposed surface and water inter-phasing. If there is a way that this fluid body left over from the boiling process can be utilised in the cooking, then a certain amount of water-soluble vitamins and some minerals can be recovered in the diet.

The table presents a typical value of nutrient losses as compared to the raw foods. Another table is presented which reflects the losses in minerals upon cooking, however, the losses are not as significant as that of vitamins. As evident from the second table, the losses in minerals are mostly encountered from cooking and also draining of the fluid from cooking, e.g., in the boiling process, etc. Heat processing does not have any significant effect and nor does freezing. Since the cooking and draining are enriched with nutrients both vitamins and minerals, many nutritionists believe that reusing the drained fluid in our dietary variety such as in soups will provide us with a lot of additional nutritional goodness.

So, the bottom line is whatever way you cook your food or whatever may be your preference, cooked or raw please understand the benefits and drawbacks. Do not set your mind in one direction; variety is the spice of life and enjoy a healthy meal.

Table: Maximum Vitamin Losses (as compared to raw foods)

Vitamins	Freezing	Dry processing	Cooking	Cooking and draining	Reheating
Vitamin A	5%	50%	25%	35%	10%
Vitamin C	30%	80%	50%	75%	50%
Thiamine (B1)	5%	30%	55%	70%	40%
Riboflavin (B2)	0%	10%	25%	45%	5%
Niacin (B3)	0%	10%	40%	55%	5%
Pyridoxine (B6)	0%	10%	50%	65%	45%
Folic Acid (B9)	5%	59%	70%	75%	30%
Cobalamin (B12)	0%	0%	45%	50%	45%
Beta-Carotene (Pro-vitamin A)	5%	50%	25%	35%	10%

(Ref: A Glance at Nutrition. By Mostafa Waly and Vickie A. Vaclavik December 2019)

Unlike vitamins, which are more prone to the application of heat during cooking, minerals are more stable nutritional component of foods. The next table offers some published data to confirm mineral stability. Most mineral losses occur during prepping of foods where minerals leach out in the water applied; e.g., washing blanching, etc. To minimise the loss, it is best to wash vegetables whole or uncut.

Table: Maximum Mineral Losses

Minerals	Freezing	Dry-process	Cooking	Cooking and draining	Reheating
Calcium	5%	0	20	25	0
Iron	0	0	35	40	0
Magnesium	0	0	25	40	0
Phosphorus	0	0	25	35	0
Potassium	10%	0	30	70	0
Sodium	0	0	25	55	0
Zinc	0	0	25	25	0
Copper	10%	0	40	45	0

(Ref: A Glance at Nutrition

By Mostafa Waly and Vickie A. Vaclavik December 2019)

In a publication in J Nutr Sci Vitaminol (Tokyo) 1990; 36 Suppl 1:S25–32; discussion S33, the authors Kimura and Itokawa reported their study results and suggested that there is a significant loss of minerals in foods from cooking. The study included analysing losses of minerals (sodium, potassium, phosphorous, calcium, magnesium, iron, zinc, and manganese, copper). The authors reported following:

1. When compared with raw or un-cooked food the mineral content of cooked food was about 60–70% low.
2. The losses in mineral content from vegetables were significantly high.
3. Cooking methods had a lot to do with the percentage losses; e.g., mineral losses were much higher in cut and prepared vegetables after boiling and soaking in water followed by the process of frying stewing, etc.
4. The lower the application of heat in the cooking process and less use of water during preparation stages were considered to help with the preservation of the nutrient content.

My extensive search on the correlation between nutrient losses and cooking methods lead to some important findings. There is no denying that preparing any produce be it of vegetation origin (fruits, vegetables, etc.) or animal origin (meats, eggs, fish, etc.) for cooking will lead to nutrient losses, only the degree of loss is dependent on preparation steps and cooking procedure.

Some Preliminary Effects of Cooking on Vitamin Stability

Vitamins	Effect of Water	Effect of Heat (potency loss)	Additional Information
Thiamine (Vitamin B1)	Leaches out	Yes over 100°C	Water-soluble and heat sensitive
Riboflavin (Vitamin B2)	Slightly less leaches out	Yes over 100°C For longer time	Water-soluble but less heat sensitive
Niacin (Vitamin B3)	Leaches out	Yes over 100°C	Water soluble, losses if cooked for longer time
Pantothenic Acid (Vitamin B5)	Leaches out	Yes over 100°C For longer time	Water soluble, losses if cooked for longer time
Pyridoxine (Vitamin B6)	Leaches out	Yes over 100°C	Water-soluble and heat sensitive
Folic Acid (Vitamin B9)	Leaches out	Yes over 100°C For longer time	Water soluble, losses if cooked for longer time
Cobalamin (Vitamin B12)	Leaches out	Yes over 100°C	Water-soluble but lesser heat sensitive
Biotin (Vitamin B)	Leaches out	Yes over 100°C	Water-soluble and heat sensitive
Ascorbic Acid Vitamin C	Highly Soluble	Yes, less than 100°C	Water-soluble and heat sensitive
Retinol (Vitamin A)	In-soluble	Less sensitive	Slight losses
Calciferol (Vitamin D)	Very slight Solubility	Yes, but less sensitive	Slight losses
Tocopherol (Vitamin E)	In-soluble	Yes, may cause Food rancidity	Strong anti-oxidant Losses with rancidity
Phylloquinone (Vitamin K)	In-soluble	It is heat stable at 100°C for short cooking duration	Sensitive to cooking medium ph. and is light sensitive

An interesting question many nutritionists have faced at some time or other is how to reduce nutrient loss during cooking. By nutrients, we are primarily targeting vitamins, as minerals and other macro-nutrient such as proteins, amino acids essential fatty acids and others such as herbs, etc., are more or less stable in the range of temperature applied for cooking; only be careful when preparing the produce for cooking.

It is important to understand what the common factors which affect vitamin stability are, e.g., heat, water, light and air. All can have de-stabilising effect to some degree.

1. In many vegetables and fruits, the outer layer, i.e., the skin has the concentration of nutrients, so, prepare your cooking with skin on if that is possible and does not pose any threat to the cooking process itself. For example, a soup with onion skins on will not taste very nice. But each to themselves, some like its skin on, some skin off. Skins of some soft vegetables (Zucchini, Carrots, Cucumbers, etc.) and tubers (potatoes, parsnips, turnips, etc.) if left on can be pleasant to eat and also increases the fibre content.
2. Minimise the use of water in the cooking process. If you must then make sure that the residual water is used up in your preparation as it contains a good portion of nutrients which have leached out.
3. Do not store cooked portions as leftovers; cook enough for same-day consumption. Storage may have oxidative damage from air, light and other environmental factors.
4. Where possible shorten the cooking time, and also try to apply slow cooking process at a much-reduced temperature.

These basic procedures would go a long way to preserve the nutritional goodness of your home-cooked meals.

We started this section of the chapter by claiming that vitamin deficiencies are not rare. Looking at the published statistics we can say with some confidence that the statement is very true, judge for yourself.

There are a number of reputable publications which over the years have highlighted this issue; even the developed nations are not immune to this. Deficiencies especially in Vitamin A, elemental iron and iodine are still of major concern. However, due to a wide intake of vitamin supplements due to the availability and affordability of vitamins, deficiency in most developed nations is now declining, however, occasionally there are certain pockets of people caught in the statistics where deficiency of certain vitamins is still highlighted.

It has been reported that in the USA alone irrespective of socio-economic status almost 92% of the population is suffering from at least one mineral and one vitamin deficiency based on the Dietary Reference Intakes (Ref: https://

thebiostation.com › bioblog › Nutrient IV Therapy). This is quite significant and worth taking note of it.

Furthermore, in the USA, according to the CDC and the US Department of Agriculture (USDA).

7 out of 10 are deficient in calcium.

8 out of 10 are deficient in vitamin E.

50 percent of Americans are deficient in vitamin A, vitamin C, and magnesium.

More than 50 percent of the general population is vitamin D deficient, regardless of age.

90 percent of Americans of colour are vitamin D deficient.

Approximately 70 percent of elderly Americans are vitamin D deficient (Ref as above).

This is an alarming statistic for a well-developed nation. Now let's look at some of the available statistics for UK and Australia.

In 2021, a survey was conducted by UK Statistics on Vitamin and Mineral Deficiency 2021 (Ref: https://vitall.co.uk/health-tests-blog/statistics-vitaminmineral-deficiency-uk) to determine the deficiency status of UK residents. It was found that approx. 22% of the people had vitamin D deficiency while less than 5% were deficient in the vitamin B12 and B9.

In Australia, one in 4 (around 25%) are vitamin D deficient. In a 2018 report published in Chemical Pathology, in a small sample of 309 pre-operative general surgical patients, 21.4% were vitamin C deficient.

The importance of vitamin C deficiency has been recognised in Australian adults not only in clinically healthy patients but also in Intensive Care Units (ICU) and hospitalised in-patients. According to a survey (2017) by Flinders University (Australia) almost half of the 149 patients in the survey admitted to Flinders Medical Centre were vitamin C deficient.

Australia's Health 2018 (www.aihw.gov.au › indicators-of-australias-health) it was reported that as many as 93% of Australian Adults were not eating enough fruit and vegetables and therefore likely to be deficient in certain essential vitamins and minerals and should take supplements on regular basis.

It is also of concern that with the abundance of sunshine, a significant ratio of Australian adult population is deficient in vitamin D. Among the population those who are at a higher risk level are older citizens, people who are hospital in-patients, convulsing and in rehabilitation and in general people who spend most of their time indoors and have limited exposure to sunlight.

Other vitamin deficiencies occur with Folic acid, and vitamin B12 but due to a mandatory fortification in certain daily foods, e.g., breakfast cereals the deficiencies are not as prevalent as in the past.

Table: A Summary of the Functions of 8 Essential B-Group Vitamins in Cell Metabolism.

Thiamine (Vitamin B1)	Forms Co-enzymes and assists in glucose metabolism. Also, it is involved in the synthesis of RNA, DNA and ATP molecules in the body.
Riboflavin (Vitamin B2)	Helps in the metabolism of Glucose, and other carbohydrate molecules and also fats. Also, acts as an electron carrier to assists in the activity of other B-group vitamins. It also forms pre-cursor of co-enzymes (FAD and FMN) which is required in many enzyme reactions in the body including activation of other vitamins.
Niacin (Vitamin B3)	Also, forms precursor of coenzymes called NAD and NADP and Assists in Glucose, Fats and Protein metabolism. It is also an electron carrier.
Pantothenic Acid (Vitamin B5)	Vitamin B5 in addition to Glucose, Fats and Protein metabolism also helps in cholesterol metabolism and is involved in the biosynthesis of neurotransmitters. It forms a precursor of coenzyme A and is essential for the metabolism of many molecules formed during energy metabolism processes in the body.
Pyridoxine (Vitamin B6)	Helps in the conversion of Glycogen a carbohydrate which is stored in the liver and muscle into glucose and energy. It also helps in bio-synthesis of amino acids, haemoglobins and neurotransmitters. It also acts as an important coenzyme in several bio-chemical processes.
Biotin (Vitamin B7)	It helps in the metabolism of Glucose, Fats and Proteins and amino acid bio-synthesis. It is a coenzyme for carboxylase enzymes, needed for synthesis of fatty acids and in gluconeogenesis
Folic Acid (Vitamin B9)	Acts as a co-enzyme and assists in bio-synthesis of DNA, RNA, amino acids and Red Blood Cells. Folic acid is also required in many enzyme reactions for amino acid synthesis and vitamin metabolism.

Cobalamin (Vitamin B12)	Acts as a co-enzyme, assists in Fats and Protein metabolism, bio-synthesis of Red Blood Cells and folate function. A coenzyme involved in the metabolism of every cell of the human body

It is interesting to note that all B-group vitamins have important functions in the role as co-enzymes in biochemical reactions. B-group vitamins bind with several enzymes in numerous enzymatic reactions to enhance enzyme functions and to speed up the reaction.

These co-enzymes can also be carriers of electrons in a biochemical process, which simply means that the electrons generate electrical current and impulses which enhances the reactions and provide energy. Now, it may seem that the biochemistry is as simple as my oversimplified explanation but it is not. The human body is a very finely tuned machine where every biochemical reaction is precision driven and the biochemistry behind it, very complex.

Several B-group vitamins are also involved in the biosynthesis of important components in the body which are responsible for the formation of important life-giving molecules such as red blood cells, haemoglobins, neurotransmitters (e.g., dopamine, serotonin noradrenaline and the hormone melatonin, etc.).

Without an efficient network of neurotransmitters important messages cannot be transferred or conveyed to the appropriate destinations of the body for specific tasks; e.g., if the muscles do not receive chemical signals on time, then the specific muscle or a group of muscles will not be able to conduct specific movements necessary for the body to perform in due time. In the table above, there has been reference made to certain co-enzyme molecules such as FAD, FMN, NAD, NADP and important biochemicals DNA and RNA; but, what are they?

They are complex molecules which participate in advanced biochemical reactions and have significant functional effects on our body systems. Such as neurotransmitters are carriers of messages or signals from the brain to various or specific parts of an organ or a body system to carry out specific functions. I hope the following description also will simplify the understanding of those complex molecules mentioned above.

FAD, is short for Flavin Adenine Dinucleotide and is formed by the reaction of riboflavin (vitamin B_2), and phosphate group of ADP molecule (adenosine diphosphate) which we are familiar with from our encounter with the Krebs cycle.

FMN (Flavin Mono Nucleotide), this molecule together with FAD are a part of the 90 or so Flavo-proteins which in simple terms are essential to the human genome encoding mechanism. Both FAD and FMN essentially require vitamin B2.

NAD (Nicotinamide Adenine Dinucleotide) is a coenzyme central to all metabolism. They are found in all living cells; NAD is called a dinucleotide because it consists of two nucleotides joined through their phosphate groups.

One nucleotide contains an adenine nucleobase and the other nicotinamide (vitamin B3). Without the availability, this co-enzyme cannot be formed.

NADP (Nicotinamide adenine dinucleotide phosphate) also requires vitamin B3 for the formation of the co-enzyme which is important for metabolic reactions such as the Calvin cycle and lipid and nucleic acid syntheses. It is used by all cells both plant and animal life.

The **Calvin cycle** is a process by which all plants and vegetation including algae use carbon dioxide from the atmosphere and convert into food, e.g., into sugar.

All living organisms on planet Earth depend on the Calvin cycle for energy and food due to inter-dependence on the food chain such as, herbivores eating plants and vegetation, carnivores eating herbivores and finally we humans at the top end of the chain derive our food supply both from herbivores and the plant sources for our energy, and nutritional needs to survive.

For his work, **Melvin Calvin** received the unshared Nobel Prize in Chemistry in 1961.

The other two complex molecules referred above are DNA and RNA with which most of us are now familiar with to some extent.

DNA, short for deoxyribonucleic acid, is the molecule that contains the genetic code of all organisms includes animals, plants, bacteria and all other forms of life.

Every cell of an organism contains the same DNA and is hereditary meaning it is passed on from parents to the off-springs. DNA has a very characteristic double helix structural configuration which carries all genetic instructions, the coiled double helix structure of DNA is very recognisable. The **1962 Nobel Prize** in Physiology or Medicine was shared by **James Watson, Francis Crick and Maurice Wilkins** for their discovery of the molecular structure of DNA, which helped solve the mysteries of our genetic coding.

RNA, Ribo-Nucleic Acid is a complex polymeric molecule made of long-chain sugar molecules linked together by phosphate groups. Its essential functions in our body are like a messenger to DNA to transfer proper genetic instructions to ribosomes which then are involved in the synthesis of protein molecules by combining correct amino acids in proper sequence. RNA is also involved in various biological roles, for example, in coding, decoding and regulation of genetic expressions as instructed by DNA. The proper analogy is, if the DNA is the General Manager of Body Corporate, then RNA is the Works Manager carrying out all instructions from the General Manager and getting them done.

For this discovery and work on RNA, the **Nobel Prize of 2006** for Physiology was shared by **Andrew Fire** and **Craig Mello.**

DNA (A Double Helix Structure)

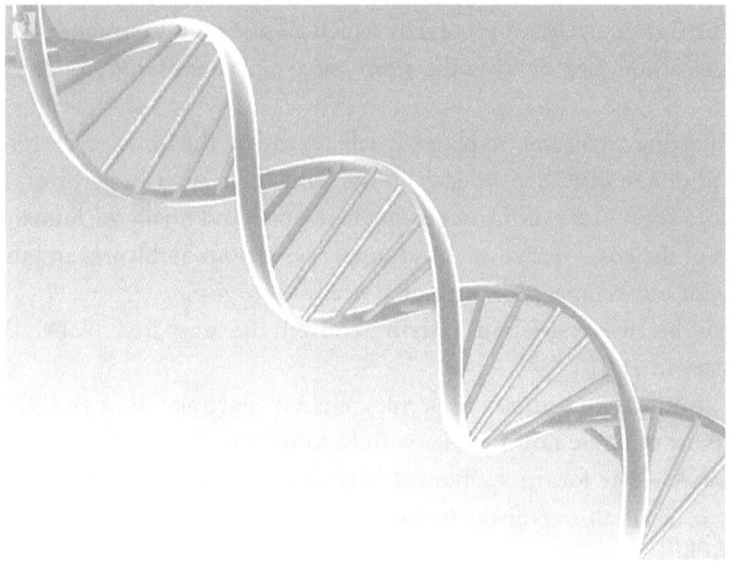

Vitamin-Derived Co-Enzymes and Co-Factors in Nutrition

Coenzymes and cofactors are complex molecules which help specific enzyme to function efficiently. Co-enzymes are organic molecules that are bound with an enzyme at the enzyme active sites during a bio-reaction while co-factors are not necessarily bound to the enzyme during a reaction. Co-factors are more or less molecules which assists a reaction to be carries out effectively and efficiently. These co-factors can be either organic in nature combined with an organic molecule such as a vitamin, or they can be inorganic in nature and be bound with an inorganic element such as zinc, copper and other like elements.

All B-group vitamins are co-enzymes which combine with specific or several other enzyme systems to participate in biochemical reactions for energy production.

There are hundreds of bio-chemical reactions that are happening every moment within our body's cellular structure which involve vitamins bound as co-enzymes, and, or co-factors. Processes such as blood coagulation, hormone production, collagen synthesis, specific proteins required for specific functions as instructed by our DNA and those instructions carried out to completion by our RNA, etc. These instructions and many more could not have been processed if our body lacked a specific or a combination of vitamins.

All B-group vitamins are necessary and are important components of co-factors and co-enzyme formation; all have specific tasks to perform either in our cellular metabolism and also take part in numerous life-sustaining processes happening in our bodies without which we cannot survive. Some of these important metabolic functions are set down in the table below. And, therefore, it is absolutely essential to include foods rich in B-group vitamins and also for our supplementation on a daily basis. But again, I say overuse or overdosing with your vitamin supplements may be unwise, your body is the best judge, listen to your body check out the signs of deficiencies and use in moderation.

Later in the chapter, we will touch upon vitamin sources and deficiency signs.

The Metabolic Functions of the B-Vitamins and Principal Deficiency. Ref: (David A. Bender, Jack R. Cooper in selected Topics from Neurochemistry 1985)

Vitamin	Metabolic Functions	Deficiency Disease
Vitamin B1 (Thiamine)	Pyruvate, 2-oxo-glutarate and branched chain Oxoacid decarboxylases, transketolase	Beriberi: ascending symmetrical peripheral neuropathy, Wernicke's encephalopathy, Korsakoff's psychosis.
Vitamin B2 (Riboflavin)	FAD and FMN coenzymes in oxidases	Angular stomatitis and cheilosis, lens opacity, cataracts.
Vitamin B3 (Niacin)	NAD and NADP coenzymes in redox reactions	Pellagra: photosensitive dermatitis, depressive psychosis.
Vitamin B5 (Pantothenic acid)	Acetyl CoA and acyl carrier protein	Nutritional melalgia (burning foot syndrome)

Vitamin B6 (Pyridoxine)	Pyridoxal phosphate: aminotransferases, amino acid decarboxylases, phosphorylase, role in steroid hormone action	Convulsions, peripheral neuropathy, secondary pellagra, depression
Vitamin B7 (Biotin)	Coenzyme in carboxylations	Dermatitis
B9 (Folic acid)	Coenzyme for one-carbon transfer reactions	Megaloblastic anaemia, various psychiatric disorders
B12 (Cobalamin)	Coenzyme for: methylmalonyl CoA mutase and homocysteine methyltransferase	Pernicious (megaloblastic) anaemia, sub-acute combined degeneration of the spinal cord various psychiatric disorders

So, what are these diseases in the table above?

Beriberi: It is an inflammation of the nerves and nerve endings causing instability, walking disability, etc., caused mainly by Vitamin B1 deficiency.

According to the Cambridge Journals of Medical History, beriberi was encountered in the British India around 1798. However, looking back into history Jacobus Bonitus a Western physician working in Java an Indonesian Island mentioned a beriberi-like disease as early as 1629. But it was not until Christiaan Eijkman a Dutch Chemist (Nobel Laureate 1929) who found the cause of the disease during his work with Vitamin B1. Beriberi comes from the Sri Lankan language Sinhalese meaning extreme weakness.

Wernicke's encephalopathy: Brain disorder, confusion, etc., caused mainly by alcoholism and Vitamin B1 deficiency.

Korsakoff's psychosis: This disease can initially start as a mild Wernicke's encephalopathy and further develop into serious memory loss, confusion and changes in behavioural patterns.

Angular stomatitis: It is a fungal and yeast infection commonly caused by Candida infection. A dietary deficiency of vitamin B2 Riboflavin is the primary cause.

Cheilosis: Is inflammation of the mouth particularly at the corners which causes pain during opening of the mouth during chewing, yawning and also talking. It is caused by B-vitamin deficiency in general and in particular a dietary deficiency of vitamin B2.

Pellagra: Pellagra is a serious skin disease characterised by vitamin B3 deficiency. It can be very debilitating if not treated correctly for the sufferer and manifest into other areas of health complication.

As we now know, vitamins are essential for the bio-synthesis of the vitamin-derived co-enzymes and co-factors.

Although it is fair to say that fresh fruits, vegetables and others as mixed diet of nuts, cereals, legumes proteins, etc., can provide significant nutrition; **but is it enough?**

Vitamin B-Complex

Our body essentially needs 13 vitamins of which 8 are from the B-group of vitamins. These 8 B-group of vitamins are collectively known as the B complex and are water-soluble and can be available from foods we eat. However, they are easily destroyed by heat (during process), moisture and humidity (during storage of foods), refinement of raw foods, e.g., refinement of rice and flour and also other environmental conditions such as UV radiation and free radical contaminants. The diagram below would demonstrate the utilisation of these vitamins singularly or in various combinations collectively as B complex in our body.

There are 8 types of vitamin B:
Thiamine (B1)
Riboflavin (B2)
Niacin (B3)
Pantothenic acid (B5)
Pyridoxine (B6)
Biotin (B7)
Folic acid or folates (B9)
Cyanocobalamin (B12).

Vitamin B-Complex in Our Body

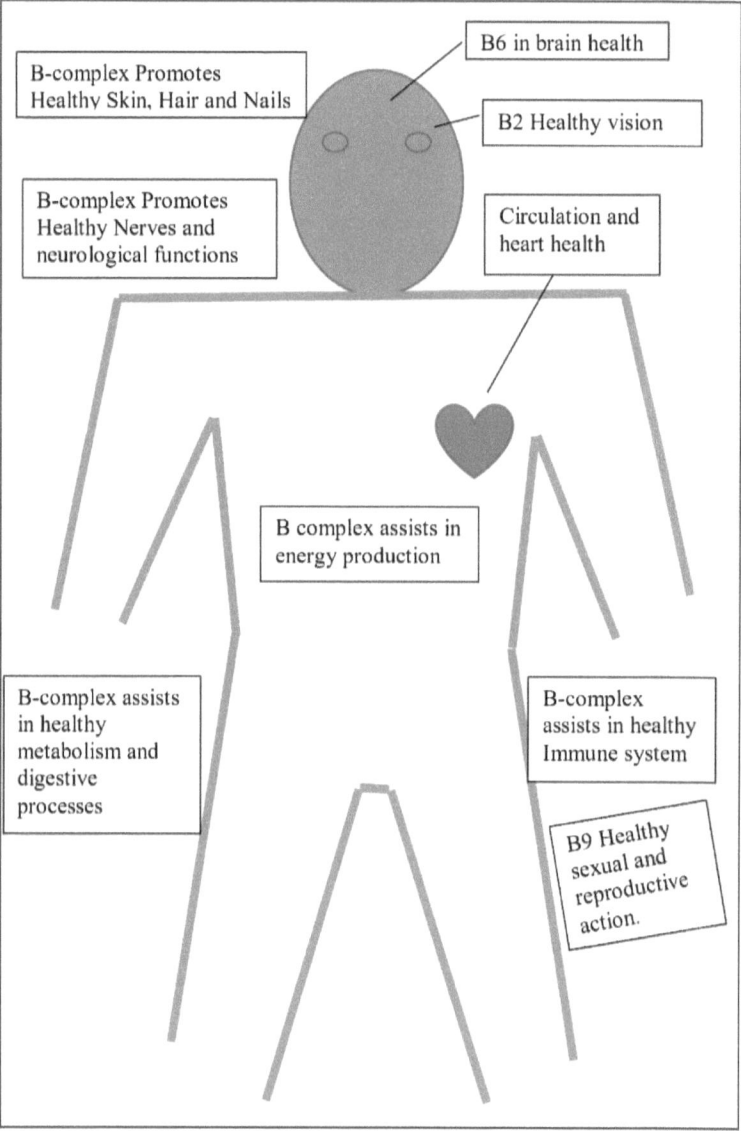

The Table Below Suggests the Basic Functions of Several Vitamins and the Food Sources.

Essential Vitamins	Physiological functions	Some Popular Food Sources	Daily Required amount
Thiamine (Vitamin B1)	Conversion of food into energy. Nervous system function.	Green beans and peas. Enriched grain products (e.g., bread, cereal, pasta, and rice), nuts, and Sunflower seeds. Whole grains. Pork.	1.2(mg)
Riboflavin (Vitamin B2)	Conversion of food into energy. Growth factors. Red blood cell formation.	Eggs, meats, poultry, seafood (e.g., oysters). Grain products (e.g., bread, cereal, pasta, rice) Mushrooms and Spinach. Milk.	1.3(mg)
Niacin (Vitamin B3)	Cholesterol production. Conversion of food into energy. Digestion. Nervous system function.	Beans. Enriched grain products (e.g., bread, cereal, pasta, rice). Beef, Pork, Poultry and Seafood. Whole grains and Nuts.	16(mg)
Pantothenic Acid (Vitamin B5)	Conversion of food into energy. Fat metabolism. Hormone synthesis. Nervous system function. Red blood cell formation.	Avocados, Beans, peas and Broccoli. Milk and Yoghurt. Poultry, Seafood and eggs. Sweet potatoes and Mushrooms. Whole grains.	5(mg)
Pyridoxine (Vitamin B6)	Immune and Nervous system function. Protein, fats and carbohydrate metabolism. Red blood cell formation.	Chickpeas. Fruits (other than citrus). Potatoes. Salmon and Tuna.	1.7(mg)

Biotin (Vitamin B7)	Energy storage. Protein, carbohydrate, and fat metabolism.	Avocados and Cauliflower. Eggs. Fruits (e.g., raspberries) Liver, Pork and Salmon Nuts and Whole grains	30(mcg)
Folic Acid (Vitamin B9)	Prevention of birth defects. Protein metabolism. Red blood cell formation.	Asparagus, Avocados. Beans, peas and other Green leafy vegetables (e.g., spinach). Enriched grain products (e.g., bread, cereal, pasta, rice). Oranges and orange juice.	400mcg
Cobalamin (Vitamin B12)	Conversion of food into energy. Nervous system function. Red blood cell formation.	Dairy products. Eggs, Meat and Poultry. Fortified cereals. Seafood (e.g., clams, trout, salmon, haddock, tuna).	2.4(mcg)
Ascorbic Acid (Vitamin C)	Antioxidant activity. Collagen and connective tissue formation. Immune function. Wound healing.	Fruit (e.g., cantaloupe, citrus fruits, kiwifruit, and strawberries). Juices (e.g., oranges, grapefruit, and tomato). Vegetables (e.g., broccoli, Brussels sprouts, peppers, and tomatoes).	90(mg)
Retinol (Vitamin A)	Growth and development. Immune function. Red blood cell formation. Reproduction skin and bone formation. Vision.	Fruits e.g., Cantaloupe Carrots, Green leafy vegetables (e.g., spinach and broccoli). Pumpkin, Red peppers, sweet potatoes etc. Dairy products and Eggs. Fortified cereals	900(mcg)

Calciferol (Vitamin D)	Blood pressure regulation. Bone growth. Calcium balance. Hormone production. Immune function. Nervous system function.	Fish (e.g., herring, mackerel, salmon, trout, and tuna) and Fish oils e.g., cod liver oil. Pork and eggs. Fortified dairy products Fortified margarine. Fortified orange juice. Fortified plant-based beverages (e.g., soy, rice, and almond). Fortified cereals. Mushrooms.	20(mcg)
Tocopherol (Vitamin E)	Antioxidant (lipids). Formation of blood vessels. Immune function.	Fortified cereals. Green vegetables (e.g., spinach and broccoli). Nuts, seeds and Peanuts and peanut butter. Vegetable oils.	15(mg)
Phytonadione Vitamin K	Blood clotting. (Coagulant factor) Strong bones.	Green vegetables (e.g., broccoli, kale, spinach, turnip greens, collard greens, Swiss chard, mustard greens). Juices.	120 (mcg)

The table represents the deficiencies caused by the inadequacies of B complex and other vitamins that we are so dependent on with our food intake or supplementation. The table also provides an important guide to the importance of most vitamins currently known to us and the food sources that we can complement in our dietary choices.

It is noteworthy that B-group vitamins are required in small quantities and perform various physiological functions either singularly or collectively.

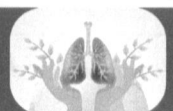

Chapter 7

VITAMIN C: THE SPARK OF LIFE

"Chemically Vitamin C is a small molecule yet larger than life; in fact, so large that it makes me wonder how come we human beings are genetically mutant in our ability to manufacture it within our body."

– Jay Das, 2007

Vitamin C: The Spark of Life

Vitamins are biochemical nutrients and are required in our body to perform many of the all-important biochemical processes essential to sustain our lives, good health and wellbeing.

With our quest for knowledge and understanding of modern advancements in global research and development in nutritional supplements, we are now beginning to understand the link between our biochemical make up and the utilisation of these nutrients and wonder why we are at the top echelon of the evolutionary chain lack biochemically in certain nutrients when the lower animals are blessed with the biochemical presence of these nutrients in their body to continue their life cycle.

One such nutrient is ascorbic acid (Vitamin C), which is arguably the most studied, researched and published vitamin and perhaps one of the most important supplements required in our daily life. It is also an essential vitamin which our body cannot biosynthesise and therefore must be supplemented on a daily basis from our dietary food intake and or supplemented in the form of tablets or powder also liquid preparations.

Let us now consider the question why is vitamin C so important for us? It is relatively easy to define and answer this question if we also look at its scientific research and developments in the context of clinical trials done.

According to Dr Pauling the only scientist to have won the unshared Nobel Prize twice "it is a biochemical an orthomolecular substance, not a drug; which is required in our body to perform various biochemical reactions to sustain life and keep us functioning day to day. It is not only essential for humans and animal species but also for plant forms."

And upon a closer understanding, the definition can be extended to consider the wide range of functions that this wonderful water-soluble vitamin has in the human body. It is an essential vitamin as our body cannot produce it yet we need it on a regular basis.

Let us now consider its commonly known and the beneficial properties as published in various scientific literatures. The categorised list below is by no means exhaustive and complete and by logging on to any number of search engines on the internet readers can find this information and many more research reports and publications on this wonderful nutrient.

1. It promotes the healing of cuts, abrasions and wounds.
2. Helps fight infections.
3. Has a protective effect on the body from irritants which are constituents of smog, tobacco smoke, alcohol abuse, illegal drugs and certain food chemicals and preservatives into cancer-causing substances.
4. It assists in dilating blood vessels by enlarging and widening them which reduces the risk of developing high blood pressure and heart diseases.
5. It helps regulate cholesterol levels.
6. It prevents the development of scurvy, a disease characterised by weakness, fatigue, anaemia, swollen joints, bleeding gums and loose teeth.
7. It has some positive effects in lowering the risk of developing cataracts and other minor eye complaints such as clouding of the lens of the eye that impairs vision.
8. It may also help protect diabetics against the deterioration of nerves, eyes and kidneys.

9. It may also help reduce the severity of the symptoms of colds and flu.
10. Also, aids in iron absorption from dietary food intakes.
11. May reduce the levels of heavy metal absorption in the blood.
12. It is responsible for the bio-synthesis of many biochemicals in our body such as Collagen, several neurotransmitters and many others which are important in our daily function as human beings.

The list goes on and on…

In the words of Dr Emanuel Cheraskin, Dr Ringsdorf and Dr Sisley In their book 'THE VITAMIN C CONNECTION' (Harper and Row 1983).

"There are more than ten thousand published scientific papers that make it quite clear that there is not one body process (such as what goes on inside cells or tissues) and not one disease or syndrome (from the common cold to leprosy) that is not influenced directly or indirectly by vitamin C."

Now there would probably be another few thousand publications added to that list since the above quote in 1983.

Historical Progression

It is very interesting to learn about the chronological development of the understanding of vitamin C throughout our history. Although vitamin C was not discovered then, looking back into history it is now clear that people then used plant materials for treatment of conditions which we today know are caused by vitamin C deficiency.

1550 BC—Ebers Papyrus
The earliest known reference to the suggestion of a treatment for a scurvy-like disease was reported in Ebers Papyrus in about 1550 BC by eating onions which we now know to contain some vitamin C.

400BC—Hippocrates
(Father of Medicine) describes the concept of vitamin C deficiency.

1497—Voyage of Vasco da Gama
Vasco da Gama during his 1497 expedition to India around the Cape of Good Hope suffered heavy casualty to a particular sickness which he recorded "Many of our men fell ill here, their feet and hands swelling, and their gums growing over their teeth so that they could not eat." Up the eastern coast of Africa, local traders traded fresh oranges with them and within 6 days of consuming fresh

oranges the crew recovered and Vasco da Gama again recorded "It pleased God in his mercy that…all our sick recovered their health for the air of the place is very good." Upon his return, voyage the crew was again affected with the same symptoms and had to resort to a fresh supply of oranges from the locals. Vasco da Gama recognised oranges as an effective cure for their sickness.

1535—Early Cures
French explorer Cartier used cedar bark and leaves as a cure for scurvy; (cedar bark and leaves are now known to contain vitamin C).

1734—Johann Friedrich Bachstrom
A Dutch scientist and writer wrote in Observationes circa scorbutum ("Observations on Scurvy") "that scurvy is solely owing to a total abstinence from fresh vegetables, fruits and greens; which is alone the primary cause of the disease." How true is this statement as we know today that the highest concentration of Vitamin C is in fresh fruits and green vegetables.

1774—Early use of citrus fruits
A British naval physician, Lind documented that there was an active substance in citrus fruits which could cure scurvy. This became the scientific rationale for the cure for the disease.

1796—Early regular rationing of citrus juices
The British navy was given a daily ration of lime or lemon juice to overcome vitamin C deficiency.

1880—Limeys
British sailors were provided with a ration of lime juice to prevent scurvy; for this practice, they were nick-named as 'limeys'.

1907—Guinea pigs fed on a cabbage diet:
Norwegian biochemists Axel Holst and Alfred Fröhlich devised an ingenious experiment to demonstrate that animals may also develop a scurvy-like disease if barred from eating certain foods now known to contain vitamin C.

Their model animal was a guinea pig and they proved that when fed on a cabbage diet, their symptoms disappeared.

1928—Vitamin C first isolated

In 1928, the Hungarian biochemist Dr Szent-Gyorgyi and independently by the American Charles Glen King first isolated vitamin C and showed it to be ascorbic acid, but it was Szent-Gyorgyi who went on to win the Nobel Prize in 1937 in medicine for his work.

1933–34—Vitamin C first produced synthetically

In 1933–34, British Chemists Walter Norman Haworth determined the structure of Vitamin C. Haworth and Sir Edmund Hirst followed by Polish scientist Tadeusz Reichstein were the first to independently produce Vitamin C synthetically. The synthetic form is identical to the natural form. For his work, Haworth won the Nobel Prize for Chemistry in 1937, however, in recognition for his work the process was named after Reichstein.

1934—Commercial production of Vitamin C

The Swiss Pharmaceutical Company Hoffmann-La Roche first mass-produced vitamin C in 1934. This made the vitamin available in a commercial quantity thus beginning the modern area of vitamin C supplementation.

1957—The missing link

In 1957, the American scientist J. J. Burns showed that the reason some mammals were susceptible to scurvy was the inability of their liver to produce the active enzyme L-gulonolactone oxidase, which is the last of the chain of four enzymes which bio-synthesises vitamin C. We humans lack this enzyme and hence cannot produce Vitamin C in our body.

1970—Dr Linus Pauling and common Cold

Linus Pauling (Nobel Prize for Chemistry in 1954 and Nobel Peace Prize in 1962 both unshared) first publishes his best-selling book 'Vitamin C and the common cold'.

1999—Irwin Stone

Published a book 'THE HEALING FACTOR' explaining the role of Vitamin C against disease.

2007—Finding the missing link:

It took scientists 50 years to isolate the missing enzyme. A team of scientists led by Dr Sean Bulley working with various kiwifruit varieties and the world's largest kiwifruit DNA database isolated the missing link and therefore discovered the final pathways for Vitamin C production.

In mammals (except us humans) which are capable of producing ascorbic acid, is produced in the liver from blood glucose. Each biochemical step is controlled by a specific enzyme except the last which is controlled by a specific enzyme called L-gulonolactone oxidase. This is the missing enzyme for us humans because we carry a defective gene and cannot produce this particular enzyme. This is the gene that mutated in a primate ancestor of ours, millions of years ago. This is the final step that is blocked from our final biochemical pathways producing ascorbic acid from glucose in our liver.

Dr Linus Pauling (1901–1994) and Dr Fredrick Klenner (1907–1984): They popularised Vitamin C as a nutritional supplement for the prevention and treatment of many diseases.

I cannot even begin to think how and why we humans at the top of the evolutionary chain have missed out on this important biochemical development, perhaps this was the impetus required to search for the elusive molecule which would deliver us from the unfortunate genetic shortfall. This elusive molecule as we now call ascorbic acid (Vitamin C) remained elusive until 1928 when Hungarian biochemist and Nobel Prize winner Dr Szent-Gyorgyi isolated it.

Up until 1965, it was assumed that all primates were unable to produce their own ascorbic acid and were thus susceptible to the disease, scurvy. It was pointed out (By Irwin Stone) that this was merely an assumption and one which had never been tested. It was suggested that the whole order of the primates should be examined for the presence of L-gulonolactone oxidase in their livers. If this was done, then the data obtained might have been useful in pinpointing the time, when the genetic mutation occurred. Thus, it might be possible to determine in which primate ancestor of man this important enzyme system was lost.

How interesting, that such a prestigious award as the Nobel Prize in Medicine and Chemistry was presented for the recognition of scientific works for ascorbic acid (Vitamin C).

In 1939, Szent-Gyorgyi wrote, "Vitamins, if properly understood and applied, will help us to reduce human suffering to an extent which the most fantastic mind would fail to imagine."

And how true is this statement as we know now that vitamins play a very important role in our cellular metabolism; and the formation of cofactors combines with enzyme systems which enter into numerous metabolic and catalytic activities happening within our body.

Now back to ascorbic acid. In many lower mammals such as goats, cows, pigs, etc., ascorbic acid is produced in the liver from blood glucose by the stepwise reactions shown in the diagram. Each step, except the last, is controlled by a specific enzyme. In the last step, the 2-keto-L-gulonolactone, once formed, is automatically converted into ascorbic acid. No enzyme is required. But in humans, the step of transforming L-gulonolactone into 2keto-L-gulonolactone as catalysed by the specific enzyme L-gulonolactone oxidase is missing due to us carrying a defective gene.

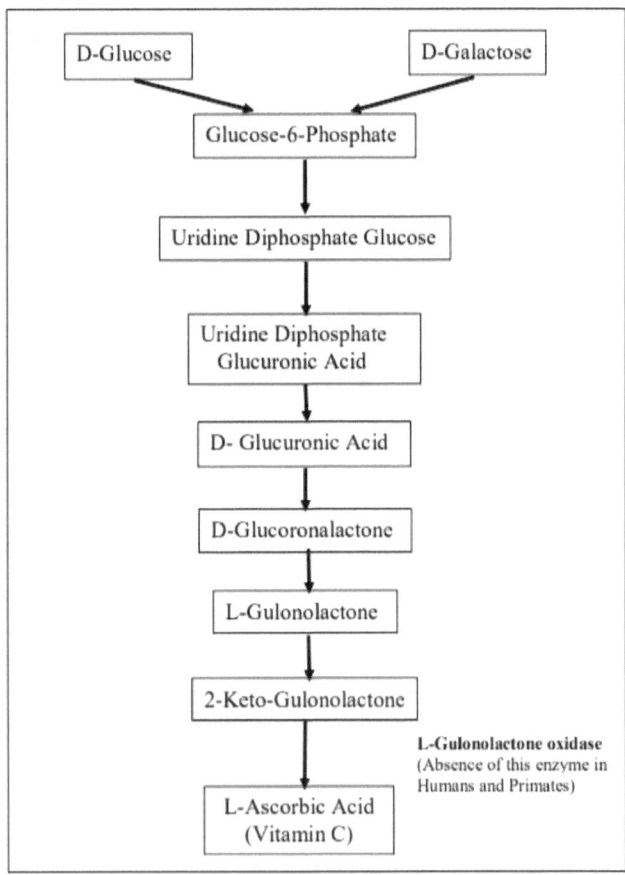

This is the gene that mutated in a primate ancestor of ours, millions of years ago. It is this step that is blocked in humans which prevents us from producing large amounts of ascorbic acid from glucose and galactose in the liver. It is very interesting that biochemists have now studied animal models and their capability in manufacturing and utilisation of ascorbic acid under stress conditions within their bodies and have come up with some great values which not only signify the importance of ascorbic acid but also theorise our requirement for it.

Although the studies were done way back in the 1970s, nonetheless still remain significant works.

Two independent studies by Chatterjee 1973 and Subramanian et al. 1973, found that an adult goat produced around 200mg/kg body weight of ascorbic acid under normal conditions but under stress the animals were capable of producing several times more of that amount.

The above findings were corroborated by (C. Long et al. Journal of Surgical Research 2003) in human trials by demonstrating that during times of stress and trauma or injury, we tend to use up a large quantity of vitamin C from our body pool of reserves which must be replenished as we are mutant in our ability to manufacture vitamin C in our body.

Vitamin C since the early days of its mass production has gained much popularity as a supplement not only for health and general well-being but also for the very established fact that we humans and the higher primates are genetically mutant in that we cannot manufacture it in our body. With this popularity came wide opposing views from the established orthodox school of thought that vitamin C offers no significant benefit to us as a supplement which to this day remains a hurdle to overcome. However, with scientific research and clinical trials being conducted around the world it is pleasing to note that views are changing.

Later in the chapter some of the publications are summarised and referenced to demonstrate the results and make good reading for those who are interested and want to further their understanding of this subject.

If we study great discoveries and ideas put forward by leading researchers of their time, we find several examples which for some reason or other were ignored at the time when those were researched or proposed. There could have been several reasons for this; they could have been very radical and advanced for their time or simply lack of funding. One such great idea was put forward by Sir Archibald Garrod (English physician in 1908) in a series of papers 'Inborn errors of metabolism'.

He claimed that certain diseases were due to the inherited lack of certain enzymes. In his original papers, he described four genetic diseases albinism (due to the lack of an enzyme used in the production of the black skin pigment melanin), alkaptonuria, cystinuria (both diseases of protein metabolism) and pentosuria often confused with diabetes and caused by the inherent lack of an enzyme for the metabolism of pentose a sugar). All these diseases are due to genetic mutation which causes a block in the formation of specific enzymes required to carry out the end metabolism process. Even though the papers published by Sir Archibald were very convincing, they were ignored at the time and perhaps forgotten until very late into 1940s when it was concluded that inborn errors of metabolism are caused by the lack of specific enzymes.

Since Sir Archibald Garrod's work, the list has now grown considerably and many more new ones have been reported. Most inborn errors of metabolisms are also caused by genetic mutation in the genetic makeup of the genes which code the enzymes. Therefore, inactivity of one or a group of enzymes will cause a deficiency in enzyme activity leading to specific disorders. Classic examples apart from those mentioned earlier are Maple Syrup Urine Disease caused by a deficiency of an enzyme called Branched Chain Ketoacid dehydrogenase (BCKD) which primarily causes neurological disorders. And, Phenylketonuria caused by the deficiency of the enzyme Phenylalanine Hydroxylase (PAH) which mainly causes intellectual disabilities.

My research into Vitamin C and its many applications although has been referred throughout this Chapter; I felt the need to put into some chronological order the milestones and achievements in vitamin C research since its discovery in 1937.

Vitamin C and Some Other Milestones since 1937

1941—Canadian cardiologist Dr J. C. Patterson reports that more than 80% of his heart disease patients have low vitamin C levels compared to other patients.

1954—Dr G. C. Willis shows that vitamin C supplementation can reduce arterial deposits. This makes the first claim that atherosclerosis is reversible.

1957—The American scientist J.J. Burns proved the requirement of dietary vitamin C to prevent scurvy in certain mammals.

1960s—Biochemist Irwin Stone and others recommend increased dietary vitamin C supplementation to improve health.

1967—Boris Sokoloff studied the effect of 13 gm of vitamin C, on a group of 60 people aged over 60 years with CVD. Not a single vascular event during the yearlong study period was noted.

1970—Dr Linus Pauling publishes his first book on vitamin C.

1970s—Vitamin C consumption in the US rises by 300%. Mortality from heart disease decreases by 30% in the US the only country with a significant drop in heart disease fatalities.

1983—Dr Emanuel Cheraskin, Dr Ringsdorf and Dr Sisley wrote the book 'THE VITAMIN C CONNECTION'.

1986—Dr Pauling summarises the evidence for vitamin C against heart disease and other diseases in his book *'How to Live Longer and Feel Better'*, which becomes a bestseller.

1989—Dr Rath and Dr Pauling discover that optimum dietary vitamin C prevents the deposition of lipoprotein in artery walls.

1991—Dr Rath and Dr Pauling publish *'Solution to the Puzzle of Human Cardiovascular Disease'*. This scientific paper explains (a) that vitamin C deficiency is the direct and most frequent cause of heart attacks, (b) how plasma risk factors lead to atherosclerotic deposits in arterial walls, (c) why humans suffer from heart attack and stroke but rarely from failure of other organs, and (d) why animal species who are able to produce their own vitamin C in the body do not develop heart disease.

1992—Dr Enstrom and colleagues (UCLA) show that in over 11,000 Americans, increased intake of vitamin C reduces the death rate from heart disease by nearly half and prolongs life for more than six years.

1993—Dr Pauling tapes a video lecture on heart disease.

1998—The Vitamin C Foundation submits grant proposal to the US National Institutes of Health to study Pauling's claim.

In 1957, the American scientist JJ. Burns (Burns and Evans J. Biol. Chem 200, 125 (1953)) and Burns et al. Science 124, 1148 (1956) showed that the reason some mammals were susceptible to scurvy was their <u>inability</u> to synthesise the active enzyme L-Gulonolactone Oxidase, which is the enzyme required in the last step in the chain of sequences synthesising vitamin C.

Unfortunately, we also fall into this category.

I now quote American Biochemist Irvine Stone's famous quote in his book.

'The living factor', vitamin C against disease.

"We can surmise that the production of ascorbic acid was an early accomplishment of the life process because of its wide distribution in nearly all present-day living organisms. It is produced in comparatively large amounts in the simplest plants and the most complex; it is synthesised in the most primitive animal species as well as in the most highly organised. Except possibly for a few microorganisms, those

species of animals that cannot make their own ascorbic acid are the exceptions and require it in their food if they are to survive. Without it, life cannot exist. Because of its nearly universal presence in both plants and animals, we can also assume that its production was well organised before the time when evolving life forms diverged along separate plant and animal lines."

Vitamin C and Requirement

Just summarising the requirement of vitamin C in our daily supplementation, we need to remember that we humans are incapable of bio-synthesising it and hence require it on a daily basis.

Various animal studies have shown that storage of vitamin C is depleted quite rapidly from stored organs and if not supplemented on a regular basis, then deficiency signs and symptoms can show up. Our brain, liver, Lungs and adrenaline glands are the main body organs that store vitamin C. It is also known that our muscle fibres lose vitamin C rapidly and therefore adequate intake must be maintained. Our skeletal muscle stores the most vitamin C reserves.

Vitamin C requirements are higher in women during pregnancy. Lactation increases the vitamin C requirement of women, to satisfy the vitamin needs of the infant's normal growth.

Smokers with lower plasma vitamin C values require an increased intake due to increased oxidative stress.

Vitamin C supplementation may be effective for improving the health status of patients who are considered at high risk of viral infections (Ref as below):

- Hemilä H. Vitamin C and infections. *Nutrients* (2017) 52:222–3
- Matthay MA, Aldrich JM, Gotts JE. Treatment for severe acute respiratory distress syndrome from COVID-19. *Lancet Respir Med* (2020) 8:433–34

There are many reputable references which points to the fact that vitamin C is important to uplift our immunity and strengthen our immune system; although it is a bit early to conclusively link vitamin C with its positive effect in COVID-19 infection the early reports are very encouraging. The jury is still out on this issue as clinical trials with vitamin C is being conducted in a number of research facilities. But in the meantime, an adequate dose of vitamin C as a daily supplement can only help.

ClinicalTrials.gov lists the clinical trials that are and have been evaluated on the use of vitamin C in patients with COVID-19. A few examples are listed below.

High-dose intravenous Vitamin C (HDIVC) as adjuvant therapy in critical patients with positive COVID-19. A pilot randomised controlled dose comparison trial.

Administration of Intravenous Vitamin C in Novel Coronavirus Infection COVID-19 and Decreased Oxygenation.

Acute respiratory failure due to COVİD-19 pneumonia has poor prognosis and high mortality. Studies suggest that high-dose vitamin C treatment reduces mortality in patients with sepsis (body's response to acute infection) and acute respiratory distress syndrome (ARDS), and may also be beneficial in COVİD-19 disease.

(Ref: US National Library of Medicine, Clinical Trials.gov ClinicalTrials.gov Identifier: NCT04710329).

A similar trial (Ref: ClinicalTrials.gov Identifier: NCT04682574) initiated Nov. 2020 and anticipated completion in March 2022 of latter may offer some insight into vitamin C use.

Vitamin C May Increase the Recovery Rate of Outpatient Cases of SARS-CoV-2 Infection by 70%.

Reanalysis of the COVID A to Z randomised Clinical Trial (Ref: Front. Immunol. 10 May 2021), Vitamin C and COVID-19 observational studies conducted at the University of Otago Christ Church NZ March 2022 indicated that patients with COVID-19 have significantly depleted vitamin C status.

Considering the anti-inflammatory, immunomodulatory, anti-oxidative, antithrombotic and antiviral properties of Vitamin C (ascorbic acid) it is not unusual to link vitamin C's beneficial impact in patients suffering from sepsis and acute respiratory distress syndrome (ARDS) and many other respiratory conditions like pneumonia. It may be years before such a positive link is proven beyond doubt, but in the meantime, unless proven otherwise I feel Vitamin C therapy has a place as an adjunct.

Vitamin C has been known to enhance many biochemical reactions acting as biochemical catalysts involving elements e.g., iron and copper which act as coenzymes. Particularly important are fatty acid transportation, the bio-conversion of the amino acid tryptophan to serotonin a neurotransmitter molecule and the bio-conversion of cholesterol into bile acids.

Vitamin C is also involved in the synthesis of collagen molecules and in activating the B-group vitamins and folic acid.

The importance and involvement of Vitamin C is never-ending and has a flow-on effect into numerous other biochemical processes. Vitamin C forms cofactors for multiple enzymatic systems including dopamine, another important neurotransmitter molecule carnitine helping mitochondria in energy production processes. Several human studies in recent times have suggested that Vitamin C may have an immunomodulatory role therefore offering some benefit as a supplement in viral infection.

What happens to vitamin C after it is consumed orally?

As a water-soluble vitamin, the absorption is much easier and simpler. It does not get stored in the body for long, rather it is transported to the organ tissues through circulation. The extra amount after tissue requirement and saturation is excreted in the urine. The following schematic diagram will be helpful. It is reported that the vitamin C concentration in the body can be around 300mg–2000mg (Ref: Jacob RA, Sotoudeh G. Vitamin C function and status in chronic disease. Nutr Clin Care 2002; 5:66–74). 300 mg is a minimum requirement to prevent scurvy.

In another report, it is mentioned that the average adult body pool is 1.2g–2.0g; (Ref: Sauberlich HE. Ascorbic acid. In: Brown ML, editor. Present knowledge in nutrition. Nutrition Foundation, Washington DC; 1990). Because it is so highly water soluble, it cannot be stored for long and therefore must be replenished in our food intake or supplemented daily.

The average half-life of ascorbic acid in an adult human is about 10–20 days, with a turnover of 1 mg/kg body and a body pool of 22 mg/kg at plasma ascorbate concentration of 50 µmol/L (Ref: www.ncbi.nlm.nih.gov › articles › PMC201008).

Half-life is the time taken for Vitamin C in the plasma to be reduced by 50% of its intake concentration.

Vitamin C and Stress

It has now been researched that several animals for example goats which are capable of producing Vitamin C in their bodies under normal conditions (up to 13g/day) can also produce a significantly higher amounts of Vitamin C (up to 13 times more) under stress conditions. A monkey our closest evolutionary primate is administered around 55mg/kg body weight a day for routine health maintenance (Nutrient Requirements of Laboratory Animals Fourth Revised Edition, 1995 National Research Council (US) Subcommittee on Laboratory Animal Nutrition. Washington (DC): National Academies Press (US); 1995. Whereas our RDA is only 75mg/day for women and around 90mg/day for an average adult male. The current RDA levels were set a few decades ago and are vastly inadequate. According to the scientist at Psychology Today Australia (Ref…

https://www.psychologytoday.com/au/articles/200304/vitamin-c-stressbuster) people who have high levels of vitamin C do not show the expected mental and physical signs of stress when subjected to acute psychological challenges and should be considered as a part of stress management.

Vitamin C's Distribution in Our Body:

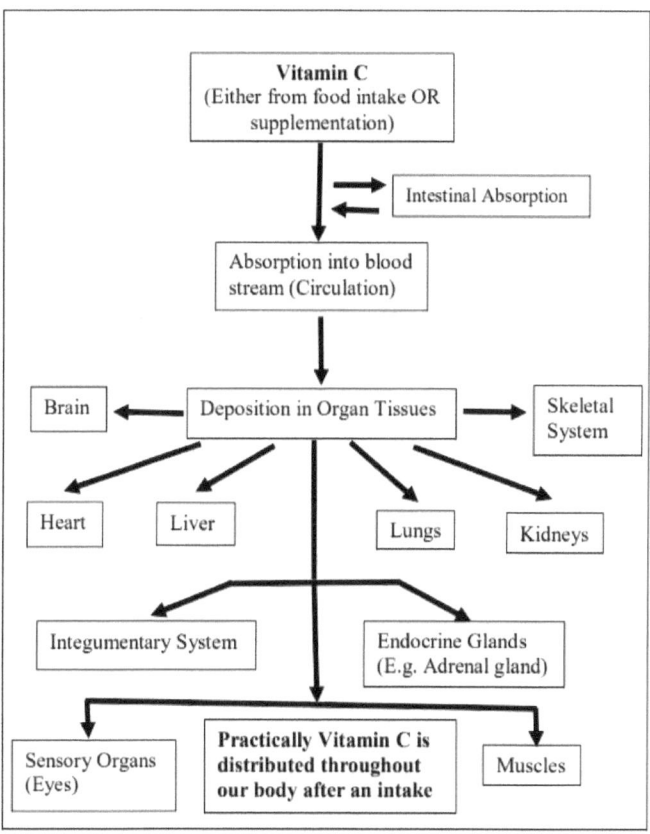

According to Mayo Clinic, the recommended daily amount for vitamin C is 75 milligrams (mg) a day for women and 90 mg a day for men. During pregnancy, 120 mg a day is recommended. The upper limit (**UL**) for all adults is 2,000 mg a day; (Mayo Clinic).

Vitamin C is perhaps the most studied, researched and versatile vitamin of all the known and currently used vitamins. Besides being used as a daily supplement in the form of tablets, liquids and powders its use as a topical supplement for anti-ageing has in recent times become very widespread. It is a significantly active anti-oxidant and finds use in topical dermatology as a preventive form of treatment in photo-ageing, hyper-pigmentation and in many other minor skin blemishes. Till recently one of the difficulties in the use of vitamin C topically had been the compound's instability in an aqueous medium, but, now with enhanced stabilisation and newer delivery methods for skin penetration and absorption, its use has increased.

Numerous studies and research findings have outlined a number of benefits of the topical use of vitamin C which are summarised below.

Benefits of Vitamin C (and Its Derivatives) in Topical Dermatology

- Assists in protecting skin against Sun's harmful radiations. May have some value in sun-screen preparations.
- Actively promotes collagen synthesis which increases skin elasticity, reduces skin sagging and visible signs of skin ageing.
- May also have some positive effects in smoothening the ageing skin wrinkling.
- Helps reduce hyper-pigmentation.
- May reduce redness of the skin due to sunburn and promotes skin brightening.
- Promotes wound healing.

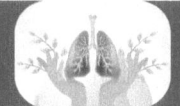

Chapter 8

MINERALS AND HERBS

Our health and well-being are in the hands of Mother Nature. She provides all that we need; vitamins from fresh produce, Minerals from the Earth and herbs from Her own garden.
— Jay Das, 2022

Minerals in Our Health and Well-Being

Let me begin this chapter by quoting Arthur Young (b. 1741, London, d.1820, London), an English writer:

"God sleeps in the minerals, awakens in plants and thinks in man."

My own quote is absolutely true providing we can go back to basics and forage for the fresh ingredients we need and eat them raw. But one thing we forget to consider is our taste buds, our modern fast life and living and also our love for convenience.

I hope I have adequately given you enough awareness on vitamins in earlier chapters, so now let us look at minerals and herbs and their importance in our dietary consideration.

Our body consists of a significant portion of minerals which include salts, and the natural elements found on earth and in our foods. Out of the total body mineral composition consisting of almost 100 minerals, only 6 elements oxygen, Carbon, Hydrogen, Nitrogen, Phosphorous and Calcium constitute almost all (approximately 96%) of the minerals and the rest consists of trace elements such as iron, zinc, iodine, sodium, chlorides, chromium and others. Our body minerals can be grouped as essential and non-essential and other elements. Essential elements are the ones which are necessary for our body and vital physiological roles and must be either taken in with our food and, or supplements. It is believed that there are around 20–25 essential elements that our body cannot synthesise; in fact our body cannot synthesize any mineral as such so all elements must be supplemented. The essential elements can also be categorised into 3 areas according to their requirement and amounts in our body.

The non-essential elements do not have any major specific roles to play, many of these are simply useless and thought to have entered into our body as contaminants and other processes. Also, there are a significant number of elements which are toxins and undesirable for our general health and well-being. There are other elements also found in our body such as traces of Lead, Arsenic, Cadmium, Strontium and Mercury, etc., which are poorly absorbed and also considered non-essential for life. These elements are highly toxic even at a very low concentration.

Apart from these, there are some other nonessential elements which are required from time to time in some biochemical processes such as gold and silver. Gold in the human body is approximately in the order of 0.22mg in a person of 80kg body weight; this amount is almost negligible and although some claim therapeutic benefit the mainstream science does not. Gold supplements are unheard of but gold jewellery is very popular and liked by both men and women of several cultural backgrounds. Our body composition varies largely from individual to individual depending on their physical attributes, BMI, etc., so let us look at a generalisation of what our mineral composition looks like.

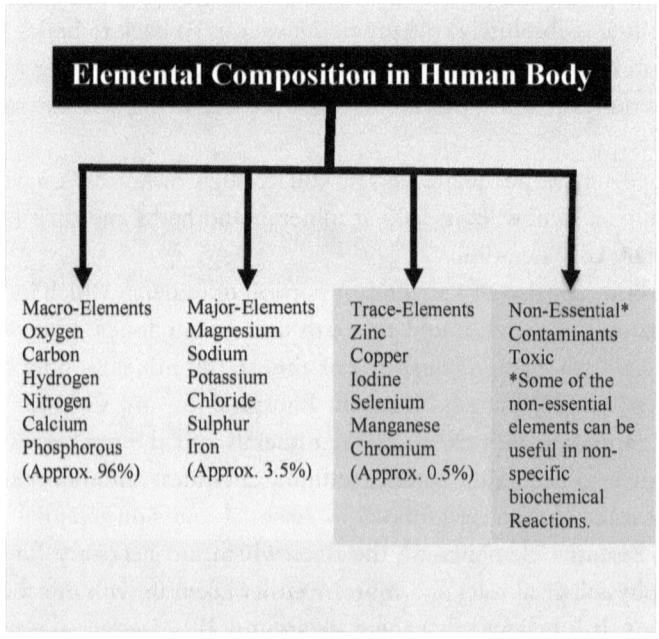

Macro-Elements	Major-Elements	Trace-Elements	Non-Essential*
Oxygen	Magnesium	Zinc	Contaminants
Carbon	Sodium	Copper	Toxic
Hydrogen	Potassium	Iodine	*Some of the
Nitrogen	Chloride	Selenium	non-essential
Calcium	Sulphur	Manganese	elements can be
Phosphorous	Iron	Chromium	useful in non-
(Approx. 96%)	(Approx. 3.5%)	(Approx. 0.5%)	specific biochemical Reactions.

We are organic beings composed of elemental oxygen, carbon, hydrogen, nitrogen, calcium, phosphorous, etc. We have distinct skeletal structures, bone tissues and others, e.g., blood, brain, synovial and joint fluids, etc., and a complex body system network which gives us a very unique evolutionary configuration.

If we make a slight assumption, that our body composition is 50% water and 50% other solid matter, and knowing fully well that water is composed of oxygen and Hydrogen, and other solid matter such as protein, fats and Lipids, carbohydrates, etc., are all organic matter and composed of oxygen, carbon, hydrogen, nitrogen and our blood has iron as the central element of haemoglobin and the skeletal structure is mainly composed of calcium, magnesium, zinc, phosphorous, etc., then an approximate composition of the human body can be derived as per the table below.

Oxygen is the most common element followed by carbon, hydrogen, nitrogen, calcium, etc.; the table below summarises this point. All these elements except strontium are essential. I have not included several other elements in the list such as boron as the amount contained in the body is near negligible and truly in trace amounts.

Oxygen is the most abundant element in our body and is mostly contributed by water. In a person of 70kg body weight with 50% water content, oxygen alone accounts for more than 31kg plus the contribution from other matter would be very significant as well. The next most abundant element is carbon as it constitutes the framework of all organic organisms. Hydrogen is the next abundant element and similar to oxygen the majority comes from the water content of the human body. So, it follows on, till we get to the trace elements which appear to be quite small in terms of the amounts but they have significant biochemical involvement in our body.

(Approx. elemental composition of an 80kg human body)

Elements	Amount (80Kg) %	Elements	Amount (80Kg) %
Oxygen	52kg 65	Copper	0.08g
Carbon	14.0kg 17.5	Manganese	0.0136g
Hydrogen	7.6kg 9.5	Molybdenum	0.0104g
Nitrogen	2.4kg 3	Chromium	Very small amount
Calcium	1.2kg 1.3	Selenium	Very small amount
Phosphorus	0.88kg 1.1	Cobalt	Very small amount
Sulphur	0.2kg 0.25	Vanadium	Very small amount

Potassium	0.2kg	0.25	Lithium	Very small amount
Sodium	0.12kg	0.15		
Chlorine	0.12kg	0.15		
Magnesium	40g	0.05		
Iron	4.8g	0.006		
Fluorine	3.0g	0.00375		
Zinc	2.6g	0.00325		
Strontium	0.37g	0.0005		
Iodine	0.0128g			

Minerals play an important role in our biochemical processes which keeps us alive. Just like vitamins, minerals also take part in various metabolic functions, e.g., they combine with various enzymes to form co-enzymes and participate in the energy-producing reactions, in the growth and maintenance of our body, in healing processes, as adjuncts to vitamins and also facilitate the uptake of vitamins by the cells. They are also involved in the maintenance and repair of our cellular structure. Trace elements function as co-factors to regulate enzymatic reactions. All trace elements are important for our health and well-being, e.g., iron is required for co-factoring many metabolic enzymes; copper is necessary to neutralise toxins by co-factoring with several liver enzymes and magnesium co-factors with about 300 enzymes for energy-producing reactions where ATP is the main energy-producing molecule and many more.

Zinc plays an important role in the metabolic pathway for glycolysis of sugars (fructose) by co-factoring with certain liver enzymes and Aldolase. Zinc is also an important co-factor for many other enzyme systems such DNA and RNA polymerases involved in the metabolism of nucleic acids. Another trace element which is required in a very small quantity is Molybdenum which co-factors with a group of enzymes called oxidase enzymes necessary for purine nucleotide catabolism. Molybdenum is also important for the detoxification of residual sulphur-containing compounds (sulphates) by co-factoring with the enzyme sulphite oxidase in the metabolism of sulphur-containing compounds such as amino acid cysteine.

The dosages of elements particularly trace elements required as supplements are very important as there is not much margin between the safe dose and the therapeutic dose. Too much may cause toxicity and too little may not have significant clinical benefit.

The macro-elements such as oxygen, carbon, hydrogen, nitrogen, etc., are all involved in the bio-synthesis of hormones, steroids, proteins, essential fatty acids, etc., while the trace minerals or the trace elements are involved in the manufacture of red blood cells, haemoglobin (iron), hydroxyapatite (calcium), adenosine triphosphate (phosphorous), glutathione (sulphur), thyroxine (iodine), etc. These are bio-molecules which are ineffective in the absence of relevant trace elements.

Trace elements are found in varying amounts in living tissues, they are not required in bulk quantities as the macro-elements and are nutritionally sufficient in minute quantities to perform essential biochemical tasks assigned to them naturally or physiologically. The main function of these elements is to act in conjunction with specific enzymes as biological catalysts and ensure the efficient completion of those biochemical reactions.

Unlike vitamins, trace elements are stable entities and have a high threshold to heat and humidity meaning, they are quite stable and therefore maintain their nutritional value effectively.

If ingested in higher dosages, trace elements can be toxic and side effects such as gastro-intestinal disorders, nausea, vomiting, cramps and other specific discomforts related to specific trace elements may be encountered.

Mineral Chart

Minerals	Physiological functions	Some Popular Food Sources	Daily Requirements
Calcium	Blood clotting. Healthy Bone, teeth and skeletal structure. Muscle and blood vessels Constriction and relaxation. Hormone secretion. Nervous system function.	Canned seafood with bones (e.g., salmon and sardines). Dairy products, Tofu. Fortified ready to eat foods and beverages. Green vegetables	1–1.3 (g)
Magnesium	Blood pressure regulation. Energy production. Immune function. Cardiovascular health Nervous system function.	Fruits Avocados, bananas and raisins. Beans. Peas, Potatoes, etc. Dairy products, whole grains. Green leafy vegetables, nuts and pumpkin seeds	320–420 (mg)

Iron	Energy production. Immune function. Red blood cell formation. Reproduction. Wound healing. Also, helps in the energy metabolism.	Beans and green vegetables, Fruits (e.g., raisins and prunes). Eggs and Poultry, Meat, Liver, Seafood. Nuts, Seeds, whole grain. Iron enriched foods	8–18 (mg)
Zinc	Growth and development. Antioxidant, immune function. Nervous system function. Sexual health and reproduction. Wound healing. Co-factor in many enzyme systems.	Beans and peas. Beef and Poultry. Dairy products. Fortified cereals and whole grains and nuts. Shellfish.	8–14 (mg)
Copper	Antioxidant. Collagen and connective tissue formation. Energy production. Iron metabolism. Nervous system function. Co-factor enzyme system	Chocolate and cocoa. Crustaceans and shellfish. Lentils, nuts and seeds. Organ meats liver kidney whole grains.	1.2–1.7 (mg)
Sodium	Acid-base and Fluid balance. Blood pressure regulation. Muscle contraction. Nervous system function. Cellular structure integrity.	Breads and cereal Cheese. Cold cuts and cured meats and Chicken, Eggs. Hot dogs. Snacks (chips, crackers, etc.). Soups, fried foods, fast foods.	2300 (mg)
Potassium	Blood pressure regulation. Fluid balance. Muscle contraction. Nervous system function. Has similar function as Sodium. It is the major cation inside the cell fluid while Sodium is outside.	Beans and vegetables (e.g., potatoes, sweet potatoes, beet green vegetables). Dairy products Fruits (e.g., bananas, dried apricots). Seafood (e.g., clams and salmon). Tomato and products.	4700 (mg)

Manganese	Carbohydrate, protein, and cholesterol metabolism. Cartilage and bone formation. Co-factor enzyme system. Role in bone health, antioxidant, fats and carbohydrate metabolism.	Beans, Spinach, Sweet potato. Nuts and whole grains. Pineapple.	2.3 (mg)
Chromium	Insulin function. Protein, carbohydrate and fat metabolism. Regulation of blood glucose	Fruits (apples and bananas), Green vegetables, Broccoli Juices (e.g., grape and orange). Spices garlic and basil. Meat and Turkey. Nuts and whole grains.	35 (mcg)
Selenium	Antioxidant and Anti-Inflammatory. Lowers oxidative stress Immunity and reproductive function. Thyroid function.	Eggs and Poultry Meats and seafood. Nuts (e.g., Brazil nuts) and seeds. Whole grains. Enriched pasta and rice.	55 (mcg)
Phosphorus	Bone Health. Healthy teeth. Energy production and storage. Hormone activation. It helps maintain body's acid-base balance and is a part of every cell with in the body.	Beans and peas Dairy products. Meat, Poultry and Seafood. Nuts and seeds, whole grain, Enriched, and fortified cereals and breads.	1250 (mg)
Chloride	Acid-base and fluid balance. Conversion food into energy. Digestive functions Nervous system function.	Olives, Vegetables (e.g., celery, lettuce, and tomatoes). Seaweeds (dulse and kelp). Table salt and sea salts.	2300 (mg)

Sulphur	Build and repair DNA structure. Healthy skin, ligaments and tendons. Required in bio-synthesis of proteins and amino acids. It is a natural anti-bacterial agent.	Leafy green vegetables, onions garlic, leaks, radish and shallots. Nuts, seeds, grains, and legumes. Meats, eggs, fish, turkey and poultry.	No daily Requirements have been set.

Ref: (US Food and Drug Administration (FDA); www.fda.gov/nutritioneducation Interactive Nutrition Facts Label • March 2020

www.fda.gov/nutritioneducation Vitamins and Minerals Chart 1) and Mineral Therapy (Important functions and minimum daily required amounts) dietaryguidlines@nhmrc.gov.au or info@health.govt.nz.

Please note that there are many other references and most have variable data reported; however, the data in the chart above must be verified and are only for reference purposes.

Some elements work biochemically in groups or clusters; for example, elements sodium, potassium and chlorine are important elements in the body fluids. Sodium and chlorine are ions in the extracellular fluid while potassium is inside the cell fluid, intracellular and responsible for maintaining the osmotic pressure between the cell membrane, i.e., from within and from outside so that the integrity of cellular shape is maintained.

If the shape of our cells is not maintained to its right configuration, then nutrients and oxygen carrying capacity as in red blood cells (aided by haemoglobin) will be impaired causing disruption to the body's homeostasis which is the ability of a living organism to maintain body's internal environment to a condition of continued survival.

Sodium, potassium and chlorine in their ionised forms (cations, a positively charged ion and anion a negatively charged ion) assist in maintaining body's homeostasis state.

Iron and sulphur also form a stable alliance within the body with unique properties which makes them particularly useful in biochemical reactions involving electron transfers due to their ability to store electrons and release them when needed. Therefore, both are important co-factors in many vital enzymatic reactions such as participating in NADH dehydrogenase, Coenzyme Q and cytochrome-C enzyme systems.

Iron as a trace mineral is also important in forming co-factors with other specific enzyme systems in partnership with Phosphorous and Iodine.

The functions of metals that catalyse biological processes as metal-enzyme complexes: It is estimated that in excess of 25% of all enzymes in our system form complexes or co-factors (Metalloenzymes) to catalyse numerous biochemical processes.

In these metal-enzyme complexes, the metal ion is firmly bound to the enzyme active sites and functions both as electron donors and acceptors. Several metal ions such as magnesium, iron, zinc, copper, manganese, molybdenum, etc., form complexes which have important roles in human biochemical functions.

The table represents examples of minerals which act as co-factors in various enzymatic systems; this table by no means is exhaustive and there are numerous other examples of the Metalloenzymes in our system part-taking in our daily biological processes.

Metal-Enzymes Complexes

Elements	Enzymatic System	Functions
Magnesium	Glucose6-phosphate Hexokinase: DNA polymerase:	Hydrolyses Glucose 6-phosphate to free glucose Phosphorylates hexoses, forming hexose phosphate. This enzyme catalyses the synthesis of DNA molecules from nucleoside triphosphates.
Iron	Catalase: Hydrogenase: Aconitase:	This enzyme catalyses the decomposition of Hydrogen Peroxide into water and oxygen. It catalyses the reversible oxidation of molecular hydrogen. This is the enzyme system that catalyses the isomerisation of citrates to isocitrates.
Zinc	Alcohol dehydrogenase: Carboxypeptidase: Aminopeptidase:	These are dehydrogenase enzymes and participate in the metabolism of alcohols, aldehyde and ketone molecules in our diets. It is a protease enzyme which hydrolyses the peptide bond at the end of a protein or peptide containing carboxyl terminal. While the Aminopeptidases does the same thing at the Nitrogen terminus.

Copper	Cytochrome: oxidase: Laccase: Nitrous-oxide reductase: Nitrite reductase:	Its basic function is to reduce molecular oxygen to form water which helps in ATP production. It is multi-copper containing enzyme with diverse biological profiles. It breaks down harmful phenolic compounds, it is also eco-friendly. It is also multi-copper enzyme which reduces the green-house gas Nitrous Oxide to nitrogen gas and denitrification of certain bacteria, e.g., *E. Coli*. This enzyme catalyses the reduction of Nitrites to ammonia/ammonium ion. Nitrites can be harmful as they can damage the cells and form nitrosamines which are carcinogenic.
Manganese	Arginase:	Arginase is a manganese containing enzyme which is the final enzymatic system of the urea cycle. It converts Arginine to urea and amino acid ornithine.
Molybdenum	Nitrate reductase: Sulphite oxidase: Xanthine oxidase:	Nitrate reductase are molybdenum containing enzyme system which reduces nitrates to nitrites. This enzyme system oxidises sulphites to sulphates. These enzymes catalyse the oxidation of hypoxanthine to xanthine and also catalyse the oxidation of xanthine to uric acid. These enzymes play an important role in the catabolism of purines in humans.

Although minerals are inactive substances, they account for 6% of our body weight and play an important role in our health and well-being in combination with various protein structures.

Summarising their major roles, the following immediately springs to mind:

Metal-Enzyme Complexes; this has been discussed briefly above.

Bio-complexes; e.g., Haemoglobin (containing iron) for the transportation of oxygen to our tissues, metallo-proteins which are formed as a part of metallic elements and protein structure and it is estimated that almost half of all proteins in our body contain one or multiple metals. Zinc is also found in the hormone insulin.

Zinc-finger proteins are one of the most abundant groups of proteins and have a wide range of biochemical functions as these are able to interact with DNA, RNA, PAR (poly-ADP-ribose) and other proteins.

Tissue Mineralisation and Tissue Salts: Many minerals are a part of our soft tissues and form a protective layer. Important examples are bone and teeth tissues (calcium and other minerals). Our skeletal structure has mineralised tissues.

The concept of tissue salt was developed by the German medical doctor Schuessler (b.1821–d. 1889). He maintained that to keep a normal balance among the vital tissue salts we must take in the deficient mineral salt in a homeopathic form which will rapidly assimilate into the bloodstream and be deposited into the tissues. There are 12 Schuessler salts.

Schuessler's salts:

(Ref: https://www.healthline.com/health/tissue-salts)

Schuessler's salts	Chemical Name	Health Benefits
Calc. Fluor	Calcium Fluoride	Strengthens tooth enamel and bones, restores tissue elasticity, helps haemorrhoids; helps hernia pain.
Calc. Phos	Calcium Phosphate	Restores cells, heals fractures, helps the digestive system.
Calc. Sulph	Calcium Sulphate	Purifies blood and reduces infection, treats skin disorders such as acne, prevents sore throats and colds.
Ferr. Phos	Ferrous Phosphate	Anti-inflammatory; reduces fever, accelerates healing reduces bleeding.
Kali. Mur	Potassium Chloride	Purifies blood; treats infection, reduces swelling aids digestion.
Kali. Phos	Potassium Phosphate	Supports nerve health, lessens anxiety, irritability, and fatigue; relieves headaches, aids memory.
Kali. Sulph	Potassium Sulphate	Heals mucous membrane; heals skin balances metabolism conditions your pancreas.

Mag. Phos	Magnesium Phosphate	Eases cramps and pain, reduces spasms, relieves tension headaches.
Nat. Mur	Sodium Chloride	Balances bodily fluids, reduces water retention, aids digestion treats eczema.
Nat. Phos	Sodium Phosphate	Neutralises acidity and aids digestion, relieves seasickness, treats arthritis.
Nat. Sulph	Sodium Sulphate	Cleans pancreas, cleans kidneys and liver, treats cold and flu
Silica	Silicon Dioxide	Conditions skin, conditions connective tissue, cleanses blood, strengthens hair and nails.

Electrolytes and electrolyte imbalance: There are three major elements Sodium, potassium, and chlorine which regulate the fluid balance in our body. Calcium and phosphorus also have an important role to play. The concentrations of these elements must be at a certain required level to function optimally. When the concentration of these elements is not at their desired levels, then there is a shift in the balance resulting in electrolyte imbalance. Although, the kidneys are entrusted with the task of regulating the balance. Body's electrolyte balance must be within a narrow range of compliance for the body to function adequately.

One of the most important functions of electrolytes is to maintain the integrity of the cellular structure, any compromise will cause lack of fluid balance in the intra-cellular (controlled by potassium) and the extra-cellular (controlled by Sodium) fluids and the osmotic pressure through the cell membrane which maintains the shape of the cells. If the shape is compromised in anyway, then the transportation of nutrients and oxygen will be seriously disrupted leading to health complications. Besides this, there are many more reasons why the electrolyte balance should be maintained at all times.

It controls normal blood pressure and blood pH within the required range. Important for the growth of new tissues and to maintain their health and nourishment. It regulates the nerve and muscle activities. Electrolytes generate and carry electrical charge in the body, you can say they work in similar fashion as a real battery. This electricity is used by our nervous system to send signals to our brain which sends messages via the neurotransmitters to various body organs to function; a classic example is the beating of the heart, the voluntary muscle actions and some of the sensory actions and many more. If the electrolytes did not generate electrical current, then our body may not function the same as a car would not run on flat batteries.

There are several reasons which can cause an electrolyte imbalance in our system. One of the prime reasons is sweating excessively which causes loss of fluids and electrolytes from our body. Other reasons are vomiting, not drinking enough water and metabolic disorders which cause large urinary output. Kidney dysfunction is also an important reason along with a lack of Anti-Diuretic Hormone (ADH) can be a serious cause. An important solution is to drink plenty of water, keep hydrated with electrolyte drinks especially during hot weather when we tend to lose body fluids in the way of excess sweating and frequent urination. Especially at risk are elderly seniors, convulsing and infirm patients.

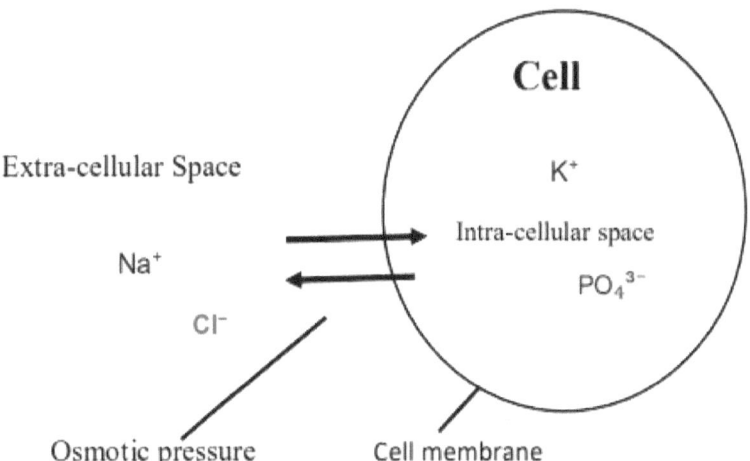

Distribution of Electrolytes in Cellular environment (A spherical shaped cell with higher surface area to maximise Oxygen and Nutrient carrying capacity).

Health Benefits of Commonly Used Herbs

Herbs unlike vitamins and minerals occur naturally as plant materials and in vegetation. They are applied in many ways in human health and general well-being. Some herbs are used in our cooking to enhance the taste and flavour, some are used as infusions and teas, and many herbs have been scientifically processed to define the active ingredients which are found to be of therapeutic value. These herbs have been processed to an end usable form called dry herbal extracts with an assayable quantity of the active ingredient. Multiple herbs and/or their extracts are manufactured into distinct dosage forms (tablets, capsules or liquid) for use in various diseases. If prescribed in a correct manner, then herbs can be of significant value and at par with vitamin and mineral therapy.

Herbs have been used since time immemorial, these are plant matter which have wonderful healing properties and were used in ancient times unwittingly not knowing their effect on human physiological and psychological status. It was trial and error and we can say a self-conducted and managed clinical trial.

Today we know a lot about herbs and medicinal plants, and, from their early knowledge acquired we in modern times are successful in building up a repository of knowledge for our general health and well-being.

My first introduction to herbs in a scientific and academic way was when I came across a book on herbs by Nancy Beckham in the early 1980s which rekindled my interest in herbs and their application in human health. Rekindled, because my earliest encounters with herbs were very early in my life when my mother either used them for culinary purposes and, or, applied them for our little nicks and bruises and other minor ailments which were quite regular when we were growing up.

Later in life, I was introduced to a book written on the scientific use of herbs which really gave me an in-depth view on the application of herbs in alternative medicine. However, it is common knowledge that over the years many orthodox medicines have made use of herbs in significant ways, especially in respiratory and abdominal medicines which have become common members of many household medicine chests.

The use of herbs in human health dates back to many generations; I have noted that its application in ancient Greek, Chinese and Indian traditional medicines dates back to many centuries. Reference have also been made to almost 20,000 BCE with discoveries of cave paintings suggesting that the use of herbs in that prehistoric time era was not uncommon.

The credibility of herbs began when traditional Chinese and Indian medicines evolved around 2000–3000 years ago and still to this day their traditional use have been quite strong.

A Greek physician by the name of Pedanius Dioscorides wrote the first book on herbal plants and medicine, 'De Materia Medica', a 5-volume encyclopaedia around 65 AD which remains one of the earliest reference books on herbs that still survives to this day.

It would be unfair of me to simply ignore the earlier traditional physicians such as the early Sumerians who practiced traditional herbal medicines even before the great Greek Philosophers and Scholars became interested in this subject matter. Hippocrates in the 5th century BCE, revered as the father of modern medicine in one of his chronicles listed more than 400 herbs and their traditional uses.

As I have mentioned earlier, herbs have also been very widely used in culinary art. Foods cooked with herbs not only tasted good but also had some health benefits. When I was growing up, coriander and curry leaves were extensively used in Asian cooking, particularly in South East Asian cooking. Now, we know for a fact that coriander and curry leaves have tons of interesting health properties.

Let's look at both of these common household culinary herbs used in Eastern dishes primarily the sub-continent and places like Malaysian, Singaporean, Indian and Sri Lankan dishes.

Coriander: Botanically known as *Coriandrum sativum*, coriander may lower blood sugar by activating certain enzymes. Coriander contains antioxidants which have demonstrable immune-boosting effects. Coriander may also protect heart health by lowering the bad cholesterol (LDL) and increase the good cholesterol (HDL) levels. Antioxidants in coriander may reduce brain inflammation, helping to reduce anxiety symptoms and improve memory.

It also exhibits antimicrobial properties and may reduce the effect of *Salmonella* (Salmonella is a pathogen and is responsible for food poisoning). Antioxidants in coriander have been known to protect skin from sun damage if applied topically.

When ingested, coriander herb is quite safe and has been known to have been used in cooking for generations and in significant quantities.

Coriander seeds and oils are also used in culinary applications and in some cases limited topical applications.

The herb may also have some positive effects on digestive discomforts.

(Ref: Surprising Health Benefits of Coriander—Health line https://www.healthline.com › nutrition › coriander-bene…and also Webmed)

Coriander Herb (Comparison, fresh and dry herb seeds)
(Ref: Nutrient composition of coriander leaf and seeds as per USDA National Nutrition Data base, 2013).

Nutrients	Coriander leaf/100g	Coriander seed/100g
Water	7.3g	8.86g
Energy	279 kcal	298 kcal
Protein	21.93g	12.37g
Total Lipids (Fats)	4.78g	17.77g
Carbohydrates (by difference)	52.10g	54.99g
Fibre (Total dietary)	10.4g	41.9g
Calcium	1246mg	709mg
Iron	42.46mg	16.32mg
Magnesium	694mg	330mg
Phosphorous	481mg	409mg
Potassium	4466mg	1267mg
Sodium	211mg	35mg
Zinc	4.72mg	4.70mg
Vitamin C (Total ascorbic acid)	566.7mg	21.0mg
Thiamine (vitamin B1)	1.252mg	0.239mg
Riboflavin (vitamin B2)	1.50mg	0.290mg
Niacin (vitamin B3)	10.707mg	2.130mg
Vitamin B12	-	-
Vitamin A I.U	5850	-
Vitamin D	-	-
Total saturated fatty acids	0.115g	0.990g
Total monounsaturated fatty acids	2.232g	13.580g
Total polyunsaturated fatty acids	0.328g	1.750g
Cholesterol	-	-

Curry Leaves: Botanically known as *Murraya koenigii,* curry leaves contain heaps of antioxidants which may help in stress release and reduce the effects of free radical damage.

May improve heart health by reducing cholesterol and triglycerides. Topically curry leaves can be applied for the effective treatment of burns, bruises and skin eruptions.

The leaves have many pharmacological activities such as anti-diabetic, cholesterol-reducing properties, antimicrobial activities, etc.

It is also noted for its anti-ulcer and anti-oxidant activities.

It is good for digestion.

(Ref: Sinha Parul, Akhtar Javed, Batra Neha, Jain Honey, Bhardwaj Anju, Curry Leaves-A medicinal herb. Asian J. Pharm Res. 2 (2): April June 2021 p. 51–53). AND Curry Leaf Benefits and Uses—Healthline.

I have personally read these publications and feel comfortable with the properties of these two herbs. However, in order to get due credit and be accepted as a mainstream herbal reference guides, further trials are needed. I have also found some nutritional data on these two herbs as presented below which I felt was also important to establish the credibility of their application.

Curry Leaves, Nutritional value per 100g (Data sourced from USDA)

Parameters	Values
Energy	108kcal
Protein	6.1g
Fibre	6.4g
Phosphorous	57mg
Calcium	830mg
Iron	0.93mg
Magnesium	44mg
Carotene	7560mcg
Riboflavin	0.210mg
Niacin	2.3mg
Vitamin C	4mg
Folic Acid	23.5mcg

Parsley and Coriander are sometimes confused to be the same herb as the broad leaf parsley and coriander look similar. Apart from the fundamental difference in the odour. Parsley is an exceptionally rich source of Vitamin K which is K1 (Phylloquinone) and vitamin K2 (Menaquinone) a group of fat-soluble vitamins particularly important for human dietary needs due to its role in blood clotting and bone metabolism.

Parsley finds extensive use in Western food preparations mainly in salads and soups and has a pleasant taste and flavour.

There are some good evidences in favour of parsley for our general health and well-being.

It helps to improve calcium absorption and also our bone density status. Research has demonstrated that myricetin present in parsley helps in the treatment and prevention of diabetes.

It also possesses some anti-inflammatory properties and may be capable of reducing circulating fats from blood.

Nutritional analysis of Parsley (30g)

Parsley is rich in vitamin K which is important in our dietary needs.

Calories: 11 calories
Carbs: 2 grams
Protein: 1 gram
Fat: less than 1 gram
Fibre: 1 gram
Vitamin A: 108% of the Reference Daily Intake (RDI).
Vitamin C: 53% of the RDI
Vitamin K: 547% of the RDI
Folate: 11% of the RDI
Potassium: 4% of the RDI

Nutritional Data for all the three herbs mentioned above reflects a significant nutritional content for minerals, fibre and protein and would make an ideal supplement for addition to our culinary delights.

Apart from coriander and curry leaves there are 12 culinary herbs of my choice that are commonly used in most kitchens. The table below indicates some of their most sought-after health benefits.

Herbs and Spices	Common Botanical Name	Clinical Benefits
Holy Basil	*Ocimum basilicum*	Anti-bacterial, anti-fungal and boosts immunity
Turmeric	*Curcuma longa*	Anti-inflammatory

Garlic	*Allium sativum*	Immunity and blood pressure control
Ginger	*Zingiber officinale*	Nausea and anti-inflammatory
Fenugreek	*Trigonella foenum-graecum*	Blood sugar control
Cinnamon	*Cinnamomum verum*	Blood sugar control
Peppermint	*Mentha piperita*	Anti-nausea, calming effect
Parsley	*Petroselinum crispum*	Rich in vitamin K, important in bone health.
Rosemary	*Rosmarinus officinalis*	Anti-allergic and anti-inflammatory
Sage	*Salvia officinalis*	Memory and brain function
Thyme	*Thymus vulgaris*	Thyme is good for bacterial, viral, fungal, and parasitic infections.
Chives	*Allium Schoenoprasum*	Helps in common digestive problems.

The list above can easily be extended by the addition of several more commonly used culinary herbs, these include Dill (*Anethum Graveolens*), Fennel seeds (*Foeniculum Vulgare*), Oregano (*Origanum Vulgare*), Lemongrass (*Cymbopogon Citratus*) and many more.

Apart from their culinary use to enhance taste, these herbs also have mild to significant health benefits as mentioned; the intake quantities vary in order to extract the therapeutic benefits.

There are also herbs which are used as teas (aqueous infusions) offering quite a valuable health benefit.

I have picked a few for our understanding and to evaluate the scientifically proven benefits, and what the scientific communities say about some of these herbal teas.

The first tea that comes to my mind is **Jasmine** (*Jasminum officinale*) tea which is invariably served at the conclusion of a Chinese cuisine. Looking up at some of the scientific information I found that Jasmine tea is packed in nutritional goodness. It is rich in polyphenol antioxidants which have been linked with a reduction in heart disease risks and also reduces the oxidation rate of bad cholesterol (LDL) thus preventing our arteries from clogging. It boosts our metabolic rate and increases the rate of fat burning by 10–16%. I think this is why Jasmine tea is served in most good Chinese restaurants after meals.

History would have it that it was introduced into China from South Asia during the Han dynasty (206 BC–220 AD) but its actual use first originated in Fuzhou in Fujian Province during the Song dynasty (960–1127 AD).

Camellia Sinensis: is a green tea and has been used for several centuries for its medicinal properties. It is the common tea as we know it today and comes in many varieties, e.g., black tea, green tea, white tea, etc.

The important health benefits come from the content of bioactive phenolic antioxidant compounds catechins, caffeine and also amino acid L-threonine. The primary health benefits of drinking *Camellia Sinensis* are for heart health, reduction of LDL, lowering of blood cholesterol, triglycerides and blood pressure. Drinking this tea also helps lower the anxiety and stress levels and also improves immunity.

Echinacea (Angustifolia and Purpurea): Echinacea is also high in antioxidants and bioflavonoids which have many proven health benefits; if the tea is drunk on a regular basis, it has the potential to improve our immune function, lower blood glucose, inflammation, and stress and anxiety levels. Several studies published in trusted journals suggest that Echinacea may also help fight infections and viruses and help recover faster from illness.

Chamomile: When you need peace and tranquillity, suffering from depression and need a good night's sleep you immediately think of Chamomile tea. It also contains an antioxidant called apigenin which has been known to promote sleep and it has also been found that drinking Chamomile tea may improve the quality of sleep.

In a 2016 study (Ref: J Adv Nurs 2016 Feb; 72 (2):306–15), the effects of an intervention with drinking chamomile tea on sleep quality and depression in sleep-disturbed postnatal women was studied, it was a randomised controlled trial and the conclusion was that Chamomile tea may be recommended to postpartum (the period immediately after child-birth) women as a supplementary approach to alleviating depression and sleep quality problems.

In a December 2019 study published in the Journal of Pharmacopuncture, it has been suggested that Chamomile tea may be helpful in women with PMS (premenstrual syndrome).

Chamomile tea is a very refreshing, healthy and safe to drink beverage. It also has a pleasant taste and an acceptable aroma and flavour and therefore a cup of chamomile tea can be beneficial for all particularly the senior members of our population.

Rosehip (*Rosa Canina*): Rosehip is the fruit of rose bush, and has been used throughout human history since the pre-historic times. It is also believed to be one of the oldest medicinal plants. Its reference has been mentioned about 600 BC in the writings of a Greek poet Sappho who referred to it as the queen of flowers due to the beauty of a rose flower. The ancient Chinese, Persians, Egyptians and other ancient civilisations were fascinated with the rose fruit (rosehip) and applied it in various healing medications.

Pliny the Elder, the Roman scholar and herbalist applied various preparations of rosehip for the remedy of toothaches to dog bites. It is believed that the Latin name Rosa Canina or Dog Rose came from this dog bite medication. Modern-day research has revealed that rosehip contains significant levels of Vitamin C and also other antioxidant chemicals, e.g., carotenoids, polyphenols Vitamin E and Astaxanthin, etc., and has a powerful antioxidant activity. Regularly drinking rosehip tea promotes collagen synthesis and has a significant effect on the antiaging process.

Pine needles (Latin name genus Pinus, spruce genus Picea): The story goes that in 1536, French explorer Jacques Cartier while exploring the area of present-day Gulf of St. Lawrence in Eastern Canada got stranded in the icy waters of the St. Lawrence River. Most of his crew were suffering from a mysterious disease that threatened to kill more than half of his crew. Seeing this Cartier sought help from the local Iroquois Indians who advised Cartier to drink a concoction of spruce tree needles (Pine tree) which they called the tree of life (arbor vitæ).

Surprisingly Cartier's crew suffering from the mysterious illness now we know as scurvy got better only after a few days of drinking the spruce tree needle tea. Today we know that spruce tree needles and bark contain up to 5 times more vitamin C than oranges. It also contains nutrients, e.g., polyphenols like procyanidins, catechins, and phenolic acids.

Pine needles and bark have been researched extensively and reported to offer significant health benefits in heart health, inflammation, promotes healthy ageing and in general a well-tolerated herbal medicine.

In a recent publication (January 2020 in the European Journal of Preventive Cardiology), it was found that drinking tea especially green tea at least 3 times a week may increase longevity compared with non-tea drinkers.

There are many herbs and spices which have been used for many centuries as safe herbal medicines, many of them are still in use today with scientific validations to many of the claims; some of these which are popularly used are:

Ginger Tea which has proven benefits in the treatment of Nausea and Vomiting, antioxidant properties and also anti-inflammatory. The active in ginger is Gingerol with powerful medicinal properties. Ginger is also used in cooking and in pharmaceutical preparations.

Peppermint Tea is extensively used in mild digestive ailments.

Hibiscus Tea has been known to be used in lowering blood pressure and cholesterol.

Fennel seed Tea may ease Menopause Symptoms and stimulate milk production in nursing mothers, helps with easing Flatulence, improves Digestion processes and boosts metabolism.

There seem to be herbal teas and combinations available for every mild form of common ailments that we suffer from. Some of the highly beneficial but lesser-known herbal teas are as follows which do have some scientific validation of their claims.

Passion Flower Tea: It contains flavones and bioflavonoids and helps in mild symptoms of anxiety and restlessness and may aid in a good restful night's sleep.

Liquorice Tea: It has been known to have some beneficial effects on aches and pains, mild flu symptoms and anti-inflammatory properties. It has a strong taste characterised by combining all the taste sensations e.g., sweet, sour, salty and also bitter taste.

Dandelion Tea: Dandelion tea has been used quite extensively for its positive effects on liver health. It has also been used in aiding immune-boost and fight against infection. It also has a diuretic effect helping to flush the body to get rid of toxins and improve the healing process.

Cayenne Tea: It may not be very popular as a tea on its own due to its bitter and hot stinging taste and may be acceptable to only some. But it certainly packs a punch when it is used for the relief of scratchy, inflamed and painful throats, tonsils and the general pharynx area. It can also provide significant relief in mild colds if used at the onset of the flu symptoms.

Ginseng Tea: Very popular among Asian tea drinkers and known to possess immune-modulatory properties. It contains among many important biochemical constituents, Ginsenosides and Polysaccharides which have potential immune boosting, protection against viral and bacterial infections and autoimmune diseases (Ref: Trends in Food Science and Technology volume 83, January 2019, Pages 12–30). Its use has also been proven to reduce tiredness and fatigue by increasing energy levels and also has been reported to be useful in erectile dysfunction (Ref: Asian J Androl. 2007 Mar; 9(2):241–4).

It is important to realise that herbal medicines and teas are meant to be taken on a regular basis not just as a once-off or at the height of a particular ailment hoping for a quick fix. Benefits are achievable on a regular timely use. Also, before using herbal medicines it is absolutely necessary to have a proper guidance of a qualified herbalist and to follow directives given in relation to the use of such products.

The use of herbal medicines in the past few decades has shown a wider public acceptance and consequently, their use in various forms, e.g., in tinctures, liquid extracts, tablets and capsules, teas and infusions and also in plain crushed dry herbal powders has increased in primary healthcare or as an adjunct to orthodox medicines. It is now estimated that around 80% of the world-wide population have used herbal products in some form in their normal course of preventive or primary healthcare regime.

With increasing use, comes an increased responsibility of the herbal medicine manufacturers, regulatory bodies, herbal medicine practitioners and above all us the consumers for its safety, efficacy and also drug-herbal interactions. Herbal preparations have been used in human society for many centuries and have also been believed since the dawn of modern human society in their earliest beginning. In general, their safety has long been established; however, with the advent of modern drugs (medicinal products) many of which are synthetic in nature pose a real threat to drug-herbal interactions. Simple preparations such as tinctures or herbal teas may not pose any serious risks or threats of interactions if used in moderation and with a common sense approach due to the dilution factors.

Herbal teas are calorie-free like water.

But when used in much higher concentrations and laced with impurities the risk or threat can become a real issue and often the concerns are worth noting.

A trip to the local health care services or centres may be useful. Like any medication, herbs and their preparations if used with caution and with a sensible approach can provide significant benefits and work side by side with the orthodox medicines, but, with carefree use without heeding qualified directions, there can be many negative effects such as; diarrhoea, in some cases constipation, nausea and vomiting, headaches, allergic reactions and skin rashes, asthma and respiratory problems and also sleeplessness. These can initially show up as mild complications.

Usually, self-administration of herbs, poor quality preparations with contamination and impurities in the form of adulteration and prescription of wrong herbs for wrong symptoms can manifest as above-mentioned complications. It is always important to check with your herbalist and make sure that your symptoms match with the prescription; and it is a good idea to seek the services of a qualified and a registered herbal practitioner. In cases of pregnancy and lactating or nursing mothers, additional caution is required and if need be, re-confirm or have a second opinion if in doubt and at the first sign of discomfort stop using the medication and seek qualified help.

This is true not just only for herbal medicines but also for orthodox medicines. There can be interaction of prescription medicines and herbal medicines if both are taken at the same time. Unless there are some known interactions of concern it is best to space both forms of medications well between dosage administrations so that both may be able to deliver the full physiological effect and the user gets a chance to experience the best of both forms of medication. Should there be known interactions then it is best not to take them in conjunction and avoid a harmful consequence.

The table presented below briefly outlines the interactions that herbal medicines can have with a drug molecule or a prescription medication and vice versa. Many of these medications and interactions have a low to moderate adverse or interactive effect and therefore a consultation with your professional health care adviser before taking an herbal medicine or a prescribed medicine will be a distinct advantage.

In order to learn more about these interactions, interested readers may look up the following website and make themselves aware of any side effects that they may possibly encounter when taking a prescription and herbal medicine together.

(Ref: Drug Interactions Checker—Medscape Reference https://reference.medscape.com › drug-interaction checker https://www.karger.com/Article/Fulltext/334488)

Herb/Drug Interactions

Herbs	Drugs	Interactive effect
Ginkgo	Anti-convalescents (anti-seizure anti-epileptic) Thiazides (Diuretics) Acetaminophens (Pain relievers)	May increase the episodes of seizures. May lead to hypertension. May cause bleeding in the brain causing increased pressure on the brain.
Garlic	Anti-hypertensive Aspirin and Warfarin Hypoglycaemic	May decrease blood pressure May lower blood sugar level

Ginger	Blood thinning medications (Aspirin and Warfarin) Diabetic medications	May increase the risk of bleeding May lower the blood sugar level
Chamomile	Blood thinning medications (Aspirin and Warfarin) Tranquilliser/Sedatives/ant	Increases the risk of bleeding Reduce the effect of the drug.
Rosehip	Blood thinning medications (Aspirin and Warfarin) Interaction with Oestrogens Anti-psychotic drugs	May slow the blood clotting process. May increase the effects and side effects of Oestrogens. May reduce the effects of the drug.
Cranberry	Warfarin	Increased anti-coagulant effect
Echinacea	Caffeine Midazolam	Reduction in blood caffeine concentration Increased bioavailability of the drug
Evening Primrose	Fluphenazine	May bring about seizure
Fenugreek	Warfarin	Increased anti-coagulant effect
Milk Thistle	Warfarin, Diazepam, Phenytoin, etc.	Decreases the effect of medication by lowering their concentration

Early History of Herbs

Turmeric is probably one of the oldest plants that has been used both as herbs (top plant part) and spice (the root and rhizome) which is still widely used in most kitchens around the world and also used as a medicinal herb. In ancient India, around 4000 BCE (about 6000 years ago) there are mentions of various applications of herbs and plants, medicinal preparations from minerals and also concoctions derived from animal sources. The Ayurvedic system of ancient medicinal practice is still in use today in some form which specialises in the use of traditional herbs and plant parts using roots, barks and leaves. The early Mesopotamians and the Sumerians also made use of herbs and medicinal plants and inscribed the study of herbs on clay tablets which dates back to 5000 years.

Archaeological findings in China suggest that in the Bronze age-period (3300 BCE–1200 BCE) herbs and herbal medicine practices were quite active. It is also known that the earliest emperor of ancient China, Shennong is believed to have written the first Chinese Pharmacopoeia '*Shénnóng Běncǎo Jīng*' or The Divine Farmer's Herb-Root Classic, one of the first-ever almanacs detailing the herbs used in Chinese medicine.

The original text '*Shénnóng Běncǎo Jīng*' has long been lost, it mentioned some 365 herbs and entries made on their safety and efficacies as a result of emperor Shennong's self-administering of the herbs which eventually was the cause of his death. It is believed that he died after consuming a toxic weed bearing yellow flowers perhaps Tansy (*Tanacetum Vulgare*) which contains alkaloids poisonous to humans.

In ancient Greece and Rome, there have been a number of pioneering figures starting from Hippocrates of Kos who was known to be the greatest physician of his time and presently known as the **Father of Modern Medicine**. Born around 460BC, his teachings and philosophies were compiled into a collection known as **'*Corpus Hippocraticum*'** which gave an early account of the medical work by Hippocrates in ancient Greece. Hippocrates had made reference to 250 or so herbs and plants to treat different diseases and ailments which grew in his native island of Kos mentioned in the Corpus Hippocraticum.

Galen, was a Greek physician around 130AD–210AD who became the greatest physician and Surgeon of ancient Rome during the time of Emperor Marcus Aurelius. Galen's writings are compiled in **'The Galenic Corpus'**. Galen's work on herbal medicine was very impressive and to this date certain herbal preparations are known as 'Galenicals'. Galen described in excess of 347 herbal remedies which earned him the title of 'Father of Pharmacology'.

Galen's teachings had a profound influence on **'Unani Medicine'**.

Pedanius Dioscorides was a Greek physician, pharmacologist and a botanist who authored a 5-volume encyclopaedia known to the western world as De Materia Medica about herbal medicines and other related medicinal products.

The **'De Materia Medica'** written between 50AD–70AD consisted of more than 1000 medicines containing herbal products, minerals and from animals.

Dioscorides's Materia Medica became the standard for all modern pharmacopoeia. Dioscorides evaluated more than 600 herbal and medicinal plants and classified them into groups by their characteristics; e.g., appearance, tastes, sharpness and other qualities of herbal parts roots, stems leaves and their aromatic properties. Several herbs such as the use of parsley having diuretic properties, fennel for improving milk flow, the herb horehound with honey as an expectorant and many more were all foretold by Dioscorides.

There are many Greco-Roman physicians who practiced herbal medicines and wrote treaties on medicines from herbs and plants which many of us still use to this day.

Ebers Papyrus of the ancient Egyptians dates back to around 1700 BCE some of which still survives today and mentions herbs like garlic, juniper, opioids, myrrh, thyme, cannabis, frankincense, fennel, etc., used by Egyptians who lived in those antiquated times. These herbs have been used for some 4000 years and were revered for their medicinal purposes and on important cultural occasions. It is now known that Ebers Papyrus listed over 850 herbal medicines many of those are used in today's herbal medicines.

The Indian **Ayurvedic** system of herbal medicine combined the simple essence of life; **Ayur** meaning life and **Veda** meaning knowledge and shifted the responsibility of health and well-being to the individuals. The earliest Ayurvedic texts are believed to have been composed by the ancient Munis, Rishis and the ancient practitioners of healthcare with knowledge passed on through generations and through self-experimentation of wild plants that grew around them. The earliest Ayurvedic shlokas (poetic verses in Sanskrit an ancient spoken language in India) depicting herbs and their properties were written around 3000 BCE–2500 BCE which makes them about 5000 years old. In successive generations of Ayurvedas, texts like **Charaka Samhita** and **Sushruta Samhita** were composed around 400 BCE–200 BCE to give the Ayurvedic system a more modern aspect of the traditional herbal medicinal practice.

In more recent times, Bhava Prakasha Nighantu was written in the 16th century AD by the renowned Indian Ayurvedic herbal practitioner Bhava Mishra who gave a more comprehensive meaning to the old scripture and introduced modern herbs. Throughout the ancient period Before Common Era (BCE) since the advent of the original Ayurveda, transformations have taken place and future authors have added specifics to enhance herbal knowledge as a modality for health care. Authors such as Susruta, Nagarjuna in the 5th century AD, 10th century authors Rangacharaya and Chandranandana followed through to Bhava Mishra all contributed in a big way for the future generations to marvel upon.

The beauty of Ayurveda is that it is still evolving to this day with the additions of Priya Nighantu, Dravyagunakosa, and Bedi Vanaspatikosa, etc., all written in the late 20th century (1980s–1998s). Ayurveda has not only provided insight into the ancient 5000-year-old philosophy of healing with natural medicine in particular native herbs available then, but, additions of contemporary herbals by subsequent generations of dedicated authors have enriched it with modern herbs and contemporary Ayurvedic practices. Many of the herbs described in the ancient Ayurvedic texts such as *Withania somnifera* (Aswagandha), Holy Basil (Tulsi), Bacopa (Brahmi), Turmeric (Haldi) etc. have all now become part of the commonly applied herbal remedies.

Herbal medicine has come a long way since the cave-dwelling early Homo sapiens (earliest reference about 60,000 years in cave paintings), followed by **Shénnóng Běncǎo Jīng** in the Bronze Age, ancient **Sumerians** (5000 years ago), ***Ebers Papyrus*** (1700 BCE) followed by the Islamic (Unani Herbal Medicines) in the medieval age and the Greco-Roman physicians **Hippocrates** to Pedanius Dioscorides the Greek author and many more who contributed to herbal medicine for generations to come. The Ayurvedic System of Herbal medicine possibly having the earliest roots of origin (5000 years) still continues to expand the horizons of natural and holistic practices of healing and health care.

In the last 5000 years of recorded history of medicinal herbs (herbs that have been used for human health and well-being), there has not been a single incidence of awarding a Nobel Prize directly for herbs and herbal medicine even though there has been a significant number of drug molecules extracted from herbs and plants which have served the human society admirably in the area of health care. So, when I heard that the Nobel Prize for Medicine (there is no category for herbal medicine) for 2021 was awarded to China's Tu Youyou for extracting an anti-malarial drug from an herb mentioned in a traditional text of Chinese medicine.

The herb concerned is Sweet Wormwood (*Artemesia annua*) which has its origins about 4th century BCE. Tu Youyou isolated Artemisinin from Artemesia annua which has proven to be an effective pharmacological active drug as an alternative to standard Chloroquine. Could this precedence be the prelude to more Nobel Prizes for herbs and herbal medicine in years to come, I certainly hope so as many herbal practitioners, and researchers from either side of the healthcare spectrum (alternative and orthodox) have dedicated their lives to working with herbs and plant species to extract pharmacologically active molecules for the general health and well-being of the humanity at large.

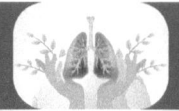

Chapter 9

MOVEMENTS, ENERGY EXPENDITURE AND SOME BASIC EXERCISE GUIDES

Body movement is the art of synchronising our body, mind and soul; our body benefits from movement and activates our inner healing processes.

– Jay Das, 2021

By allowing our body to move by way of physical activities, we are integrating our body functions with our motor control and skills and therefore sharpening our physiological and psychological parameters to a state of continued readiness and alertness.

Our human body is designed for movement and activity, with a consistent need for refuelling. Rest and relaxation are important pit stops along the way. Movement exercises are of more value in our advancing age. Due to natural loss, our ability and capacity for coordination between our physiological and psychological parameters diminish, movements and exercises become more necessary and important. We need to find a balance between age-related lag and normal requirements to enjoy a moderately active lifestyle.

This can be provided by good nutrition and regular exercise.

Below are some movements in the form of simple exercises which can be performed by all especially seniors to keep fit and keep moving so that stiffness in the joints arms and legs which are the most common causes of inactivity or inability to move freely can be helped.

Why do we need to do exercises?

There are many scientifically validated reasons why exercising helps. But remember some people have the ability to endure more workout pain and stress than others and so there are no hard and fast rules or strict time parameters.

The US Centre for Disease Control and Prevention (CDC) has recommended that we should do at least two and a half hours of moderate cardio-activity or one and a quarter of an hour of vigorous cardio exercises every week. Additionally, they have also recommended a 2-day strength training. This will obviously involve a reasonable amount of weight training, brisk running, and well-structured gym sessions. For our purposes to keep a target of achieving a reasonable level of fitness, simple exercises can be a good start. But by all means those who have the basic level of fitness, graduating to the next level as per the CDC's recommendation can be a good thing. But prior to undertaking vigorous cardio-activities, you must have a medical appraisal and also consultation from a cardio-activity instructor. Now let us look at some of the benefits of exercising.

Exercise enhances endurance and energy levels.

Doing exercise has been validated to assist in lowering the risk of chronic diseases.

Regular exercise has been shown to improve cognitive skills.

Exercise can also improve the sleep patterns.

Exercising can assist in weight loss in obesity situations which has positive benefits in obesity-related lifestyle diseases.

There are many more reasons why we should undertake to do some form of exercise on a regular basis. Although, it is not guaranteed that positive benefits will be evident soon thereafter; one thing is certain that these simple exercises as pictorially depicted in this chapter and others will assist in improving the movements and general activity level.

Better Health Channel Victorian Government, Australia (Ref: Physical Activity-its important-Better Health Channel www.betterhealth.vic.gov.au) in their better health publication recommends that we all should do at least 30 minutes of daily physical activities.

A minimum of 30 minutes activity can help minimise diabetes, cancer and cardiovascular diseases and can improve our quality of life.

According to the above reputable publication, regular physical activity may help and may even provide a long-term benefit in the following health conditions:

Reducing the risk of a heart attack.

Manage and improve weight control.

Assist in lowering blood cholesterol levels.

Lowering the risk of type 2 diabetes and some cancers and blood pressure.

Also, **strengthens bones, muscles and joints and lowers the risk of developing osteoporosis.**

Lowering the risk of falls.

Shorten the recovery time of hospitalisation or bed rest.

May also improve the energy levels, better mood, relaxed feeling and better sleep patterns.

Although all the above are important to senior's health and well-being, the last few highlighted benefits are worth noticing.

Several benefits cannot be quantified in terms of actual disease states, but it is a proven fact that continuity and regular long-term benefits of exercising are quite significant, particularly in the area of state of mind e.g., depression, stress levels and mood swings. Also, often we ignore the flow of benefits such as improved social contacts and an increase in self-confidence. This is particularly important for us seniors many of whom are restricted and confined in old age homes, infirmaries and long-term hospitalisations.

It is reported (Ref: www.healthline.com › health › depression › exercise) that endorphins and many other neurotransmitters are released during exercise. Physical activity also stimulates the release of dopamine, norepinephrine, and serotonin. These brain chemicals are essential for regulating our mental health and well-being.

Another additional benefit of regular exercise is that it reduces the levels of the body's stress hormones, such as adrenaline and cortisol. These hormones are produced by the adrenal gland located on top of the kidneys and are responsible for our fight-or-flight response. Both adrenaline and cortisol are stress hormones responsible for elevated blood pressure, heart rate and stress levels.

Exercise can be fun and interactive. Many seniors are joining social groups or clubs and dance classes which is a marvellous way of fulfilling regular basic exercise needs and also social interaction.

Let Your Organs Breathe

1. Standing in an upright position, & variations of this exercise.

Before you start working out any of the exercises mentioned here please read them carefully and check if these are within your do-able and comfort zone. If in doubt consult your healthcare practitioner and or a physical trainer.

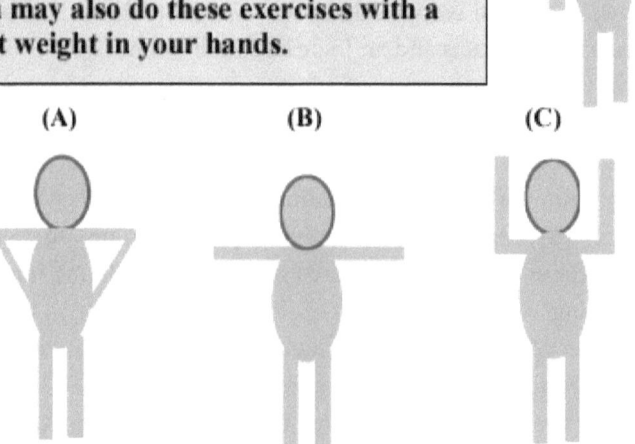

Upright Position:
Standing straight; you may have your legs slightly apart for better support and balance.
You may also do these exercises with a light weight in your hands.

(A)   (B)   (C)

A. hands firmly planted on your hips
B. Arms horizontally stretched out
C Arms raised above your shoulders
Standing in a comfortable position, legs slightly apart for stability, stretch & sway side to side & front and back.
Do these moves 1 – 2 minutes each.

2. Standing upright knee lift Exercises.

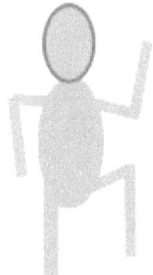

Lift knees horizontally of the ground as high as it is comfortable for you. First lift right knee then left in a marching configuration, being stationary in one position. This exercise can also be done with hands on your hips
Do this exercise to a count of 10

3. Simple Bending Exercises

Bend keeping legs firmly in position and straight as possible. Do not strain as it could be painful. If you can't bend low enough to touch feet or ground then hold your hips for balance, or legs apart.
Do this posture for the count to 5 then straighten up gently.

Another one to try is kneeling alternate right knee then left knee from upright position. The upper torso when kneeling position must be as upright as possible This strengthens the calf muscles and improves the hip movement and overall posture. Seniors must not overdo, bend only if your body permits and that to only to the limit of bending down which offers you ease and suppleness.

4. Simple Stretching Exercises

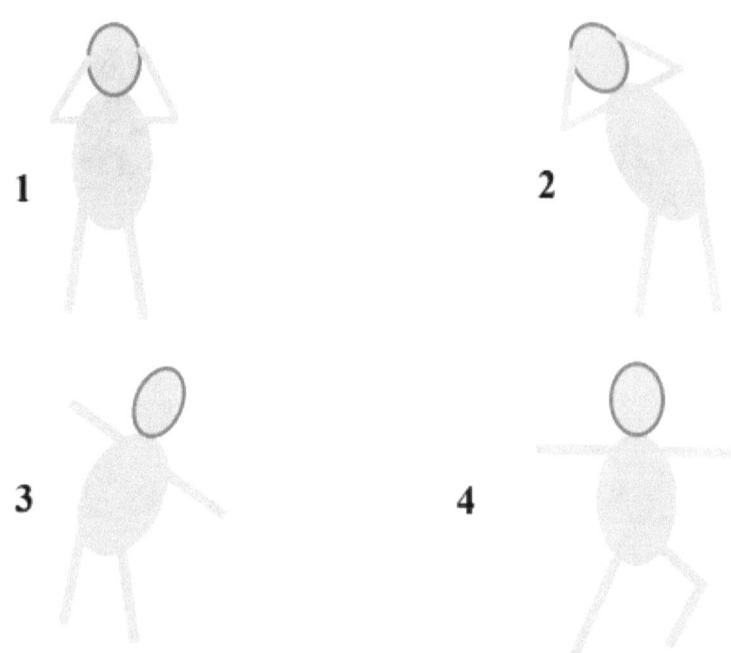

A set of 8 simple stretching exercises are presented which are suitable for all, including seniors without much strenuous efforts.

1. Legs apart hands firmly at the back of head. Gently move your head and neck side to side, front & back. Gently does it without any jerking motion or movement. Do it only 5 times without straining your neck.
2. Legs apart hands firmly at the back of head and stretching; alternate between right to left.
3. Legs apart, hands spread stretching from right to left.
4. Legs apart, knee bent arms spread horizontally. Stretch from right to left.

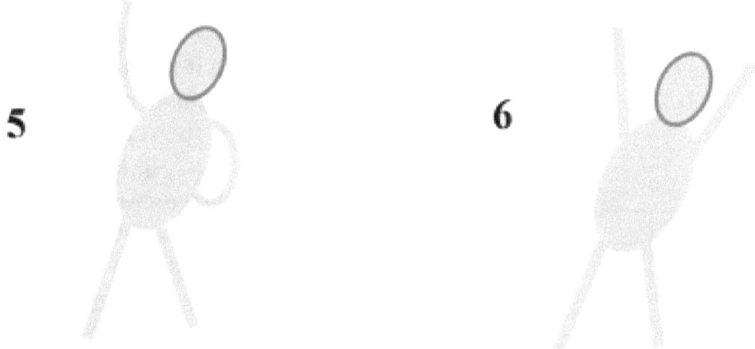

5. Legs apart, one hand on hips the other vertically above head. Stretch right to left with arms alternating between hips.
6. Stretch with legs apart, hands vertically above head.
7. Both hands on hips, stretch left to right with slow circular motion.
8. Stretch and bend on alternating knees and rest your hands on your thighs for support.

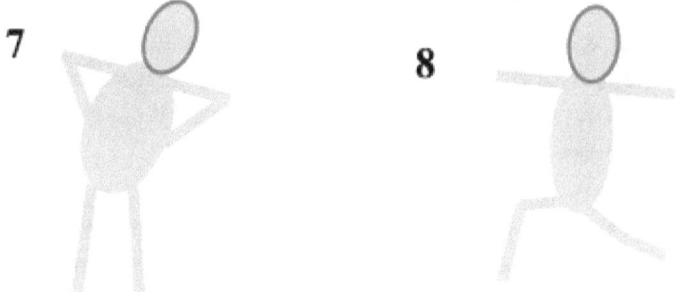

All these movement exercises can be repeated within your comfort zone.

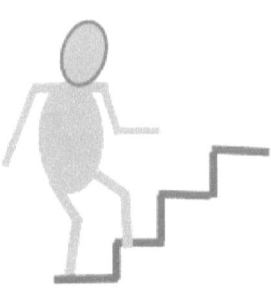

Climbing Stairs:
If you have an access to a staircase and if it is not too cumbersome then try climbing up and down the stairs. All you need, is to climb up and down only half a dozen rungs of the stairs rather than the whole stair case. If you want to, you can go the full distance but not necesseary.
This will improve posture, balance and strength in your leg muscles.

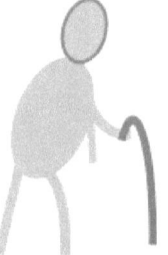

For balance and stability, it may be helpful to use a Walking stick during some of these exercises; most importantly the bending exercise where partial weight of the body may be supported by the stick.

CAUTION:
It is always a very good idea to be careful and exert a bit of caution when undertaking any physical activity.
At the first sign of discomfort, breathing difficulties please stop and have a rest and sip a glass of cold water slowly. If complications persists seek medical advice.
Please follow KIS principle; Keep It Simple.
Use commonsense approach and enjoy the simple exercises that should give you a good deal of benefit and some degree of freedom of movement.

Free-hand exercises can be varied according to one's capability, endurance limit and comfort zone. Try to move all moving parts of your body especially joints, like the elbow and knee joints. Our ability to move freely declines with age and so it is important to keep up with the free hand exercises.

Push-ups, squatting and lunging forward are some of the very common free-hand workouts that can be done within your comfort zone. It will provide both sweat-off and mild cardio boost.

More advanced versions can also be applied in your exercise routine such as one hand push-ups, Spiderman push-ups and many more depending on how innovative and energetic you are.

Start with a traditional press-up or push-up position, both are same.

A six-step simple push-ups for beginners:

Start with a clean firm area on the ground or a smooth plank. Safety is of utmost concern, do not compromise it.

Your palms should be flat on the ground.

Position yourself getting down on your hands and knees. Straighten your legs and put them together while hands stretched wider but straight for stability and comfort. You may bring your feet slightly apart for extra stability.

Lower your body horizontally to the floor but without touching the floor while inhaling push your body up gently to the original start position exhaling.

Repeat several times.

There are several variations of simple push-ups that you can try according to your endurance limits and strength, for example:

Back lift where you raise your back as a start position; good for the back muscle.

Sphinx position, literally position yourself as the mythical creature 'The Sphinx' of Egypt as your original start position.

The knuckle push-ups where you start with support from your knuckles, not open palm. It can be a bit painful.

All such variations come with a degree of difficulty and therefore more effort may be needed to perform and although the end benefit is very similar some may offer extra strengthening of the muscles involved. At the same time threshold of pain may increase to bear, but as they say "No Pain No Gain." It is sometimes important to get some professional help to start you off, as some of the variations need a bit of a doing. These push-ups if done properly will allow your body mainly the upper part for example your chest, shoulders, arm muscles and the back muscles to firm up and strengthen; and also good for the posture.

Exercise with Equipment

The scope of this chapter is just within the maintenance of simple easy-to-do exercises which we all can do in order to enhance our fitness and activity level without strenuous and regimented involvement. We are only limiting ourselves to a familiar environment, no capital outlay and involving in activity sessions which are full of creativity. Make it enjoyable and purposeful.

Previously we outlined some basic freehand exercises which may be modified to suit your limits of persuasion determined by your fitness levels, age, confidence levels and capabilities. Many seniors among us who are willing subjects, but due to their advancing age are a bit reluctant to undertake vigorous and rigorous routines offered by various professional institutions or entities. It is therefore a good start in your home at your comfort level and within your limitations.

Remember in our scheme of things there are no hard and fast rules and you modify as you go and make changes to whatever tickles your fancy. These are just a guide and basic examples, especially for seniors who can spend a bit of time and get away from the monotony of daily repetitive activity or in-activity and engage in a quality me-time guaranteed to produce at least some benefit in physical fitness.

I do not want to go into the therapeutics of it but experience has it that any light workout is beneficial for all of us.

So, what are the equipment; use a strong chair you are comfortable to sit on; firm enough to withstand gentle pressure exerted during exercises and most importantly the frame is stable with no squeaks and crackles.

A sturdy footstool could be handy if you have got one.

The other piece of equipment we need is a couple of lightweight dumbbells and nonslip surface. We are now well set; all we now need is a soothing music or a light hearted music playing in the background to give our home gym a bit more ambience.

Dress casually but tangle proof to minimise accidental trips and falls.

Ok, we are now set and ready to go.

Set the chair in a sunny ventilated area. If outdoors make sure the chair must be firmly planted on a level ground to offer maximum stability.

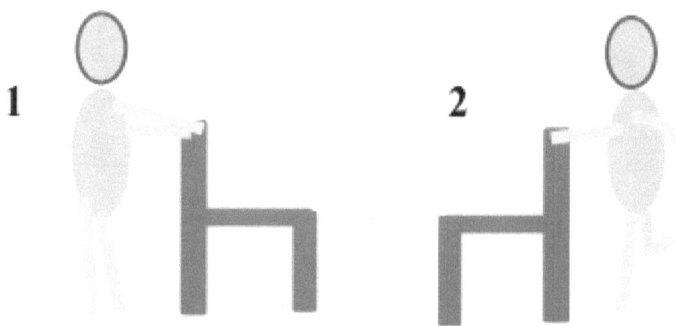

1. Standing behind a chair to adjust your posture and balance, before you start.
2. Standing behind a chair, alternate between bending right and left knees stretched. Hold feet with hand for support.

CAUTION:
All the exercises mentioned in this chapter are meant to be done with care.
All including seniors must decide if these exercises are suitable for you within your comfort zone. Before commencing please read the procedures carefully and if in doubt please have a physical appraisal done. Always maintain a balance so you do not fall. At the first sign of pain or discomfort felt you must stop and re-evaluate.

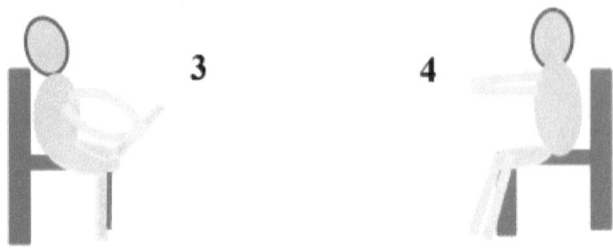

3. Sitting straight, stretch your legs as high up as you can. Support the thigh or calf with hands for balance. Alternate right and left legs without losing your balance preventing any falls.
4. Sit up straight, stretch your arms out as horizontally as possible and hold to a count of 10. Variation of this is to raise arms vertically and stretch.

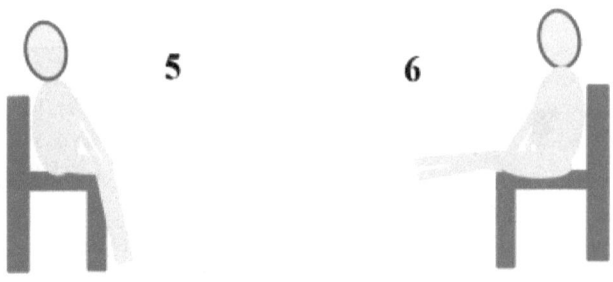

5. Sit up straight, chest stretched out take a deep breath and hold for a count of 10, exhale and repeat this 5 – 10 times.
6. Sit up straight, lift up both legs as high as you can horizontal to your seat and stretch, keeping straight to the count of 5. Again inhaling and exhaling as in exercise 5 above.
For support place hands on your knees.

Movements, Energy Expenditure and Some Basic Exercise Guides

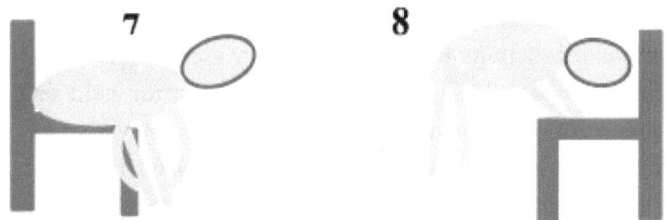

7. Sitting on a chair leaning forward and bending to touch the feet or lower part of the leg. Anyone with a weak back should not attempt to do this exercise without proper supervision. If done properly may help strengthen the back muscles.
8. Leaning forward holding the chair seat or handle for support, stretch forward and backwards then standing straight taking deep breath. Repeat this exercise exhaling when reverting to the standing position.

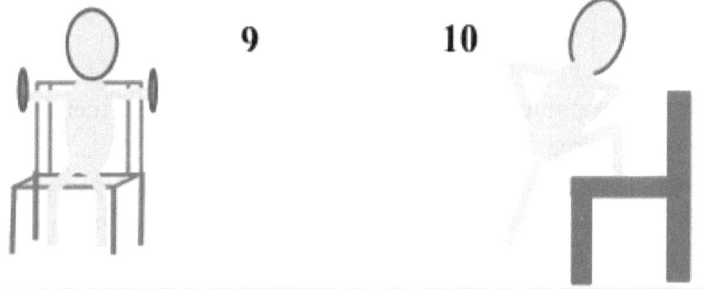

Exercise steps 9 & 10 are basic steps to which variations can be applied as desired to make it more exciting and user friendly.
9. In sitting down position using weights (dumbbells) stretch your arms then gather them in front on stretch position. Repeat few times and then vary the move by lifting your arms upwards with the weights; again repeating the move few times; add variations if desired.
10. With arms in a firm position at your hips, step up with your left leg on the seat of the chair; alternate left leg followed by right leg. These moves can also be varied as desired within your comfortable zone. This is also stretching moves which will strengthen leg & thigh muscles and also strengthen your ankles and balance.
Lifting weights can be difficult if you do not have steady hands, be careful and never overdo your exercises. Use common sense approach and at any time if you feel uncomfortable have a rest and Seek professional advice.

I suggest that these sequences be carried out up to 30 seconds to one minute each. This will take you about 5–10 minutes all up. If you wish, you may adjust the times on your needs and convenience basis.

Finally in this freehand series of simple and easy-to-do exercises I want to include one more little activity which could be very useful.

Squeezing softballs which will allow firmness in your hold or grip; do this sequence 4–6 times alternating hands. There are many variations such as sitting on an exercise ball for balance and stability. Always remember not to exceed your endurance limits and do not do these exercises if you have any impairments: Seniors exercising with equipment, especially dumbbells of lighter weight can be of significant benefit as it provides strengthening of the muscles and with proper nutrition the age-related wear and tear can be eased which will help towards body toning and improve endurance and body fitness.

Skipping is another form of a popular workout commonly practiced and is good for losing weight by burning extra calories.

There are some basic procedures that need to be followed before you get going with your skipping routine.

Start with a good quality but simple skipping rope with a handle and a level, softer but firm ground which would be able to absorb the shock and jolt created by the skipping movements. If this is not available, then lay a shock absorber mat or a rug.

Attire appropriately; wear proper footwear with a flexible sole which can absorb the extra pressure or shock generated from the jumping motion. Grip the rope handles firmly, put your feet together or slightly apart pointing the direction of the skipping motion.

So, you are all set to start.

Position the rope behind you and begin with a gentle pace extending your arms away from the body to create a rope arc when jumping in the forward direction. Jump with both feet above the ground clearing the rope as if you are jumping over a low hoop. Look forward, because if you keep watching your feet you are likely to get tangled and off balance. Try to keep a straight posture and steady as she goes.

With steady practice, your skill levels should improve for you to move into undertaking more difficult moves. Don't try seriously complicated moves unless guided by an experienced person or an instructor and until you have mastered the basic moves.

Reverse Skip: Try reverse skip which is very similar to forward skip, making certain that you are skipping with your arms and legs moving in a synchronised fashion to each other's movement.

Criss-Cross Skip: Now try this move; it is very similar to the normal skipping movement and when you get your rhythm then you cross your arms in front of you and jump through the arc created by the rope. Revert back to the normal skip position by uncrossing your arms and continue. You may cross-over at will and as per your convenience. Criss-cross skipping when done properly can prove to be quite effective cardio and total body exercise and tones up all the moving parts of your body and muscles involved in various degrees e.g., calves, chest, arms, shoulders, etc.

There are several other versions that you could try, Cross-Leg Skips, Single-Leg and Alternate-Leg Skips these are also powerful exercise routines which will enhance your endurance, power, posture and stability. All these variations start with the normal skipping routine.

With every skipping exercise routine, your confidence level improves; you do not need to include every move in your daily exercise repertoire but alternate them to get the best out of every move to add to your overall improvement for general health and well-being.

It has been estimated (Ref: www.aqfsports.com › blogs › news › jumping rope) that skipping exercises can burn around 20 calories every minute, so working out for only 10 minutes you can lose 200 calories more if you are able to manoeuvre complicated moves.

Illustrations of Some Skipping Positions

Skipping is a simple form of exercise but one that provides a lot of benefits in terms of burning unwanted calories:

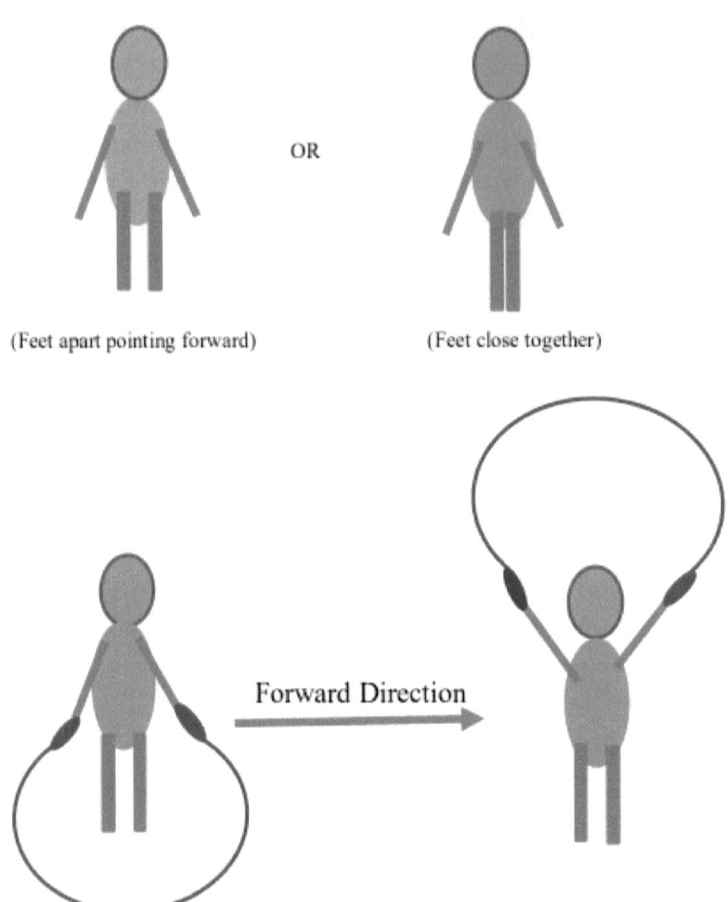

(Feet apart pointing forward)   (Feet close together)

Forward Direction

Movements, Energy Expenditure and Some Basic Exercise Guides

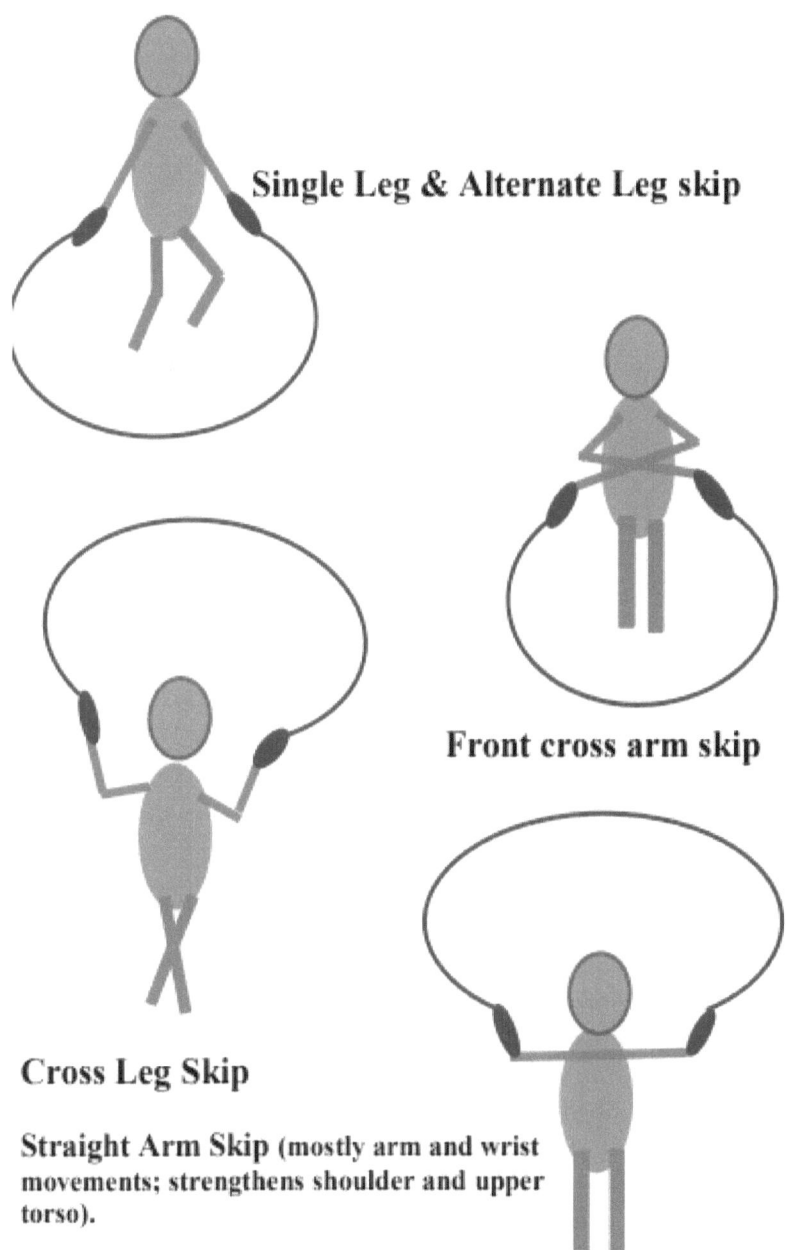

Single Leg & Alternate Leg skip

Front cross arm skip

Cross Leg Skip

Straight Arm Skip (mostly arm and wrist movements; strengthens shoulder and upper torso).

Squats are another form of safe exercise which is easy to perform.

There are few movements that we all can do, by all, I mean even seniors. Simply start by standing in an upright position with arms straight by your side and feet comfortably apart for stability but firmly planted on the floor. Bending your knees, hips pushed out, arms in front with folded palms lower yourself in a squatting position. Gently breathe in as you go through the movement motions.

Get back gently to the original position; first arms straight by your side but knees still bent slowly acquiring the original position as you breathe out.

Heels firmly planted to the floor at all times.

These squat exercises can also be done with both hands on the hips.

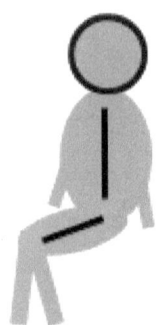 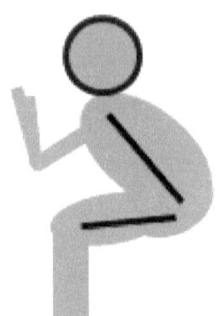 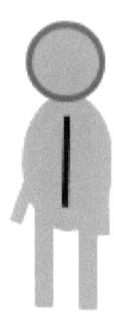

Variations to squatting are very many, you can be inventive and introduce several variations to your routine. In all cases, feet must be firm on the ground. **Wall Squats:** it is similar to regular squats, only difference is that it is performed leaning upright against the wall. It may be good for seniors as the wall could give the support and stability that they may need. I call this slide squat.

Split Squat: Follow the basic squat position upright with legs comfortably apart. In the next move, set one foot (can be either right leg or the left leg) forward in front of the other leg.

Vary the movements this time with other foot in front.

Side to Side Squat: this is a simple variation of the split squat. Extend or stretch one leg to a comfortable position then lean your basic squat movements in that direction, feet firmly on the ground. After stretching on one leg, change position on to the other leg.

Jump Squat: Similar basic movements; with every movement straighten your body making sure your legs are vertically straight when you jump back to the basic upright position. Arms can be firm at the hips or folded in front of your chest.

Squats with dumbbells: start with light weights; you can either stick to the basic squat moves with the dumbbells in each hand or just one dumbbell held in both hands in front of your chest. In this case, clutching the dumbbell end to end.

Movements, Energy Expenditure and Some Basic Exercise Guides

Controlling your breathing in and out at specific intervals will be of benefit.

Squatting exercises offer several health benefits; they offer strength and conditioning to the leg muscles including the most important hamstrings, calf muscles, and quadriceps.

It provides strength to the knee joints and improves mobility.

It strengthens the lower back.

It improves body flexibility, particularly in the lower back part of the body. It promotes weight loss.

(Journal of Strength and Conditioning Research: August 2002—Volume 16, Issue 3. p. 428–432, reports the benefit of squat in maintaining balance, mobility and strength).

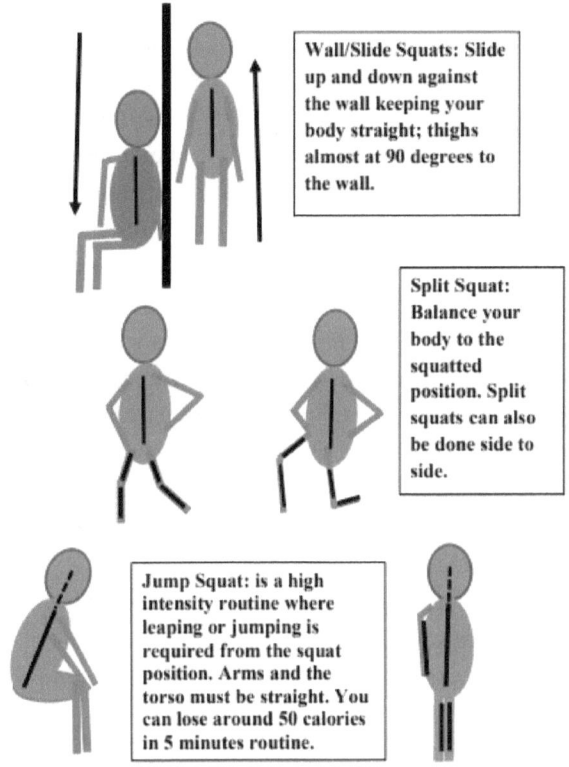

(The lines indicate the straightness of the contour)

These exercises are just guides, it is important that for any strenuous routine, a careful evaluation of your suitability must be done by professional intervention. If done correctly and regularly, a lot of health benefits can be achieved. Also, energy burned calculations are based on performance by an average adult with around 75kg weight.

Seniors and Stretching Exercises

When attempting, the basic exercises as demonstrated in this chapter it is very important that you have a clear understanding of the postures and positions. It may also be necessary that seniors do consider their level of fitness and activity before starting. A quick professional health appraisal may help. It is an important assertion that seniors do get a lot of benefit from stretching exercises particularly those who have age-related joint and mobility issues. With aging, the lubricant within the bone structure especially bone joint cavities called the synovial fluid starts to dry out and the buffering action of the synovial fluid declines. This causes friction within the skeletal structure resulting in joint aches and pains and loss in muscular activities, muscle tension and soreness.

To overcome this impairment regular movement exercises of just 10–20 minutes daily improve the circulation, availability of synovial fluids in the joint cavities and also reduce tension and soreness in the muscles. The overall benefit is a marked improvement in senior's activity and lifestyle and perhaps increases their longevity and quality of life.

Walking, swimming, light free hand exercises with some additional light-weight such as dumbbells and also slow rhythmic dancing moves have been known to improve the general activity levels and moods.

Another significant benefit of regular exercise performance by seniors is the improvement in their concentration and confidence which results in a lesser number of random falls. This leads to fewer injuries, improved mobility maintenance and enhancement in the quality of life.

Please evaluate all the movement exercises as suggested, try and improvise to suit your capabilities and give it a go.

Let us now itemise the real benefits of exercise in senior's population:

1. Several studies have reported that regular exercise improves the cognitive functions among seniors which lowers the risk of dementia and other memory loss functions.
2. Regular exercise enhances the activities of the feel-good hormones, endorphins, and improves the mental capacity. The extra physical activity due to exercise and stretching also has a positive effect on sleep patterns

which improves mental health, relieves stress and improves overall general health and well-being.
3. Regular exercise helps in preventing many negative health conditions. The Australian Bureau of Statistics (ABS) reported that more than 70% of seniors in our community in general suffer from at least 1 (one) of as many as 8 (eight) chronic illnesses such as cardiovascular, respiratory, and diabetes etc. Regular exercise helps to manage these conditions and in many instances under proper medical care helps in quicker recovery.
4. Group exercises undertaken by many seniors improve their social interactions and help them to recover from loneliness and depression.
5. Exercise improves the stability and balance in seniors and therefore helps minimise incidences of falls and minor indoor trips and tumbles. Many incidences of falls can be serious and results in fractures and may end up in hospitalisation or seniors' care facilities.

Somewhere, in this chapter, I have mentioned that walking, swimming and light dance moves are also very helpful in improving the general health and well-being of seniors. All these together with the exercises mentioned will give seniors a good and healthy choice in determining their lifestyle. Walking is particularly healthy and offers seniors a greater flexibility of exercising and enjoying the freshness and beauty of Nature and if walking with a companion also helps pass the time quicker and effortlessly. Choose your own pace mild to a steady pace for a longer or shorter duration; up and, or, down the hill within your level of fitness.

Walking will help strengthen your leg muscles, improve your posture if you try to walk steady and upright and also improve your balance and steadiness. It will also improve your arthritic condition in conjunction with your medication as prescribed by your physician.

Swimming also is an important tool for maintaining senior's general health. Just simply splashing in water with movements in arms and legs can only mean one thing; more strength and agility. Swaying with music in light dance or aerobic moves is another arm in a senior's armoury which improves coordination and motor control which regulates reflexes through the central nervous system.

Any form of exercising is good for seniors, providing it is doable without causing any stress, strain or any mental anxiety. Exercise should be enjoyable however, involved or simple easy to go it may be. At the end of each session, the person doing the exercises must have the feeling of achievement and look forward to the next session. This is the only way goals can be achieved and the fruits of your labour can be harvested.

It is important also, to understand that every movement that we make expends energy; where does this energy come from? From the foods we intake, therefore, it is necessary to look at our dietary practices and review them to see if we are getting enough energy input in the 24-hour period to compensate for the energy output that we expend.

For seniors, this balance between input and output is a lot less than a younger age person because of the difference in the metabolic rates. A younger person is more active and hence requires more energy input to balance the output.

In the next chapter, we will look at senior's nutrition and dietary practices. Energy intake and energy output is a simple equation. The ideal scenario in health management is that the daily energy input should be equal to the energy output or expended. The extra bit of energy which is not expended gets stored as fat; and if not utilised this ends up in fat build up in the body resulting in overweight and, or, obesity.

Now, **Energy-In** is the result of energy produced by consuming foods and drinks. Typically, our diet can be broken down into carbohydrates, proteins and fats and few others such as fruits and nuts, etc. For drinks, we consume water, fruit juices and alcohol (in moderation). All have energy components within themselves and in the body breakdown into measurable units of kcal or Joules.

Per gram of carbohydrates provides approximately 4 kcal.

Proteins provide approximately a similar amount of energy.

While Fats provide the most energy approximately 9 kcal per gram.

Alcohols also provide a significantly high amount of energy around 7 kcal per gram, but it is important to note that alcohol is not a food as such as it does not provide the body with any extra nutrients but rather has an opposite effect in that it neutralises vitamins and minerals in the body and therefore consumption of alcohol increases the demand for vitamins and minerals in the body. Fruit juices provide energy in varying amounts due to the composition of the juice. Some energy values have been reported in Chapter 4.

Energy-Out is the amount of energy that our body burns to compensate for all the metabolic processes within our body and also the physical activities we need to carry out daily in order to survive. Our energy consumption largely depends on many factors such as gender, age, growth and development factors and also the level of activity that we need to go through on a daily basis.

In general, the body follows a simple equation:

Energy-In = Energy-Out

As I have mentioned earlier that every movement we make, such as running, talking, yawning, clapping or any movement activities you can think of is associated with an energy expended value. It is also surprising to know that even when we are in a rest or sleep mode not doing anything, we also use up energy.

Our body needs energy for all the metabolic processes that are happening within our body which is keeping us alive.

According to Harvard Medical School's published calories burned chart, an average 70kg person will burn around 45 calories in an hour. Similarly, just for the privilege of breathing an 80–85 kg person burns 56 Cal while a 55–60 kg person is likely to burn off only 38 Cal per hour; interesting.

On a similar note, energy spent in sitting and standing reflects a significant difference. When standing, as much as 100–200 calories may be burned off while sitting consumes around 60–130 calories per hour. The margin or the range is due to the allowance calculated for gender, age and various physical attributes. So, if you are looking to lose weight standing up rather than sitting for extended period of time could be an option to consider but if you are trying to preserve your weight, then sitting down has a distinct advantage over standing up.

But remember for seniors standing up for longer than necessary is not advisable due to several temporary lapses which can cause discomfort such as dizzy spells, feeling weak, headaches, aching legs, etc. As per the examples above every metabolic process happening in our body to sustain life is spending or burning off calories; some of these metabolic processes are as we have discussed respiration, digestion, circulation, elimination of wastes from the body such as sweating and eliminating excrements, and even the process of tissue repairs, growth and development of cellular structure, blood circulation, etc., all require energy to function. Some processes utilise more energy than others.

The rate of our metabolism is calculated by the sum of total energy used by all our body functions. It is the sum of total energy spent in 24-hour day and can be categorised as energy spent under the following conditions:

Tables provided generalised energy requirements with various age groups and also some daily activities undertaken and energy expended by a 70 kg adult. However, it is true that any movement incurs burning off calories no matter how large or small the calorie value may be. In generalisation, our energy is used up in the following manner.

- The energy spent at rest for carrying out bodily functions such as breathing, blood circulation, and several internal biochemical reactions happening continuously, is known as the Basal Metabolic Rate (BMR).
- Energy is spent during food ingestion, digestion and transportation of nutrients. This activity spends the least amount of energy which is estimated to be around 5–10% of our total energy spent.
- Energy is spent by our regular physical activities such as daily chores, physical movements and other recreational activities such as playing sports, etc.

Our BMR requirement is heavily dependent on our age, gender, BMI, our body's internal energy requirement and many other factors. The total requirement is estimated to be around 1200 calories in 24-hour period which is known as the Base or Basal Energy Expenditure (BEE) and is about 60% of our daily energy requirement. Besides this, our body has a need for additional energy to perform physical activities such as walking, talking, and running and other daily chores that are required for us to carry out on a regular basis. It is estimated that our daily **Energy-In** requirement is around 2500–2000 calories and reflects the bare essential daily requirement of the gender and age group represented in the table with no heavy or strenuous activity undertaken and as explained above these values are estimates only and may be influenced by body mass index (BMI) and level of activities undertaken etc. The heavier the level of activity undertaken, the requirement for energy intake becomes more.

(Minimum Daily Energy-In requirement in Calories Ref: National Health and Medical Research Council, Australia)

Age group	Male	Female
12–15 years	2100	1900
19–30 years	2500	2000
51–70	2200	1800
Seniors over 70s	2000	1700

Under very basic, normal circumstances the energy input from dietary sources must be similar to the energy burned off in order for weight stabilisation; any less will result in weight loss and any surplus energy will be converted into fat leading to weight gain.

Energy Expenditure table for popular leisure and domestic activities; may be used as a basic guide for calculating daily energy outputs.

Calories burned in 30 minutes. Ref: www.health.harvard.edu/diet and *medicalnewstoday.com/articles/319731).

Activities	Energy Burned in 30 minutes by a person about 70kg
Dancing slow steps	108
Moderate walking	136
Brisk walking	140
Aerobics (slow)	252
Vacuuming*	70
Washing Car	165
Bowling	110
Playing Golf (using a cart) Playing Golf (carrying the clubs)	126 200
Sleeping	22
Doing Laundry work*	70
Sitting and reading book	40
Standing	35
Jogging moderate (5 mph)	280
Running (10mph) fast	565
House work, cleaning (Moderate Level)*	105
Swimming (Moderate)	210
Moderate walking (3.5mph)	135
Gymnastics	145
Weight Training (moderate)	108
Gardening	162
Yoga*	140
Cooking	70
Lawn Mowing manual	200
Bicycling (moderate)	250
Shopping for Groceries (using a cart)	106

The daily chores can be categorised into 4 levels, graded according to the activity levels; Light, moderate, hard and strenuous. This is not to confuse with the do-ability of the chore but simply the level of activity involved which will determine the calories we need to burn off.

Grading of Daily Activity levels

Our daily chores can be categorised into 4 levels, graded according to the activity levels; Light, moderate, hard and strenuous. This is not to confuse with the do-ability of the chore but simply the level of activity involved which will determine the calories we need to burn off.

Activity Grading	Daily Chores	Calories Burned in 30 minutes. (70kg Body Weight)	
		Male	Female
(Light)	Light domestic chores Such as cleaning, cooking, Washing and ironing, Light gardening and Light office (desk) duties.	Up to 100	Up to 80
(Moderate)	Lawn mowing (manual), Gardening weeding, pruning, planting, etc. Heavy house work. Cycling (5mph or more) Carry heavy load.	200+	150+
(High)	Swimming fast laps, various Martial Arts, cycling fast (15mph), Playing various sports, Squash, skipping rope, etc.	350+	300+
(Strenuous)	Uphill skiing. Running up the stairs, running (10 mph or more) Heavy gym workout and weight lifting.	550+	500+

Researchers at Mayo Clinic have estimated that in order to lose around half a kilogram of body fat we need to burn off 3,500 calories.

How can we estimate our daily energy requirement (EER)? It is very important to have a general idea as to how much energy we need in order to maintain a steady body weight for our good health and well-being. I found an extremely good article (Ref: Balancing Energy Input with Energy

Output-Medicine... https://med.libretexts.org ›... › 4: Metabolism and Energy) this publication does offer some insight to the above question and many more.

The fundamental issue here as we have touched upon before is that the energy intake must be equal to the energy output, otherwise the extra energy can be converted into body fat and contribute to weight increase.

The above publication offers a simple formula for calculating EER for both adult males and females which takes into consideration age, gender, height and weight and also the physical activity level (PA).

Adult Male:

EER=662- [9.53×age(y)] +PA× [15.91×wt (kg) +5.39.6×ht (m)]

Adult Female:

EER=354- [6.91×age(y)] +PA× [9.36×wt (kg) +726×ht (m)]

Source: Health Canada. 'Dietary Reference Intake Tables'. Last modified November 29, 2010.

Activity Level	Physical Activity (PA)		Activity description
	Adult Male	Adult Female	
Sedentary	1.00	1.00	No significant activity other than basic daily living
Low	1.11	1.12	Equivalent to walking 2.5–5km per day
Moderate	1.25	1.27	Equivalent to walking 5–16km per day
High	1.48	1.45	More than 16 km per day

(This table is only applicable to average-weight adults with no underlying medical causes, pregnancies, obesity, etc.).

A further table has been provided which may assist in understanding the EER requirement, however point to note is that an estimate is only for an average person. Values are likely to vary in pregnancy or lactating situations and in obesity. For more information please check out the reference.

Table showing EER requirement

Sex	Age (years)	Sedentary	Moderate	Active
Child (male & female)	2–3	1000–1200	1000–1400	1000–1400
-	4–8	1200–1400	1400–1600	1400–1800
-	9–13	1400–1600	1600–2000	1800–2200
-	14–18	1800	2000	2400
Female	19–30	1800–2000	2000–2200	2400
-	31–50	1800	2000	2200
-	51+	1600	1800	2000–2400
Male	19–30	2400–2600	2600–2800	3000
-	31–50	2200–2400	2400–2600	2800–3000
-	51+	2000–2200	2200–2400	2400–2800

(Ref: US Department of Agriculture. 2010 Dietary Guidelines for Americans. 2010 http://health.gov/dietaryguidlines/dga2010/DietaryGuidlines2010.pdf).

Body Mass Index (BMI)

BMI is a measure of an individual's health and fitness. It is calculated by considering the height and weight of a person to determine an index to predict if that index is in a healthy range and also, to predict on an ongoing basis any risks of developing diseases that could be a real issue in that person's life. BMI can be easily calculated by taking the body weight of a person as lightly clothed as possible in kilograms and then measuring the height in metres at the same time as accurately as possible.

So, you now have two readings; one for your weight (kg) and one for your height (m).

$$BMI = kg/m^2$$

Body weight (kg) divided by the square of body height (m^2)

Example: for a body weight of 70kg and height of 1.7m

The BMI should be around 24.2 kg/m^2

The table below provides some values for BMI and significance.

BMI (kg/m^2)	Classification
Less than 18.5	Underweight
18.5–24.9	Healthy weight range
25–29.9	Overweight
30 and over	Obese

(Ref: Body mass index (BMI) | Healthy Weight Guide—Australian… https://healthyweight.health.gov.au)

Another important parameter helpful in risk prediction is the waist circumference. For men, it is acknowledged that this value should be less than 94 cm while for women less than 80 cm. Any higher can suggest obesity-related chronic disease state. The higher the number the risk factor increases. These values only apply to healthy adults under normal situations and not under pregnancy and underlying health conditions.

If you are obese, you will need to reduce or control your weight, exercise more and try to bring your BMI in line with your general body weight and physique. If you are a smoker, you will need to cut down on your smoking patterns or better still don't smoke at all. If you are a regular consumer of alcohol, then drink in moderation or better still not at all, and please have regular medical appraisals.

Increased health risks associated with increased BMI; although BMI is not a definitive parameter for risk prediction, it is generally considered that for inactive individuals with a higher than 25kg/m^2 BMI there is a real possibility of the development of chronic life style diseases in later life. These may include cardiovascular diseases, liver function impairment, hypertension, arthritic conditions, depression, etc.

Being underweight at lower end of the BMI scale (less than 18.5) could also have significant health issues such as mal-nourishment, lack of immunity or low immune function, digestive and respiratory issues, low bone density and or osteoporosis. Adult women and men both are at risk. For children and young adults, the BMI calculated are interpreted in a more specific way taking into consideration of age, gender physical structure, ethnicity, etc., and best left to the professionals for a proper evaluation of health and, or, risk factors.

Waist Circumference (WC) is also an important body measurement which has been used as a predictor of disease risk factors. It may not apply to every individual but has been known to provide vital information as used by professionals in assessing a patient's health condition.

For men, it is acknowledged that this value should be less than 94 cm while for women less than 80 cm. Any higher can suggest obesity-related chronic disease state. The higher the number the risk factor increases and we should be extra aware and cautious of these values in relation to our general health and wellbeing. These values only apply to healthy adults under normal situations and not under pregnancy and underlying health conditions. According to the health department, Australian Government publication (Waist Circumference healthy weight guide Australian. https://healthyweight.health.gov.au) the above values may only apply to adults of normal body constitution and do not apply to pregnant women.

Also, these measurements are not universal and may be dependent on ethnicity, genetic disposition, cultural habits and practices and hereditary circumstances. WC above the normal parameters for those to whom it may be applicable may provide an early sign of Cardio-metabolic risks, hypertension, diabetes, hypercholesterolemia and most diabetic and obesity-related diseases. A higher circumference means an uneven distribution of body fat and should be taken seriously as an early sign of obesity and Cardio-metabolic related diseases. The initial appraisal of BMI and WC parameters should be evaluated by a health professional or by your general practitioner.

Predicting our weight consistencies is not a simple task, there are many uncertain factors involved along the way; importantly, our future socioeconomic factors, health, psychological and mental issues and our willpower and discipline are all significant factors.

Although it is a commonly held view, that BMI and WC are good indicators of a preliminary assessment of whether an adult is in a healthy weight zone or not (BMI Classification); recently it has been argued that this may not be applicable to the certain categorisation of subjects. Such as:

Many ethnic populations around the world particularly in the Pacific Island regions the Polynesians with their elegant physical appearance with large body structure, population from South Asia China Japan, etc., where weight due to fat or muscle cannot be estimated with a certain degree of accuracy. Other groups of people that may also be subject to inaccurate estimations are, Athletes, bodybuilders, weight lifters, etc., again in this category with a distinctive body shape with narrow waist it is hard to estimate the real measurements.

Pregnant women, elderly citizens, people with medical disorders, people with natural and extreme obesity may also be the subject of inaccurate measurements.

BMI and WC measurements in general do not apply to under 18 age groups.

In recent times, there is another parameter that has come into play, and this is the waist circumference (WC) in relation to the height. Researches have shown that by keeping your WC to less than half your height is a good indicator of good health. This ratio has proven to be more applicable and adjusts well in the case of most ethnic groups of people and also for children under the age of 18 years. But to every collective observation, there are exceptions.

The combination of BMI and WC can be a more acceptable identifying factor for predicting weight-related issues than a single measurement alone. Based on available knowledge there have been various conclusions and recommendations made and reported in various publications.

It has been strongly suggested that WC and BMI should be a regular part of clinical examination as vital parameters for obesity and certain other weight-related health problems. It is also important to consider other simple parameters discussed here to be monitored for a more conclusive prediction of cardiovascular diseases (CVD).

BMI and WC are both important predictors but individually they have certain limitations:

- BMI assessments seem incomplete as it does not consider certain individual bio-data such as lean body mass, the proportion of fat content, gender, etc.
- It does not differentiate between the older adults in the population who tend to have a higher percentage of fat compared to a younger adult with similar BMI.
- Issues with a muscular individual who may have a higher BMI due to higher muscle mass are not addressed as this may allow an incorrect prediction for future obesity-related complications such as cardiovascular diseases (CVD).
- Another interesting fact could be the possibility of women with similar BMI carrying higher body fat.
- Also, BMI calculations during pregnancy circumstances are highly incorrect.

Bone density which can also shed some light on the individual body mass should also be considered as a part of the overall assessment.

Measurement inaccuracies in both BMI and WC parameters can often lead to a marked change in the prediction scenario. For example, for WC measurements if the participant has a skinfold around the waist, then accurate measurement may not be possible.

According to WHO (World Health Organisation) the Waist Circumference (WC) of more than 94cm for adult males and more than 80cm for adult females could have an increased risk of metabolic complications. The risks increase with the increase in the measurement numbers.

Over the years several other measurements have been developed which have helped to increase the accuracy of prediction and thus given the health workers a better profile of their patients and therefore facilitating a smoother pathway to better health and well-being.

Waist Hip Ratio (WHR)

Waist Hip Ratio is the circumference of the waist divided by the circumference of the hips and offers a quick prediction of our health through fat distribution. Normally fats should be evenly distributed throughout the body but people who support more weight around the middle part of their body than hips may have a higher risk of developing obesity-related health issues.

A generalised waist-to-hip ratio chart is provided below suggesting a tolerable limit which must be adhered to, however, it is strongly suggested that WHO guidelines be maintained.

Degree of Health Risk	Adult Male	Adult Female
Low	0.95 or less	0.80 or less
Moderate	0.96–1.0	0.81–0.85
High	1.0 or higher	0.86 or higher

According to WHO classification The WHR parameter of less than 0.90 indicates moderate in men and less than 0.85 indicates moderate in women.

(Ref: WHO Waist Circumference and Waist-Hip Ratio: Report of a WHO Expert Consultation Geneva, 8–11 December 2008)

Impact of WHR parameter on health condition: In a study, it was reported that abdominal obesity increased the risk of cardiovascular disease and cancer (Ref: Circulation 2008 Apr 1; 117(13):1658–67). Study 2, found the WHR predicted cardiovascular disease more effectively than BMI or waist circumference (Ref: Eur J Epidemiol 2011 Jun; 26 (6):457–61).

There are many other reports published in reputable publications on the benefit of lower WHR measurements which are also worthwhile considering, (Reading Reference: www.medicalnewstoday.com/articles/319439).

One of the articles I read some time ago, considered movement to be an adjunct to medicine. But it is not a replacement for medicine. The place of medicine will always be there on our bedside drawer easy to access, and should be used when necessary and when prescribed by your physician. I do not want to be alarmist but it should be self-explanatory that if we are having strong feelings of pain in general or a specific chest pain then exercising will not do but medicine as prescribed by your physician and a trip to the medical centre can mean the difference between life and death.

Getting back to the motto 'Movement is Medicine' there are many published reports that anything from slight movements, light exercise or even just walking away periodically for a few moments from your regular workstation can mean a lot in easing the symptoms of chronic conditions.

Sifting through the published information we can summarise the following main benefits:

- Arthritic symptoms can be improved by around 40%; a report by CDC.
  (Ref:www.washingtonpost.com/news/to-yourhealth/wp/2017/03/07/arthritis-afflicts-about-1-in-4-adults-in-the-u-scdc-report-finds/).
- Symptoms and the risk of developing Type 2 diabetes is reduced significantly. Ref: University College London. 'Some is good, more is better'.
  Regular exercise can cut your diabetes risk.
  (www.sciencedaily.com/releases/2016/10/161018094926.htm)
- Walking for just 5 minutes every hour can have a positive effect on our health and general well-being.
  (Ref: https://www.nytimes.com/2016/12/28/well/move/work-walk-5minutes-work.html)
- Exercising has a positive effect on brain health. This has been particularly noticed among senior members of the population. Their cognitive impairment, memory skills and the risk of dementia have been demonstrated to reduce noticeably after a short exercise stint with light weights.
  (https://www.sciencedaily.com/releases/2016/08/160802103723.htm University of California—Los Angeles Health Sciences.)
- It is also reported that a daily 20 minutes of exercise and training is beneficial for mild inflammatory activity and also stimulates the immune system.
  (Ref: University of California—San Diego https://www.sciencedaily.com/releases/2017/01/170112115722.htm).
- Older citizens who do not have much movement in their senior years risk biological aging at a much faster rate. (Ref: University of California—San Diego.
  https://www.sciencedaily.com/releases/2017/01/170118151544.htm)

- Parkinson's disease sufferers may be able to slow the progression of their disease by doing regular exercise and body movements. (Ref: https://www.nytimes.com/2017/01/23/well/exercise-can-be-aboon-to-people-with-parkinsons-disease.html).
- Regular physical exercise and movement has been linked with a lower risk of several types of Cancers. (Ref: The JAMA Network Journals https://www.sciencedaily.com/releases/2016/05/160516115302.htm)
- It is interesting to note that sitting idle and not doing any movement for prolonged period could increase the risk of dying early. However, Harvard Health reports that as little as 25 minutes of daily moderate-level of exercise can offset the negative effects of 8 hours of sitting idle. However, a daily exercise and movement for more than 60 minutes daily can eliminate the risk of dying considerably.
  (Ref: https://well.blogs.nytimes.com/2016/03/29/sitting-increases-therisk-of-dying-early/).

Movements can mean anything from walking, simple free hand exercises or with equipment as pictorially depicted in this chapter or simply aerobic, dancing any type of movement that you can think of; all in some form or other have positive benefits to our health. So, keep moving and be healthy.

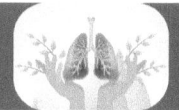

Chapter 10

SENIOR'S NUTRITION

Ageing gracefully is the new inspiration; it is a privilege that only my fellow seniors can enjoy and others can only aspire to.
— Jay Das, June 2022

Seniors in Our society?

Senior years if well cared and catered for, in my opinion, can be a wonderful time; we have an opportunity to age gracefully, we have more time to enjoy life and leisure and not to forget to reminisce the past bygone wonderful years.

I classify seniors into three age brackets which may be fitting to the present-day societal norms. I am basing my views on some of the previous community sayings that life begins at 40, and, the perception that has changed with passing of time. There is no set rule or age as to when life begins for us; is it in 40s, 50s or even 60s?

In the 30s (I mean 1930s), much before my time an American Psychologist by the name of Walter Pitkin propagated this idea in his book 'Life Begins at Forty' which heralded a new era for the young to middle aged adults of that time. One of the arguments that Pitkin put forward was that at or after the 40s people have many more years of happy life ahead.

Now, we have come a long way with technological, cultural, scientific and medical innovations our longevity has increased which I call the life quality index. Now we have many interesting things to do and look forward to which has opened up new grounds for keeping ourselves busy and active not just for ourselves but for all of us and created the awareness of healthy lifestyle and healthy living.

There are several well-known people who think life begins at 60. They base their comments on the 'feel good' aspect, plenty of opportunities that they enjoy and utilise and their awareness and the availability of leisure time to spend and make use of in their sixties.

Dr Frieda Birnbaum in her book 'Life Begins at 60' has expressed her satisfaction with life in her 60s. My favourite action star Harrison Ford has also made a comment to this effect (Ref: https://www.independent.co.uk/artsentertainment/films/news/life-begins-at-sixty-says-harrison-ford301482.html). But, it is not the comment as to who made what, rather it is the self-expectation and enjoyment what you and I can get out of life be it at any decade 40s, 50s or 60s.

We need to extract the best out of the decade which suits us most. For example, 30s and 40s are like busy setting up the base for a future good life; rearing children giving them the best possible start in life and planning for the future.

The 50s are the most venerable decade as we need to shoulder more responsibility in growing a family which matures with time, facing problems and constraints that a growing family offers. That is why the 60s can be so much to look forward to; we can only dream of the 60s in our previous decades.

Retirement for many brings joy and happiness in their 60s. For those who have been planning their future, it's time to execute; and those who are lucky enough to execute can reap the benefit, they can really live it up. This calls for good health in each of the earlier decades because if your health is not good then no amount of wealth and leisure can bring you the joy and happiness that the 60s are supposed to bring you.

Don't get me wrong I am not generalising as I know retirement also brings hardship to many as the steady stream of income dries out and a lifestyle of misery and stress can take over. Retirement can often mean loss of identity not just the loss in income; this is the time when many retirees find it difficult to cope with and adjust.

With retirement, comes an increased incidence of suicidal tendencies for older people who cannot cope well. In a recent paper published in 2020 (Ref: Social Psychiatry and Psychiatric Epidemiology, 56 (5), pp.759–771, 2020), the authors studied in detail the detrimental effect of mental health on the transition from employment to retirement and the suicidal behaviour among the older Australians. The researchers concluded that this transition is an important factor for suicidal behaviour and may be detrimental to one's mental health. The authors also concluded that initiating programmes which assist in the re-employment among seniors upon retirement may be a preventive measure.

In another significant study published in the Australian Journal of General Practice (Ref: Self-harm in their older patients-RACGP www1.racgp.org.au › ajgp › March › self-harm), the self-harm by older people was studied by a group of General Practitioners. The participating GPs identified a multifactorial reasons contributing to self-harm in their patients and concluded in part that it is through educational intervention and meeting the older patients needs through specialised and targeted services offered by specialists in the field of social and psychological trauma may be part of the solution in addition to medical intervention.

The average retirement age around the world is about 62 years while in Australia, Canada, UK, and other developed nations this age is 63–67 years.

So, my categorisation looks like this:

65 years to 74. ………………………………...... Early-Seniors
75 years to 80. ……………………………….. Mid-Seniors
81 years to the end of their life. ……………… Matured-Seniors

The first category although qualify for retirement and if eligible then for pension, and, given that the availability of appropriate nutrition and supplements to this group is adequate, they can be considered as fit and healthy; within reasons. Of course, some individual circumstances may vary which may tip the balance. Seniors in this age group may still be working and have meaningful jobs and lifestyles.

The next category of seniors is in the age bracket where many are still living an active lifestyle. But quite a few are vulnerable to ill health due to their socio-economic background and other societal reasons such as loneliness, neglect and lack of adequate care. Some may also be suffering from certain chronic ailments.

The final category, where seniors are of the age 81 years or more, it has been a common consensus that the majority may not be self-reliant and in need of some form of care regimen. They are probably suffering from old age diseases due to a decline in their lifestyle and social interaction. Looking on the bright side many seniors in this category live a very meaningful life and hence they can be the trendsetters for the rest of us seniors to follow.

United Nations Organisation (UNO) has projected that life expectancy among the world population is 72.81 years which is an increase of 0.24% from 2020. This is not taking into consideration the negative effects of COVID-19 on longevity.

It is important to realise that in developed and many developing nations there is a senior's pension scheme available for retirees, although the scheme is not universal and heavily dependent on the budgetary configuration of the country concerned. In many societies, there are family assistance and several Non-Government Organisations (NGOs) which provide some assistance which helps subsidise the living expenses and standards of many elderly retirees. This certainly boosts the morale of the needy seniors and helps them to live a contented life for the rest of their living years.

Spare a thought for poorer nations where the government lacks resources to put into senior's retirement schemes and they are left to fend for themselves. It has been reported by the World Bank that almost 689 million people (approx. 9% of the world population) live in extreme poverty.

The value of good nutrition, for all, is very important in today's society for many reasons, especially for the seniors in our society, some of which are:

- Unavailability of freshly cooked meals full of nutritional goodness which may lead to poor dietary intake.
- Lack of availability of adequate care for the senior's community.
- Socio-economic reasons preventing seniors from making the right nutritional choices.
- The feeling of loneliness, lack of confidence and forgetfulness.
- Ill health and dejections.
- Physiological changes associated with advancing age which can affect one's appetite, digestive processes, and other conditions which could stand in the way to recovery from ailments and, or, good health.
- Drug (medicine) nutrient interaction which can lead to inefficient absorption of essential nutrients from their diets. This mainly stems from a lack of awareness of drug-nutrition interaction.

All of the above and for several other reasons, many seniors in the age bracket of 81+ may not have the right facilities, means and possibly the inclination to achieve the desired nutritional outcome. It is therefore important to make use of supplements suitable to their nutritional needs to improve the quality of life as best as possible. But again, there may be an issue with affordability and awareness.

What are the most common diseases that seniors suffer in their advancing age? I have listed some basic conditions that seniors are likely to succumb to:

Sensory Changes

With ageing our sensory perceptions change significantly; hearing, sight, taste, smell and touch are the sensory parameters that connect older people to the outside world and also connect them socially. Impairment in any of the sensory faculties could cause low esteem, stress and depression and other forms of mental anguish which later may manifest in some form of major problem for the sufferer to deal with.

Sensory changes would mainly be concerned with a gradual decline in sight and hearing senses which is quite common in seniors of advanced age. These can be rectified to a certain degree by medical intervention. Certain supplementary aspects may also help such as administering vitamin A, Beta-carotene and a diet rich in carrots, leafy vegetables and yellow pumpkins.

Hearing loss can be compensated by the use of hearing aids.

Sensory perceptions and messages are taken to the brain via the sensory nerves and return back to the sensory organs concerned, e.g., finger touch, smell through the nose and taste through the taste buds in the mouth. The stronger the return message or command from the brain is, the stronger the feeling or the senses. The brain sends signals via the motor nerves to the peripheral nerve system for the activation of the sensory organs.

Neurotransmitters are the actual biochemical molecules which transmit and or carry messages from neurons to and from the brain for the actual messages and commands to be relayed to the appropriate section of the peripheral nerve system.

There are many bio-chemical neurotransmitters in our body and almost 100 have been identified of which the common neurotransmitters are glutamate, acetylcholine, glycine, norepinephrine, etc. Supplementary intake of individual or a combination of neurotransmitters can assist in a number of sensory impairments. Intake of Lecithin supplementation can improve the choline and acetylcholine levels in the body. Acetylcholine being a neurotransmitter plays an important role in muscle movement, memory function, power of thinking, and general activity of the brain. It has been reported that a low level of acetylcholine is associated with memory loss and decline in brain function; it also assists in improvement in anxiety (Ref: Br J Nutr 2013 Feb 14; 109(3), and Ref: Am J Clin Nutr. 2009 Oct; 90).

Cognitive Health

Although there may not be a cure to enhance our cognitive health after a certain age, but it has been widely reported that by making some lifestyle adjustments improvements can be noticeable.

There are a number of activities that may be considered to enhance our cognitive skills; some of these can be practiced in our old age.

- Mental Stimulation:
- Solving puzzles, simple mathematical equations, mental games which require thinking such as remembering people and places you may have visited in the distant past, birth dates etc. There can be any number of life memories that can be brought to life by the power of remembrance.
- Dietary adjustments:
- To improve blood sugar, cholesterol and triglyceride levels and controlling blood pressure.
- Avoiding abuse or misuse of alcohol, drug and tobacco.
- Try to build up social network, keeping in-touch with friends and relatives to ease loneliness and try to minimise emotional stresses.
- Light to moderate physical exercises:
- Undertake group walks or walk with a companion; a friend or a pet.
- Light physical exercises such as swimming, free hand exercises as mentioned in Chapter 5 will help to pass time, listen to music, read books, etc. All these will certainly help and lead to the path of fulfilment and enjoyment.
- Playing cards and board games in a group or simply playing alone (Patience) can be good for cognitive improvement in elderly.

In a reputable publication (The Journals of Gerontology: series B, Vol. 75, Issue 3, March 2020 pages 474-482) cognitive benefits are mentioned.

I know it is easy said than done; but a slight effort from our part could provide a meaningful benefit.

Under-Nutrition, Malnutrition and Nourishment

This is the ultimate neglect and socio-economic disaster that a senior in the higher age bracket may be trapped under. Although malnutrition can be a less prevalent and most uncommon cause of sufferance in seniors in the developed nations there have been incidences whereby few have fallen through the cracks through the systemic errors.

Another reason is that due to increasing costs of living all over the world, many seniors have to adjust with the limited resources at their disposal and resort to prioritising their needs not wants. This leads to a tendency to buy cheaper substandard food stuff to save money and to make ends meet and therefore, the use of vitamin and mineral supplements as a way for nutritional fortification is pushed way down the priority list.

Malnutrition among seniors in many under-developed and developing countries is more common as the government in those countries is not equipped to handle and deal with such eventualities. In many of these countries, the retirement age can be around 55–60 years with no pension schemes for the needy; welfare is almost non-existent and dependence on relatives and charity is crucial. In those countries, the mortality rates among seniors are quite high and may even start at the age of high 50s in some cases soon after retirement when the income stops and destitute and hardship takes over.

Lack or loss of appetite is also a reason for malnutrition. With advancing age, the urge to eat diminishes for medical or psychological reasons and it is very hard to revert back to normal conditions without medical intervention and enticement with tasty and variety of prepared meals.

Loss of Balance and Physical Injuries

Loss of balance and, or, steadiness in the frame of a senior can be linked with several health conditions and as described early sensory changes can contribute significantly.

Some common medical conditions such as Parkinson's, Multiple Sclerosis, infection in the middle and inner ears, blood pressure issues, and muscle weakness are all prime reasons for loss of balance in any age but more so in seniors. Balance problems in seniors are quite common, it is estimated that in the USA alone about 25% of seniors have reported difficulties associated with balance. It is also estimated that over 50% of seniors above the age of 75 have had a fall or likely to have a fall each year with men and women equally affected.

The Centre for Disease Control (CDC) states that the most common injury for seniors over 65 is the common fall and that more than 3 million people in the USA are treated each year. Most falls are non-fatal common falls with broken bones and fractures. Wrist and hip fractures are most common but ribs, nose, and head injuries can also be serious. Head injuries may lead to brain injuries which may prove to be of significant concern in seniors. All fall injuries are complex and will need medical intervention which may lead to hospitalisation and, or, longer rehabilitation care.

Loss of balance may also be associated with the effect of prolonged use of medications, several chronic health conditions such as dementia, respiratory conditions, cardiovascular diseases and many other health issues that seniors are likely to suffer with age and decline in their lifestyle.

Burn is also a common injury inflicted upon the old age population due to their forgetfulness such as leaving the candle or stove on after cooking and more seriously leaving the radiator or gas heaters on while sleeping with loose flammable articles lying around which are deadly sources of fire. This is most hazardous and dangerous and can be fatal.

Mental Issues

Mental issues are best tackled by experts and usually require medical intervention and care. The basic health issues under this category depression, dementia, Alzheimer's disease, and memory loss can be triggered by several life issues such as poverty, loneliness, ill-treatment, lack of good nutrition and also fear. With proper care and nutrition, most of these mental issues can be helped but not cured as almost all of these conditions are irreversible.

Care is the fundamental consideration; the feeling of security, love and respect, instilling the feeling that they are still wanted can work wonders not only for seniors but for all as these good basic human traits and comforting words can be the panacea to all cures.

Several herbs infused as teas or in combination with proteins, amino acids, vitamins and minerals as supplements can also help if administered regularly in the right dosages.

Chamomile, Passionflower, Lemon balm, Aswagandha are all tried and proven herbs which have positive calming effects. Many herbs have been used since the Ayurvedic days which dates back to around 3000 years. Other herbs such as *Ginkgo biloba*, ginseng, ginger root, turmeric, etc., are all useful herbal supplements.

Seniors and Their Dietary Requirements

First and foremost, we need to look at foods that are suitable and complimentary to the seniors' by their age group and needs.

Early-Seniors, the 65–74 age bracket are reasonably active and fit and continue to do so by being able to take care of themselves more than the seniors in the higher age brackets. This is possible due to their continued social skill and social interactions. This group of seniors also enjoy some financial security and fewer medical episodes and therefore are reasonably independent.

Many seniors in the age bracket 75–80 years (Mid-Seniors) would be less privileged than their younger counterparts and may need assistance due to their age, low mobility and health issues. This group of senior citizens along with the above 80-year-old senior members of the community are the ones we need to focus on for their welfare, health and nutritional requirements.

Many organisations in the developed nations have similar charters and are to some degree involved in the care and well-being of the seniors in this category. One important aspect of their charter is to provide cooked meals and to offer medical assistance if and when needed. Several issues reflect their nutritional needs; such as fresh foods which may not be easily accessible if these senior groups were to fend for themselves. Several other issues that may be of discussion points are food that is easily digestible and easily processed but are pre-packaged and held in cold storage for a considerable length of time with diminished food values. The idea is to offer foods which are packed with nutrition and calories to provide sufficient energy and which are not just filling. The idea is to offer prepared food with extra calories without the extra volume.

Choose safe foods which are less prone to microbiological contamination Food that can be chewed and swallowed easily to assist seniors who have dental problems and other anatomical reasons.

Adequate intake of fluids is recommended.

It is also considered helpful if meal times are consistent which allows the digestive system to cater for the food processing mechanism. Once this becomes a routine then the digestive system efficiency also increases.

Smaller portions of quality food are always better than larger meals; this is especially important in older seniors with impaired bodily functions. Overloading of the food processing system in their body may lead to several digestive issues which if not attended to timely could manifest as a major disease state.

In Chapter 4, I have mentioned sugar, salt and water being the three nutrients that our body needs and must have to function, but in moderation. These three nutrients are as natural as it gets and play an important role in our health and well-being if their intake is controlled. The same theory also applies to senior's nutrition.

So, how much sugar, salt and water are needed by seniors?

There is no fixed required quantity as it is considerably dependent upon age, gender, activity levels and body functions such as rate of urination, sweating and medical involvement for example medical interventions for diseases like blood pressure, diabetes, etc., and also daily medicinal intakes. It is important to follow the advice of your medical practitioner and stay alert about your daily intake be it meals, snacks, beverages and also medicines.

Sugar intake is very common in all ages; it is also very easy to exceed your daily requirement as all carbohydrates and proteins ingested will convert into sugars (glucose) which is the most basic molecule that gets converted into the energy molecule ATP. People of most ages except the elderly seniors can burn off the excess glucose due to various daily activities such as playing sports, walking, running, school or office works, etc. Seniors of advanced ages have limited choices of activity when it comes to burning off extra calories; however, here are some mild activities which do help seniors burn off calories.

Just standing for 10 minutes will burn 10 calories.

Walking up and down the stairs for just 10 minutes will burn off 100 calories.

Gardening for 25 minutes, weeding, digging planting will shed 100 calories.

Standard house cleaning work for 30 minutes will burn off 100 calories for you.

Playing golf for 25 minutes making sure you carry your own clubs will get rid of 100 calories.

There are many other enjoyable activities which will help burn off 100 calories in 15–20 minutes, e.g., low-impact aerobics, light swimming, walking, etc.

You will be surprised to find out how this all adds up. Let's do the calculation. Mayo Clinic has estimated that in order to lose around half a kilogram of body fat we need to burn off 3,500 calories. For people who want to lose weight, the easy way they can start burning off 100 calories each day in addition to their normal daily activities. Any of the above-mentioned activities will do. So, in a year or in 365 days, you are likely to lose 36,500 calories which is round about 5 kg of your body weight. This trimming will go a long way if you are suffering from overweight, diabetes, blood pressure issues, mild respiratory issues or many other lifestyle diseases.

This is good news indeed, as you can let yourself indulge from time to time without much of a concern. But keep in mind all health warnings and considerations must be adhered to and every bit of health advice which may be different for different people must be followed. Next to sugar, salt is also an important dietary consideration; you need it yet you don't. Sounds confusing, let me explain. Salt is very important for every animal including we humans on this planet. Salt is composed of two essential elements Sodium and chloride and more than often both get nasty reviews and ill reputation by the health and nutritional industry, yet both are essential elements and as such important in our dietary requirements.

But all criticism aside the gist is that we do need sodium and we do need chloride in small quantities for our biochemical processes which sustain our health and well-being and keep us alive. Moderation is the key word and a sensible approach to the dietary intake of salt is essential.

Listed below are only a few life-sustaining body functions that these two elements are involved in.

Sodium helps in maintaining blood volume and blood pressure by retaining fluid and maintaining fluid balance in our system.

Sodium along with potassium maintains an osmotic pressure balance from inside and outside the cell wall maintaining a perfect spherical shape of the cells which carry oxygen and nutrients efficiently.

Sodium also plays a critical role in nerve impulse conduction and muscle contraction.

Chloride, an ionized form of chlorine plays an important role in acid-base balance and helps regulate the pH of all body fluids. Chloride also in combination with hydrogen ion acts as an anti-bacterial agent in preventing bacterial overgrowth in the gastrointestinal tract.

Our body's immune system cells require chloride; also, our red blood cells require chloride to expel carbon dioxide from our body.

There are many more essential functions that both elements perform and therefore both of these are known as essential elements that our body needs and can't do without.

Even though both sodium and chlorine are essential elements, there are certain guidelines as to how much salt we should consume daily.

According to World Health Organisation (WHO) adults should not consume more than 5g (just under a teaspoon) of salt per day; the less the better. The Australian Guidelines as set by The National Health and Medical Research Council (NHMRC) also recommends use at less than 5g daily. The Food and Nutrition Board in the USA recommends a slightly lower intake of around 3g daily for seniors above the age of 70 years.

My personal opinion is that the less salt consumed by the seniors is best. My reasons are based on the following points:

Excess salt intake is associated with high blood pressure

(Blood Pressure UK

https://www.bloodpressureuk.org › healthy-eating › salt-...) and therefore increased risk of cardiovascular disease, e.g., stroke, heart attack and heart failure, etc. Seniors are more at risk due to instability in their heart condition. Excess salt can damage the lining of the stomach causing risk of infiltration of cancer-causing bacteria such as *Helicobacter pylori*. Seniors are most vulnerable as their stomach lining is already weak.

Excess salt consumption may have a detrimental effect on brain health in general, but, more so in seniors.

Older seniors are more at risk of osteoporosis. The aging process causes loss in bone density and thinning of bone structure. High salt intake has been associated with osteoporosis.

Apart from these major issues, there are other adjunct issues such as kidney damage associated with high blood pressure.

Water is an important dietary requirement for all ages with variable intake necessary to compensate for the loss of hydration due to activity levels, sweating, urinary excretion, environmental heat and humidity.

As per the guidelines from NH & MRC Australia adults and seniors should drink 3.4–2.8 litres a day depending on the gender. In general, the compliance level for all age groups except for older age seniors (75 years and above) is on a needs basis. After various activity levels, hot and humid days and under special needs, e.g., after meals we tend to drink water or other fluids such as fruit juice or alcoholic beverages such as beer to quench our thirst and to clear our food pipe.

With older seniors, the compliance level is poor as many do not adhere to their required fluid intake. This often causes dehydration irrespective of the weather conditions or activity levels. So, what are the reasons for this non-compliance?

Most important non-compliance problems come from memory loss and mobility issues. Physiological and anatomical considerations should also be rated high on the list of reasons for seniors not drinking enough water. Frail older seniors who are in care institutions can often suffer from dehydration due to several additional reasons, for example, access to independent dispensing of water is limited and availability depends on the staff of the institution offering water to drink. The other psychological reason being hesitancy to ask staff for a drink due to forgetfulness, consequence and or lack of self-assuredness.

It is absolutely necessary that seniors whether living independently or in a care situation must drink a minimum of 1.7–2 litres of fluid in 24 hours. In the seniors' care regime, it is a challenge to get them to drink this minimum quantity of fluid. So, how to achieve this? This may not be so much of an issue with seniors living independently as it is assumed that they will be able to manage with some external intervention from a relative, but for seniors under care management, this may prove to be a task in itself.

However, several solutions, each having its own merits and challenges can be trialled. This sounds like a training routine, but, if it ends up benefiting the seniors then why not.

Smaller quantities of water in an attractive container could be left in a prominent but favourite place for the senior to consume; however, they will need to be alerted or educated that it is water (or their favourite beverage) for them to drink. Replenish the container once consumed with a next lot of water or another fluid. An independently living senior can practise the same thing. Keep a tab on the number of refills.

Mix and match the refills by substituting them with different low-sugar fresh fruit juices which are preferred by seniors under the care regime.

Sometimes completely deviating from the norm may create interest in accepting a drink. For example, offer flavoured ice cubes or popsicles and even a smoothie, milkshakes, etc. This is also a means to keep seniors hydrated and provide a nutrient-enriched drink.

Extra fluid intake will be necessary on hot sweltering days and during sickness such as diarrhoea and vomiting which is a common cause of dehydration in all ages not just in the ageing population.

It is important to remember that a common cause of reluctance for fluid intake in elderly and frail seniors is incontinence. It is a major concern of carers and must be addressed adequately through psychological and, or, medical intervention.

Some of the early and common signs of senior's dehydration are:

- A strong urine with dark colour and foul odour.
- Fluctuation in blood pressure.
- Seniors may show signs of weakness and loss of balance, dizziness, etc.
- Seniors may seem to be in a state of confusion.
- Decline in the frequency of urination.

One good thing about temporary dehydration is that when adequate amount of water is administered the symptoms start to fade. However, if symptoms persist urgent medical intervention is required.

As we age our body functions, such as digestive functions also weaken. This limits our ability to absorb various vitamins, minerals, macro and micro-nutrients from the foods we eat leading to a depletion of reserves of essential nutrients. This puts more demand on the requirements of essential nutrients which may not be easily available in our foods. So, the obvious solution is to supplement on a regular basis with a good quality multi-nutrient formula. I prefer to take powder formula which has a shorter onset of activity in place of a tablet which has a longer onset of activity. The powder is more convenient and can be administered easily and stirred in water or other fluid of choice.

In the food preparation department, choose a selection of ingredients from the five food varieties mentioned in Chapter 4. There have been a number of recommendations reported in various journals and publications for seniors to consider, just to name a few:

Eat more vegetables and fruits; wash them first prior to eating raw such as fruits, carrots, radishes, tomatoes, celery, etc.

Eat more fish than red meat.

Eggs and poultry are excellent sources of protein.

Nuts are rich in essential fatty acids, unsaturated fats and proteins and make a good snack for seniors. Nuts also help preserve the lean body mass and improve the body mass index.

Use less carbohydrates in senior's diet and replace with pasta which has concentrated energy and less starch when cooked.

Lamb and beef livers have significant amounts of vitamin B12 and iron, so include this in the diet on a rotating basis.

Seafood will add variety and nutrition to your diet so include it occasionally; provided no allergic symptoms are noticed previously.

Eat complex fibre in moderation for regulation of bowel movement; oats, bran, apples, peas, lentils and beans are a good source of fibres. 20–30g fibre for older seniors per day is sufficient.

Avoid alcoholic drinks, tea, coffee or any other caffeine beverages before going to bed. A warm glass of milk if you can manage it just before bedtime will work wonders for your sleep during the night.

Now to vitamins and mineral-enriched meal planning; always try to structure your meals around healthy nutritive produce and ingredients. Steamed or boiled vegetables, salads and a third of the portion of protein will be ideal for seniors. If you are boiling vegetables, make sure that you do not drain out the liquid which is rich in vitamins and minerals from the vegetables, but make it into a sauce or gravy to top up your meal. There are several meals that you can structure such as weight gain or loss, diabetic meal plan, vegan and, or vegetarian meal plan and many more. It is a good sense that you get your meals planned on a three-monthly review by your nutritionist and move forward.

The shortlist of vegetables below can provide a guide to your choice if you are looking for and try to rotate your pick to add variety to your plate.

Sweet Potatoes: They are packed with good energy with complex fibre and carbohydrates, manganese, vitamin A and beta-carotene.

Always look for in-season produce because the likelihood of those produce being fresh is greater than off-season cold storage stuff.

Spinach and other leafy green vegetables: Rich in fibre and minerals, e.g., iron, calcium, magnesium, potassium and vitamins A, B group, C and K.

Broccoli: It should be a regular inclusion for a senior's plate. It provides a healthy amount of vitamins C and K both essential for dietary requirements for all ages and also contains compounds which may protect DNA from cell damage and also it is reported that it may help inhibit several types of cancers.

(Ref: UCLA Health https://www.uclahealth.org › news › broccoli-and-other...)

Carrots: Carrots provide an enormous amount of beta-carotene (pre-vitamin A) essential for eye health and vision. It may also have nutrients with cancer-fighting properties.

Tomatoes: This is also a fruit cum vegetable which must be in every one's plate on a regular basis due to its vitamin C, Lutein and Zeaxanthin and significant quantity of Lycopene content. These nutrients are reported to offer significant protection in age-related macular degeneration and prostate cancer. Other vegetables recommended are garlic, ginger, onions beetroots, etc., which are all healthy, but their use in moderation is recommended due to their strong taste and odour.

As I mentioned the need for a good multi-nutrient formula for inclusion in senior's daily intake is worthwhile to review; primarily the nutrients which are showing a shortage in your nutritional profile.

Calcium and vitamin D combination will assist in the strengthening of bone tissues. Vitamin D works in association with calcium to protect the bone health and structure.

Vitamin C in a multi-vitamin formulation particularly in combination with B-group vitamins is worth considering. Vitamin C is important for immunity, and B vitamins improve the cellular metabolism upon which many bodily functions are dependent on.

Vitamin E is a popular choice of seniors (55 years and above) in America as a supplement. It has been widely reported that its antioxidant activity significantly assists in age-related illnesses such as cataract, heart problems, certain types of cancers and in general minor ailments. Vitamin E in combination with vitamin A and/or Beta-carotene is also helpful in vision improvement, health of blood cells, brain and skin. Vitamin B12 is difficult to absorb at the best of times; for seniors, it is even more difficult. Choose a vitamin B complex with all the B-group vitamins with a special addition of biotin, folic acid and B12. The choice is very important and may require professional help.

Minerals are important for older seniors, older seniors may require zinc, magnesium, calcium, potassium and iron. Other trace minerals can be made available by choosing a healthy diet and frequently rotating to mix and match available nutrients and add variety to their plate. Other major nutrients required are omega fatty acids, amino acids and fish oils.

There are published reports on the benefits of omega fatty acids, fish oils and amino acids that their inclusion in senior's diet may have some positive bearing on dementia and Alzheimer's disease, rheumatoid arthritis, age-related macular degeneration (AMD), dry-eyes disease, etc. Many of the reported trials are backed up by science and many are still unclear and need further research.

Traditionally as we age our appetite decreases due to a lack of daily energy requirement for performing daily activities. It is estimated that the Basal Metabolic Rate (BMR) in seniors aged 75 and over is around 1400 Calories for males and slightly less figure of 1320 Calories per day for females. What is a calorie you may ask; a calorie is a unit of measurement for energy. When we eat food or drink, it gives us energy which is quantified in terms of calories. In a very simple scientific definition, one calorie of energy is the energy required to increase the temperature of one gram of water by one degree Celsius.

The Basal Metabolic Rate of energy requirement is the minimum energy required for all the body functions to remain active even when your body is at rest and not doing anything.

Estimated Daily energy value requirement for seniors without strenuous activities

Subject	Age Group	EER (calories)	BMR (calories)
Male	55–74	2175	-
	75+	1980	1400
Female	55–74	1820	-
	75+	1720	1320

EER: Estimate daily energy requirement and BMR: daily Basal Metabolic Rate. These values may vary slightly from one report to another depending on the method of calculation.

As we age the demand for our nutritional needs also changes, due to several of our vital functions slowing down. However, if this is not carefully monitored then there is a serious risk of nutritional deficiency and, or, a risk of overnutrition in the cases of well-to-do seniors; let me explain what this means. The capacity of our stomach to produce enough acid decreases resulting in a imbalance in the pH system resulting in a loss of digestion and absorption functions. This causes a malabsorption in the micronutrients from the food intake.

Loss of bone density can cause an excess requirement in calcium, magnesium, zinc and vitamin D as vitamin D and minerals can leach out from soft tissues where deposits of calcium are significant, e.g., bone and teeth tissues.

Muscle loss or muscle degeneration increases the demand for protein and amino acids in seniors and therefore intake of easily digestible sources such as fish, poultry, etc., may be helpful.

Dietary or supplementary iron is important for haemoglobin in blood to carry oxygen to compensate for the breathing difficulties that many seniors suffer in their advancing age. Vitamin C will assist in boosting immunity and assist iron absorption from foods.

Seniors and Their Medicinal and Supplement Requirements

Compliance is an important factor when considering the health and well-being of seniors; this is true both in independent living and community-based living situations.

There are two considerations, first, the compliance level for the access to medication in elderly citizens is poor and needs a lot to be improved if their health and general well-being is to be monitored effectively. The other consideration is that of compliance level for access to nutritional supplements. Again, the level of compliance for the intake is quite poor. There are several factors that come into play here, too many in fact, however, the following can be itemised for preliminary notification.

- The age, mental and physical health of the patient.
- Independent living or community-based care facility provided for the patient.
- Mobility and the cognitive health of the patient.
- Socio-economic status.
- Training backgrounds and interactive skills of the primary and the secondary care providers.

These are a few of the vast number of issues that need to be addressed in order for us to comply with the WHO charter that every person in every country in the world should have the opportunity to live a long and healthy life.

It is postulated that the population of seniors 60 years and above is on the rise from 1 billion in 2019 to an expected 1.4 billion in 2030 and on to 2.1 billion in 2050; this is about 1 in every 7 global citizen will be a senior according to WHO's definition; I still maintain it should be 65 years and above. In developing countries with increasing longevity, the increase will be even greater after 2050 and beyond.

I hope the relevant government departments are discussing this challenging issue and preparing themselves for the future ahead.

There is no easy solution to this, it is up to us to do our bit knowing fully well that we will be in that situation sooner than later.

One of the solutions to this global issue and challenge can come through a social network of events. Senior citizens have to be educated in societal norms of the current times not just on the healthcare aspects and how to take care of their health issues. A level of self-confidence and self-determination needs to be instilled into them so that they can feel the electricity buzzing through them.

It is true that they are the wealth of knowledge and experience in their previously chosen field and the younger generation can harness that knowledge and build their future on it. There is a view going around that in this new age of electronics and technology, it is the survival of the fittest. We all can't be IT geniuses; there needs to be a good pilot guiding our ship and make the bumpy ride much smoother.

In a family situation, who is better than a grandpa and grandma to look after the children and teach them moral values and pacify them when their parents are busy working to provide for them. There are whole heap of social issues and networks where seniors can fit in if only the present-day society will give them a chance rather than centralising the society into a nuclear family. Seriously this can be a wonderful solution among other solutions and the powers to be should consider and facilitate to make it happen. The population explosion of seniors globally as predicted requires reconfiguration and adjustment in the makeup of our society across the board.

The prime effort and resources need to be assigned to care modalities such as social welfare, health care, transport, housing, adequate low-cost accommodation, etc., which are essential and part of planning and development for the senior's friendly charter of the WHO.

In highlighting the issues with non-compliance in taking their regular medication, it is important for the caregiver to educate the senior under his/her care on the importance of the medication and the reason for taking it/them on a regular basis. Most seniors depending on their age group take multiple medicines which may pose some challenges but somehow it needs to be addressed if satisfactory compliance levels were to be achieved.

Statistically about 90% of the seniors are on one prescribed medication; around 80% are on at least 2 prescribed medications and 36% regularly take 5 or more prescription medications. Some of these medications are to improve the quality of life and some are necessity and life-sustaining medications.

Depending on the care level and the facility provided, the educational orientation may be tailor-made. Seniors who enjoy home care surrounded by their families and loved ones may or need not worry about compliance as their medication intake requirements are handled with care and diligence of the family members. Institutionalised care is very challenging indeed as one carer has a multiple charges under his/her care all requiring varying degrees of care level. It takes a special kind of person with specialised training to fulfil the role with patience and attitude to suit the situation.

When it comes to nutritional supplements, the compliance levels are bad to moderate depending on both users and the carer's beliefs about supplementation. It is important to realise that due to age our digestive capacity diminishes resulting in a weaker absorption of nutrients from our dietary intake. Supplementation is a convenient way for replenishment and most seniors are accepting to this fact if only it can be explained to them in a simple way.

There is another reason for supplementation:

Side effects of prescription drugs are quite common in every user irrespective of age. In older citizens, it is more pronounced and can manifest from a simple temporary sickness to a more noticeable and debilitating consequences. There are any number of reasons why side effects of drugs are more prevalent in older populations, e.g.:

- Older people take more medication than younger population resulting in more side effects.
- Older people have weaker digestive, absorption, and elimination systems resulting in toxin build-up which the weaker kidneys are unable to excrete in the urine. Also, weak liver function of older people is unable to or is inefficient in processing the toxins into less harmful metabolites.
- Toxin buildup in the tissues of older people can happen due to lack of water intake limiting the flush down of the tissues to be carried to the elimination processing system.

As mentioned, a good quality multi-nutrient product once a day is a good way of keeping fortified and a healthy pool of reserve. Vitamin C, D, B-complex and important elements such as iron, zinc, selenium, copper, manganese, chromium, etc., can help together with a good mix of dietary intake of greens, proteins, carbs, nuts and grains and a daily routine of light exercise can work wonders for all let alone the seniors.

But when all is said and done seniors' nutrition and welfare is a very challenging subject and requires authoritative interventions which cannot be left in a 'To Do List', or, in a 'too hard basket' as consequences can be serious if unaddressed.

We all are heading towards this elite band of population age demography sooner or later. Decisions taken today leads to the successful pathway of tomorrow.

There are many factors with healthy ageing; independent living, lack of care and motivation and also some degree of genetic influence. Other aspects which are under one's control such as physical movement, healthy eating and social grouping and interactions can be managed. All we need is a balanced life and willingness.

Self-Affirmations

Life can be very challenging as we age; so, what can we do to increase the life expectancy without compromising the quality of the lifestyle in our aging population? A big challenge indeed.

In addition to all the positives we have described in the chapter, let us look at self-motivation and uplifting experiences that seniors could practice which is likely to lead them to a graceful ageing.

How to keep busy in a meaningful way? A few pointers to think about.

- Revisit your hobbies, stimulate your past interests and join social activities.
- Renew relationships and strengthen family ties.
- Join discussion groups to revitalise your cognitive skills.
- Get involved in financial activities be it your own or assistance programmes.
- Create mentoring programmes, offer your professional and life experiences.
- Self-affirmation.

Self-affirmation can be a powerful tool to increase life span with dignity and quality. There are several publications where it has been demonstrated that positive thinking and self-affirmations can alter brain's response to health messages and subsequent behaviour change (Ref: Proc Natl Acad Sci USA 2015 Feb 17; 112(7): 1977–1982).

Another research reported that Spontaneous self-affirmation was related to positive outcomes in health contexts (Ref: Psychol Health. 2016; 31(3): 292–309).

Several other published papers which affirm that there is genuinely a positive effect of self-affirmation when practicing in a sincere and diligent way.

- Cohen, G. L., and Sherman, D. K. (2014) 'The psychology of change: Self-affirmation and social psychological intervention', *Annual Review of Psychology,* **65,** 333–371.
- Cooke, R., Trebaczyk, H., Harris, P., and Wright, A. J. (2014) 'Self—affirmation promotes physical activity', *Journal of Sport and Exercise Psychology,* **36,** 217–223.

A few affirmations that may boost self-esteem and rekindle love for life (Jay Das, 2022):

- *I have done many things in my life; I can jump the last hurdle and if needed I can jump even higher.*
- *My mind is clear, my path is steadier and my future years are brighter.*
- *I still have lots to contribute to the society, my skills, my knowledge and most of all my wisdom.*

And just one more, *"I am me; I am I and I am my positive destiny."*
(Jay Das, 2022)

The objective of an affirmation is to wipe out the negatives from the mind and replace it with positive vibes and emotions. There is no room for negatives.

Always remember in self-affirmation (exercises!) it is you in the lead role and always start with me, I am me, etc., as the lead, so give yourself the praise you deserve. Do not drag in the past but live in the present; you may bask in the glory of your past; but, let the past rest and concentrate on the present and the future. Draw inspirations from your past and use this motivation to make your present and future even more relevant.

Remember the word we have used Heal-thy-Self and use the self-affirmation tool in the management of your healing process.

I close the chapter with these words my father used to say to me "Though the path be dark as night, Trust in God and do the right" and in my version now:

"Though the path be dark as night, trust yourself and do the right."

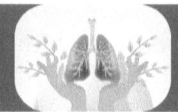

Chapter 11

COVID CRISIS

I started writing this book in December 2020 during a lockdown in Sydney, New South Wales (Australia). So, I think it is appropriate to bring out the subject of Covid-19 as it has been dominating our lives for the past 24 months and more and still continues to do so. However, the world has known of the Coronavirus since late 2019 and therefore it has been a part of our life and environment for almost 3 long years.

By virtue of my training and background in biochemistry, many of my friends and acquaintances have asked me what is coronavirus in context of the COVID-19, how did it spread and what is the future.

Before commenting on these issues, I have always pleaded ignorance as I am no longer a practicing biochemist and have not had much experience in virology and microbiology in particular pertaining to this pandemic as such to offer advice. But my interest and curiosity let me delve in this subject as best as I could with the prevailing information that was around us at the time. Take it with a grain of salt if you must, or try to read up as best as you can and put 2 and 2 together for your own interest.

World Health Organisation (WHO) and Coronavirus

One of the earliest speculations of this deadly virus was cited when the World Health Organisation (WHO) was informed of a pneumonia-like disease spreading in Wuhan City, Hubei Province in the People's Republic of China. This was in late December 2019 and gained further notoriety when the Chinese Authorities detected and identified a virus which was named as *'2019-nCoV'* a novel form of *Coronavirus*. This was on January 7th, 2020.

On 11 and 12 January 2020, WHO received further detailed information from the National Health Commission China that this outbreak originated in Wuhan through exposures in one of the seafood markets or the so-called wet market.

Since this time the virus started to spread around the world in particular among people who visited Wuhan and neighbouring areas.

As per the situation update (WHO, 20 Jan 2020) 282 confirmed cases of *2019-nCoV* had been reported from four countries including China (278 cases), Thailand (2 cases), Japan (1 case) and the Republic of Korea (1 case); all were exported from Wuhan.

Since then, the virus spread like wildfire in epic proportion in every corner of the world which led WHO to declare Coronavirus a Public Health Emergency of International Concern on 30 January 2020, followed by a pandemic on 11 March 2020. Some experts debate that WHO had made this call a little bit too late and should have called it out at the earliest possible time. Since writing this book, out of curiosity, I checked the statistics, Coronavirus (COVID-19) at a glance—31 December 2020 (an Australian Govt. Dept. of Health Report) and found a total of 28,408 cases of COVID-19 had been reported in Australia, including 909 deaths, and approximately 217 active cases.

My further check for the data to 30th June 2021 about 15 months since 11th March 2020 was as follows, a total of 30,610 cases of COVID-19 had been reported in Australia, including 910 deaths, and approximately 317 active cases. At least, due to geographical isolation and State and Federal Governmental controls, the outbreak of the virus had not been as deadly as most parts of the world especially in the developed nations. It is interesting to note that as a direct comparison according to Johns Hopkins Coronavirus Resource Centre, to June 30, 2021 total cases worldwide were 181,970,477 and the total deaths worldwide was 3,940,936.

If we compute the world population to be 7.8 billion, then the ratio of population to total cases of COVID-19 is 2.33% and for death is about 0.5% after rounding off. However, the ratio of the total number of Coronavirus cases to death is significantly high around 2.15%, whereas, this figure in Australia is 0.3% which is still 3 deaths per 1000 coronavirus cases in Australia too many.

Just to give an example, the alarming rate COVID-19 is rampant; as at 1st September 2021 almost 217,558,771 cases of the virus were detected globally with 4,517,240 deaths which equates to 2.75% and 0.57%

With 2.75% of the world's population still affected with the virus and still showing an upwards trend, it is predicted that although we have to live with this we need now is to figure out how to live our lives post-vaccination. In my opinion, until a herd immunity is achieved post vaccination which may be around 80%, we will still be struggling with the virus.

COVID-19 is caused by a highly contagious virus *SARS-CoV-2* (Severe Acute Respiratory Syndrome Coronavirus 2). It was renamed as COVID-19 by WHO on February 11, 2020 to eliminate any ambiguity associated with that name and to simplify the understanding among the general public so as not to confuse with the disease SARS which is a distinctly different virus and also to eliminate any controversy in the public health and infectious disease community.

The breakdown of COVID-19 is simply **CO**RONA **VI**RUS and 19 for the year 20**19,** the year of the outbreak.

Why the name CORONA; simply because the shape of the virus under a high-powered electron microscope is like a crown so in Latin *CORONA*.

Every reputable research laboratory around the world has been searching for a cure which had still eluded the brightest minds of our scientific community, until, due to diligent works by Oxford University scientists and several research facilities of the resourceful pharmaceutical companies we do have vaccines which have at least given us hope that we human race is still far from being decimated and extinction, and will live on to see out the future hopefully in a brighter prospective.

So, What Is COVID-19?

Is it a virus that aliens have spread, to bring human-kind to extinction so that these external celestial beings can take over our beautiful planet? No not a chance.

So, where did it come from?

To answer this let us look at some of the earliest life forms on planet Earth. Bacteria and Viruses are the creation of the evolutionary process. Just like we have been created through an evolutionary pathway. The simplest life form on planet Earth evolved as a single-cell micro-organisms called Cyanobacteria around 3.5–3.9 billion years ago which appeared as a blue green alga; its fossilised remains known as stromatolites which are the secretion of the Cyanobacteria and sediments of sand which over billions of years have shaped into layered sedimentary rock formations. Blue green algae are still around today.

Pictured here is an adaption from Ocean Park Aquarium Shark Bay Western Australia.

(Stromatolites Ocean Park Aquarium Shark Bay Western Australia).

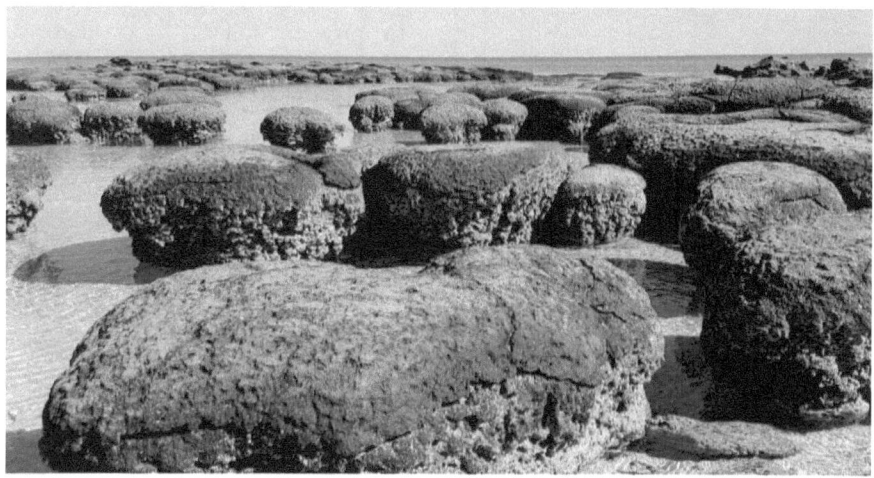

Has the world learned anything from the past epidemics or pandemics? Was the world prepared for the COVID-19 pandemic? The short answer to the first question is yes and for the second question the answer is unfortunately NO. In the last 100 years or so, the population of the world has endured several diseases and illnesses resulting in deadly consequences.

See the table below.

Diseases Known as	Virus Identified	Year of	Estimated Deaths Globally	% of Global Population
Spanish Flu	H1N1	1918	50 million as estimated by CDC	1.8 billion 2.8%
Asian Flu	H2N2	1957–58	1.1 million by CDC	2.9 billion 0.04%
Hong Kong Flu	H3N2	1968–70	1 million by CDC	3.7 billion 0.01%
HIV/AIDS	HIV	1981–	33 million	4.5 billion 0.07%
SARS	SARS-CoV	2002–3	774 (WHO)	6.3 billion (negligible)
Swine Flu	H1N1	2009–10	18,500 (WHO)	6.9 billion (negligible)

Ebola	EVD	2014–16	Approx. 25,000 (CDC)	7.4 billion (negligible)
MERS (Middle East Respiratory Syndrome)	MERS-CoV	2015–	886 (WHO)	7.4 billion (negligible)
COVID-19	Coronavirus—Unknown (possibly pangolins)	2019–	4.5 million estimated by WHO as at 7th Sept. 2021	7.8 billion 0.06%

Unfortunately, we are not done with COVID-19 yet. But as the rate of vaccinations rise among the global population and herd immunity increases there is a hope and opportunity for all of us.

Since my main aim for writing this book was to increase the awareness of nutrition and general health and well-being among the population at large and more specifically among the senior citizens, I felt that due to the extraordinary COVID-19 situation, it is befitting to just document brief sentiments regarding these extraordinary times; one in a 100-year pandemic.

Just to provide my readership a taste of some trivial knowledge, the question which came first bacteria or virus? I believe that both may have evolved at a similar time give or take a billion years long before our own evolution. Virus is a very small biological entity; it is so small and simple that it cannot function on its own and requires a living host cell to replicate and multiply. They have distinct RNA or a DNA sequencing (genetic coding material) and are covered in protein material which gives them distinctive form. So, loosely viruses can be called biological parasites.

Viruses have existed on our planet as long as the RNA and DNA molecules have been part of cells of all living organisms be it plant, animal or insects. Bacteria on the other hand is a larger infectious single-celled organism which does not require living organisms to replicate or to survive. It can multiply everywhere from adverse environment such as snow to sandy deserts and rock formations, water and even air we breathe. They also live inside all living entities as the viruses do.

There are both good bacteria and bad bacteria in our body, and it is estimated that in a human organism, there are approximately 10 times more bacterial cells than our own cellular composition. Nothing good can be said about viruses. The table below will give a quick understanding of the differences between bacteria and viruses.

Virus	**Bacteria**
Virus is not considered as living organisms and requires a living host cell to multiply.	Bacteria are living organisms and can survive independently.
There is nothing such as a good virus. Almost all viruses can cause disease.	Bacteria are both good and bad. Bad bacteria (pathogens) cause infection; good bacteria have many positive benefits e.g., helps in digestion.
Virus is many times smaller than a bacterium.	Bacteria on the average are 10–100 times larger than virus.
Virus do not respond to antibacterial agents.	Some bacteria can respond to antiviral agents.
Virus infects a host cell then multiplies to make it infected to spread the infection in other body cells eventually infecting the whole body. Systemic infection.	Bacteria works independently and is largely confined to one part of the body. Localised infection.
Viruses are contagious.	Some bacterial infections are not contagious.
Viruses are non-cellular.	Bacteria have a well-developed cell structure.

In a report recently published (Current Biology 31, 3504–3514; August 23, 2021 lead author Yassine Souilmi), it is claimed that an ancient corona virus may have infected the ancestors of people living in modern-day East Asia starting around 25,000 years ago and for millennia afterward.

In another publication *Journal of Virology*. **87** (12): 7039–45; most recent common ancestor (MRCA) of all coronaviruses is estimated to be 10,000 years or more old. The virus used bats and other bird species as a host to replicate and then transmitted to human species. It is claimed that by using different modelling of time-line calculations the origins of corona virus can be traced back to over 55 million years, more if we consider that the evolution of bats and other warm-blooded avian species co-evolved with the virus.

Modern coronavirus could be mutated versions of the ancient coronavirus with a similar mode of operation. With new mutations, it seems that the virus is forging ahead in its path to destruction. It may not be possible to fully eradicate the virus but if the infection rate is controlled then we may be able to co-exist. To date vaccination seems to be the only way out with yearly booster jabs for immunisation as we currently do for some other viral infections such as influenza, pneumonia, measles, hepatitis B, shingles, etc., in a few of these cases annual boosters are not required.

Variants of COVID-19

Since it was first acknowledged COVID-19 has mutated to several variants some variants are milder versions of the parent and some much more aggressive. The WHO has identified the variants which are of serious concern to humanity.

Alpha-first found in the United Kingdom.   Sept 2020

Beta-first found in South Africa	May 2020
Gamma-first found in Brazil	Brazil, Nov 2020
Delta-first found in India	Oct 2020
Omicron-first found in South Africa.	Nov 2021

Of these Delta strain has been the worst kind so far, while the Omicron strain seems to be the milder of the two but highly contagious. The early signs are that Omicron is overtaking the Delta variant and my view is that eventually, the milder versions of Omicron will be the predominant variant which we will have to live with as if living with another strain of flu or influenza virus and life will go on and normality will prevail. Or, we may have to perceive with the milder strains of the COVID-19 for a bit longer when hopefully the COVID-19 strains will die off and lose their power of mutation.

Anatomy of COVID-19 Virus (Simplified)

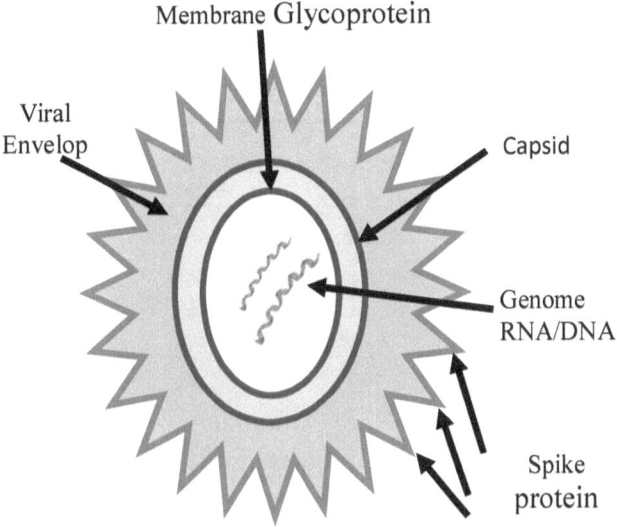

Capsid: is the protein shell encasing the viral genomes.

Viral Envelope: is an external liquid membrane protecting the capsid encasing; (Viral Envelope is not a universal feature of all viral anatomy). Genome: is the genetic coding material that all viral forms have and is made of nucleic acid. This genetic material is either DNA or RNA but not both.

This genetic material has a protective protein coating.

Membrane Glycoprotein: is the outer protein barrier which supports the spike-like structure of the virus.

Spike Proteins: the spikes, a unique feature of coronavirus protrude outside of the viral envelope giving it a crown-like feature, hence corona in Latin and is the prime site which sticks or binds to the receptor sites of a host organism to gain entry into the host body.

COVID-19 and Nutrition

Nutrition is a very important factor in combating any disease or infection be it of viral or bacterial nature. In order to examine this, we need to evaluate food categories and their effect on our immune system and immunity in general. It is a well-known fact that a weaker body is more prone to and susceptible to catching infection. We will categorise major nutrients and their role in fighting infections. It is important to keep in mind that to fight infection we all need to have a healthy body, healthy immune system and practice good hygiene. Good food mix in our dietary intake will enhances our body's reserves and therefore improves the status of good nutrients to be able to offer significant protective measures against pathogens, while poor nutritional intake with poor quality of nutrient will fail to provide the required protection. Pathogens are organisms such as bacteria and viruses which passes on the infections to its host body.

Lack of proper and balanced dietary intake have a negative impact on our immune system which effects our organs and their functions resulting in disease symptoms and illness. Primary target areas being the Respiratory System, Digestive System, Musculo-Skeletal System, Circulatory System, Endocrine System etc.; in fact, severe infections can affect almost all body organs, may be not all at once but progressive decline in body functions can be a severe life-threatening issue.

Since pathogens attack the host with immune-compromised status, it is important to increase the levels of nutritional intake. The Chart below gives some basic understanding of the utility of several nutrients that have been known to offer immense benefit during both viral and bacterial infections. Research using some of these nutrients referred in the chart and COVID-19 is emerging, and in some cases more research is needed as there are no clear evidence; but, evaluating the data available, these nutrients may serve as adjunct therapies in consort with conventional therapy provided there are no interaction, interference and hindrance from these nutrients to the conventional therapies applied.

The diagram below outlines the link between infection and lack of good nutrition in the form of a well-balanced diet.

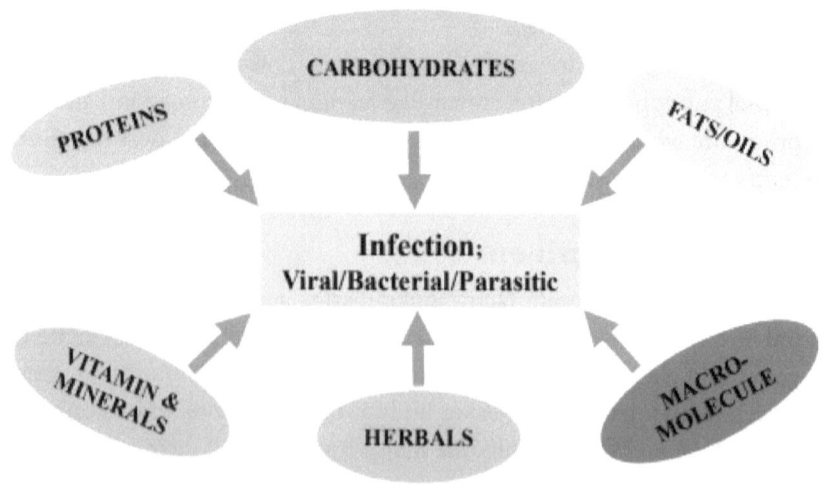

Chart: Nutrients that can Offer Benefits during Viral/Bacterial Infections

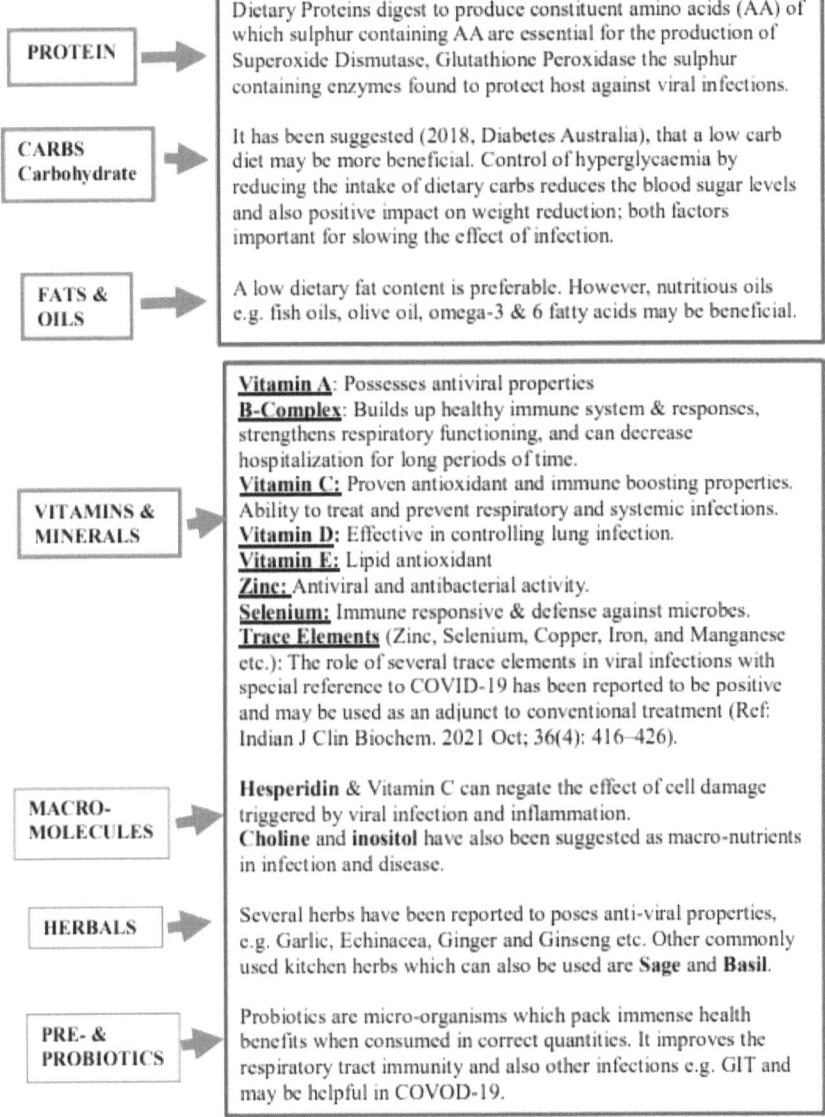

Other nutritional considerations are consumption of fresh fruit and vegetables and drinking plenty of water for the effective transportation of nutrients and flushing off the waste elimination from kidneys which as a result of filtration of the blood accumulates significant waste in the kidney tubules. Deficiencies in vitamin intake from the food or supplementary intake may have a detrimental effect on our body's response to viral infections including SARS-COV2 (Ref: An Israeli population-based study, FEBS J. 2020, 287: 3693–702).

Sulphur-based amino acids have a significant response to protecting the host immunity from viral infection and therefore an increase in the dietary intake of sulphur-containing foods is an important inclusion in our dietary makeup during viral infections; a lack of it can enhance the incidence of oxidative damage and lipid peroxidation of the cellular structure causing an increased risk to cellular immunity.

There are 5 basic steps to holistically approach any clinical therapy:

Ingestion	What we eat.
Digestion	What the body can handle.
Absorption	What the body needs.
Circulation	What the body transports to tissues.
Elimination	What the body does not want.

Dysfunction or inadequate performance in any of these five biochemical steps can manifest into a biochemical condition which if left unattended or untreated may develop into a major impairment which in time could develop into a life-threatening ailment with serious consequences. The use of proper quality nutrition which is appropriate for our dietary food intake and supplements, together, with moderate lifestyle adjustments will go a long way in achieving a desired outcome in any adverse conditions such as viral infections and other diseases we may succumb to from time to time. Medical intervention also becomes an important factor together with lifestyle adjustments in any curative undertaking bearing in mind that other therapies are also available as adjuncts if needed in particular during the healing stages or processes.

Our immune system is affected by the environmental pollution, obesity, dietary insufficiencies, general health and mental state, sleep deprivation lack of exercise, drug and alcohol abuse, and age-related insufficiencies in our organ functions and systemic failures and many other factors. Some changes and adjustments in our lifestyle management can be the key to our health and general well-being.

Since living with COVID-19 and its variants for more than 2 years and learning more about this dreaded viral disease, we can follow some very basic hygiene practices to try and keep safe as best as we can. The most simple hygienic practices we are meant to follow is to mask up in dense public places, wash our hands and arms lathering up so that the spiked protein-based virus can detach from our skin surface due to surface tension generated by the soap lather. Try not to touch the soft mucus membrane lined areas such as our nostrils, face area and mouth, etc., with infected fingers. Take no chances, assume that in public places the virus is rampant and chances of us being infected are high. It has been speculated that until communities reach a herd immunity the virus will remain a dominant disruptive influence in our lives.

At the present time, vaccination and booster shots (injections) are the main form of preventive measures that have been recommended by various Public Health Offices headed by the WHO's recommendations and ratified by individual country's health departments. It is my opinion that the virus may be swamped by a milder strain and eventually die down; the other possibility is that we may have to live with the virus taking all the precautions we possibly can. Eventually, I hope that the population can be vaccinated once every year in a combined flu/COVID jab which will keep us immune until the next 12 months or beyond. Let us not speculate, who knows our elite biochemists and specialist researchers in virology/immunology may come up with some easier and more effective way to keep us safe. Wouldn't that be something, and worthy of a Nobel Prize in Physiology?

Good nutrition is the key to strengthen our immune system so that any infiltration by the pathogens can be of milder nature and the body can offer enough resistivity to fight off the infection. It is reported that worldwide there are approximately **2 billion** people who are deficient in micro-nutrients consisting of vitamins A, B-group, C, D, and E, certain trace minerals e.g., iron, zinc, iodine, manganese, etc., which is a direct cause of poor-quality diet and malnutrition.

This may also be the cause of lack of growth in children in poorer nations, intellectual impairment, prone to diseases (viral/bacterial and other infections) which results in increased mortality. There are also several other reasons such as hygiene and lack of proper medication and a lack of appropriate health care services.

There is now a clearly established link between micro-nutrients and development of our immune system which is the first line of defence from the proliferation of pathogens. The diagram below is prepared to highlight the understanding of this issue and together with charts previously referred to could provide some awareness of this important topic.

Diagram: Expressing Relation between Biochemical Steps and Nutrition

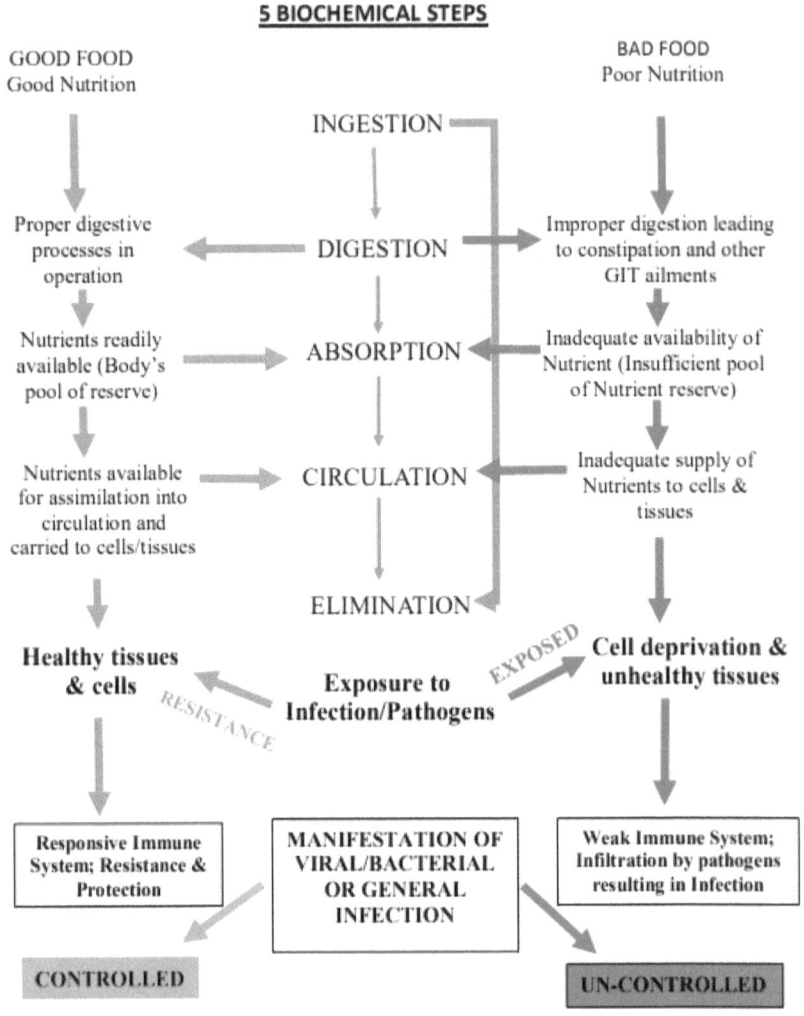

COVID-19 pandemic has disrupted many aspects of our life; it has been estimated that more than 6.4 million people have died so far and counting worldwide; amounting to less than 0.9% of global population of 7.9 billion, an estimated 560 million people have been infected causing a mortality rate of about 1.15%.

The history of human existence is full of incidences which in today's definition can be categorised as pandemics. In several cases, a significant population has died of the pandemic situation then, e.g., Black Death of 1347 it has been estimated by modern-day researchers that as many as 200 million people had perished; alarming is it not?

The table below lists some of the Pandemics in our history. The death-toll is high due to the unavailability of proper medication and patient care. Vaccines and certain anti-bacterial agents were discovered around 1796. Edward Jenner has been accredited to be the first person to use vaccinia virus (cowpox) which he later in 1798 demonstrated to offer immunity to smallpox. Since Edward Jenner's discovery of smallpox vaccine the incidence of smallpox epidemic was significantly reduced. It was not until after 100 years since Jenner's discovery Louis Pasteur discovered Cholera vaccine (around 1885). Plague vaccine was developed by Waldemar Haffkine in 1897.

After these early discoveries, the pandemic proportion of Smallpox, Plagues and Cholera were never seen in the later part of the 19th and early part of 20th centuries. Even to this day, vaccines have proven effective in protecting us against the respective diseases such as those mentioned above. The first ever Nobel Prize was awarded to Emil von Behring in medicine for his work on serum therapy for its application against Diphtheria.

Throughout human history, since records became available, we have faced pandemics of epic proportions. I found some interesting historical references which would make interesting reading (see table below).

I have selected only a handful of references from the very many examples cited in the scientific journals and reputable publications which readers if interested can easily peruse further. Few references are particularly interesting; incidences of Asiatic Cholera of 1817 which has been reported to have occurred 6 times between 1817 to 1923; other examples are that of the Great Plague of London 1665, Russian Plague of 1770, American Polio epidemic of 1916, etc., and all these pandemics for more than 2 years and caused untold deaths and suffering.

Table: Pandemics throughout Human History

Pandemic	Year	Region	%Global Population Perished.	Cause
Plague of Athens	430–426 BCE	Athens	75,000–100,000 People died	Possibly typhoid fever and Ebola.

Antonine Plague (Also, (known as Plague of Galen)	165–180 AD	First Pandemic in Roman Empire to be recorded.	5 million people died	Many experts believe that the plague was caused by smallpox virus.
Plague of Cyprian	249–262 AD	Originated in Ethiopia then spread over Rome, Greece and Syria.	Actual death toll is not known but estimated at 5000 a day in Rome only.	Still remains of unknown origin.
Plague of Justinian I	543–541 AD	Europe and the Mediterranean basin	15 million–100 million	Caused by the bacterium Yersinia pestis.
Japanese smallpox epidemic	735–737 AD	Asia, Japan	Wiped out approx. 1/3 of the Japanese Population	Smallpox virus
Black Death	1347–1351 AD	Europe	75 million–200 million	bacteria Yersinia pestis
Cocoliztli epidemic of 1576	1578 AD	Mexico and Central America	Estimated death 15 million people and a prime reason of wiping out the entire Aztec empire.	Viral haemorrhagic fever
First Cholera pandemic (there had been 6 out breaks from 1817 to 1923)	1817-1824	Calcutta, now known as Kolkata former dominion of British India and spread as far as China.	Estimates are more than one million people lost their life including all affected areas.	Contaminated drinking water

Prior to the Omicron strain, experts were trying to predict the future with COVID-19 especially with the delta strain; how much damage it will cause to humanity and what will be the aftermath of the virus. It was anybody's guess as the unpredictability factor was too great. Prior to the vaccines coming on to the scene Coronavirus pandemic was compared to the 1957–58 Asian flu caused by the H2N2 virus which had its origin from the avian influenza commonly known as the bird flu. Asian flu was a world-wide phenomenon causing more than 1 million deaths and far-reaching effects as it lasted for almost a decade.

So, what is the prognosis on COVID-19 virus and its lifecycle? The term virus originated from a Latin word meaning poison. Early in the 17th, 18th century many diseases such as Cholera, Chickenpox, and Typhoid, etc., were thought to have originated from poisons as a primary source of contamination. Progressively as scientists became more aware and acquired deeper knowledge the concepts began to change from poisonous origin to biological contaminants. Today the debate still goes on finally resting at the view that viruses are biological entities which must have a host to live on and replicate. If viruses do not have a cellular structure, how can they breathe like we do: in a very simple biological explanation there are certain definitive steps in the lifecycle of a virus.

The first step in a virus life cycle is **Attachment or Penetration** into a living host organism. This usually happens when the virus sticks to the host via a protein molecule also known as a receptor molecule on the host membrane. Specifically, in COVID-19 situation the spikes stick on to our receptive mucous membrane and enters our body. Once the virus latches on to the host cell the genome (in COVID-19 it is the RNA) is transferred or transplanted into the host cell. The next step after the viral genome is firmly planted, is the **Replication step** resulting in infiltration of the viral gene structure. The **Release** of viral genome into the host cell marks the beginning of the end of the host cell and manifestation of viral infection. The process is repeated until intervention by specific vaccine and/or anti-viral agent are applied to cause a kill factor.

During the viral incubation followed by infection, host organism is highly contagious and can easily spread the infection via the body fluids. Being a respiratory virus COVID-19 spreads via contaminated respiratory droplets e.g., breathe, cough and sneeze and saliva. Just being in the close proximity of the infected host, the virus can successfully be transmitted.

COVID-19 and Prognosis

It has been more than 2 years since the world first came to know of this once in a 100-year pandemic. Although the initial shock has passed and the population at large has overcome the fears and the tribulations, we are now entering into the co-habitation phase. Whatever the future situation may bring, we have to learn to live with it; in fact, most of the population have done so by the way of vaccinations and booster shots, even though the protective span from vaccination and booster shots is limited we need to set ourselves for the future awaiting for a long-term protective and hopefully curative measures which optimistically could be around the corner. The international population through their respective government agencies are opening up to bring about normalisation of the situation and eventually life will become normal, I guess as normal as it can be, like the seasonal flu.

Yes, the world is opening up and attempts are being made to bring back normality as in pre-pandemic conditions, this is of prime importance and target to aim for. Life can never be the same but to be protective we all will need to follow certain new sets of practices which will become the new norm for our society. Now, what will those new sets of instructions be? This can only be determined by a timeline set by various government health agencies in consultation with the WHO.

Basically, my view on this matter is a 4-step consideration:

- Vaccination and booster inoculations to provide a herd immunity; with a benchmark target of say excess of 80% of the total population above 10 years old.
- Use of masks in all public places, including public transport, densely populated venues marketplaces especially wet humid and damp areas.
- Practice of social distancing and hygiene including hand sanitisation. It is also a good practice to flush viral contaminants from our soft mucus lining (nostrils, mouth and eye areas, etc.) using a tepid warm water by way of gargling and wash-offs.
- Government intervention in the form of education and a high level of healthcare monitoring. An improvement in civic sense among the citizens and regular cleanliness checks and orderly societal activities.

These are basic common-sense issues that can easily become a part of our regular activity and a second nature. As I mentioned, initially authoritative intervention will be the key to its success but as we get set in these new-ways, life can become normal with COVID-19 becoming a seasonal viral infection like influenza with a yearly requirement of a more specialise vaccine. Since the discovery of COVID-19 in November–December 2019 the most virulent strain the Delta strain was rampant for almost 2 and a half years. Now, the Delta strain has been over lapped by the less virulent but way more contagious Omicron strain.

It is the opinion of several experts that Delta strain will be overrun by the Omicron in due course, as we are already seeing it happening now and eventually mutate to several other strains which may be more or less, same or more contagious. The COVID landscape will be ever changing and we have to adapt with those changes and eventually, it will become a part of our human ecology.

The short-term prognosis for patients who acquire the infection are as follows; fully vaccinated patients who have also been booster jabbed have a very high chance of escaping the severity of the illness, but, a notable percentage of population who have not been vaccinated at all may risk severity and complications from the infection. A small but a significant percentage of these patients may further require hospitalisation and unfortunately among these patients those who have underlying health issues may fail to recover under normal treatment and will need ICU (Intensive Care Unit) care.

Sadly, in the early days of the infection, people perished due mostly to unpreparedness of the healthcare system. Even though a lot has been learned since then, mortality among immune-compromised patients is still high. In a recent report Covid live (covidlive.com.au; July 2022 statistics) in Australia, Current Cases Admitted to Hospital was numbered to 4719 of these patient numbers 155 were re-located in ICU which is around 3.28%, but unfortunately of these patients the mortality was high (around 13%). It must be considered in context as the data fluctuates considerably.

Many patients have also passed away during home care which is not subject to the above data generated. It is alleged that many elderly people who are frail and infirm have a higher probability of getting the infection and some will pass on due to their weak immunity and other life-threatening illnesses.

Comparing with the Spanish flu of 1918, yes it had a far-reaching effect on humanity with global deaths of around 50 million, far greater in number than the current pandemic as per a July 2022 statistics (Covid-19 Coronavirus Pandemic last updated July 17, 2022) 567,348,657 people had the infection, 538,419,812 recovered (recovery rate 95%) and 6,387,224 people died. Patients who are critically ill with COVID-19 infection have a significantly high mortality rate around 25–50% globally; in several cases the mortality rate will be largely dependent on CVD (cardiovascular diseases), Chronic Obstructive Pulmonary Disease (COPD), Pneumonia and other respiratory complications. Age-related complications are also very concerning in seniors 65 years and above. We can at least hope that with the progression of the pandemic and the omicron strain taking over with herd immunity acquired the prognosis looks better and more manageable.

COVID-19 and in general Omicron is characterised with spike protein a gel-like structure which latches on to the host mucus membrane from where it penetrates into a host cell and proliferates. These spiked protein structure over time mutates and gives rise to various structural configuration which we know as variants of the original virus.

Further to these so-called variants following have now also been listed by the WHO as current variants of concern.

Lambda variant emerged in Peru 2020.

Mu variant emerged in South America in Columbia 2021.

Others worth mentioning are sub-variants of Omicron BA.1 and BA.2.

The earliest omicron sub-variant to be detected, BA.1, was first reported in November 2021 in South Africa. While scientists believe that all the sub-variants may have emerged around the same time, BA.1 was predominantly responsible for the winter surge of infections in the Northern Hemisphere in 2021.

BA. 2, a genetically distinct sub-variant which is reported to have accounted for more than half of new cases in the United States, and has become the dominant coronavirus variant around the world.

While the origin of BA. 2 is still unclear, it has quickly become the dominant strain in many countries, including India, Denmark and South Africa. It is continuing to spread in Europe, Asia and many parts of the world. BA. 2 is considered to be more transmissible but not more virulent than BA. 1. This means that while BA. 2 can spread faster than BA. 1, it might not make people sicker.

Other sub-variants BA. 4 and BA. 5 were first identified in South Africa, Europe and the US according to health experts.

The latest ones, BA 4. and BA 5, are of concern which are very closely related to the Omicron variant behind last winter's wave.

They were added to the World Health Organisation's monitoring list in March 2022 and have also been designated as variants of concern in Europe.

BA. 4 and BA. 5 appear to be able to infect people even if they've recently had other types of Omicron.

BA. 2.12.1: is a newer sub-variant, which has been spreading rapidly and became dominant in the United States in late May 2022. This sub-variant was first detected in New York State.

Omicron carries about 50 mutations not seen in combination before, including 30 mutations in the gene for the spike protein that the coronavirus uses to attach to human cells.

(https://www.nytimes.com/interactive/2021/health/coronavirus-varianttracker.html By Jonathan Corum and Carl Zimmer Updated May 24, 2022).

Lots of people have built up some immunity from past infections and vaccination, which is helping to make the disease less risky overall.

But the new sub-variants do appear to be spreading more easily.

This is partly because our immunity may be waning, and also because of the mutations the virus has undergone which makes the mutant virus more potent. Another reason for the spread is that many countries have also lifted their Covid restrictions, meaning people are mixing more, which gives the virus more chances to spread.

A wave of new infections could lead to more hospitalisations and some more deaths. But humanity is resilient and we have to arm ourselves with newer and more effective anti-viral vaccines and drugs to fight-off the dangers that these unwanted scourges impose on our society and disruption to our lives.

For interested readers, an article on COVID-19 timeline is referenced below.

A Timeline of COVID-19 Developments in 2020 (Ref: January 2, 2021 AJMC_Staff).

How Covid-19 has changed our lives

After its declaration as a pandemic (WHO March 11, 2020), Covid-19 is still rampant throughout the world. After a long and arduous two and a half years, the pandemic is still rampant but we as a humanity collectively have come to live with it. Human race is resilient it will take a lot more to put us down.

Some pundits foretell that the world will not be the same.

I am optimistic and I for one however, believe from what I have read and heard that in Australia, as we have weathered the first wave of Covid-19 which was a major unknown factor in our recent history, we have learned to be more co-operative diligent and more responsive to global adjustments. One most outstanding positive thing among many that came out is the sense of co-operation and care within our global community. The invention of vaccines and progress made in the treatment of Covid-19 has been phenomenal, even though the specificity may have been a bit more desired but nonetheless they have given us hope. The empathy with which the affluent nations have come out in helping the poorer nations has been remarkable which leads me to believe we still have hope of survival on this planet.

We mustn't lose hope come what may and better prepare for other subsequent waves.

Since writing this chapter, we as a society have moved into a more Covid-19 tolerant phase. Many parts of the world have opened up in terms of trade and travel and we are simply forging ahead into a new and more predictable territory.

Looking ahead, I see that newer strains of the virus will bring about several significant challenges in our lives within the commerce, health care, education and so-called day-to-day existence sectors which may create a profound change in our societal structure. Or, it may only exacerbate and highlight the existing societal conditions. We simply have to re-group and rethink our priorities.

We in communities have the responsibility to control Covid-19 by strenuously practicing containment and preventive measures as we would do in any other contagious diseases be it of bacterial or viral origin until a herd immunity (high percentage of population coverage) has been reached globally.

We have already witnessed adjustments to our lifestyle in so far as working from home and flexible working conditions, evolution and facilitation in telehealth services, a growing digital economy and education. All these changes and system innovations, all point to the adjustment phase that we as a global community are re-aligning to in-order to secure a safe collective future for us and our future generation. This not only redefines the current pandemic situation but also prepares us for any future pandemic which may invade our civilisation.

I think COVID-19 is here to stay and in a couple of years' time it will be just like another flu similar to as caused by the influenza virus highly contagious yet manageable. It is a challenge for virologists to invent an annual booster shot which will offer protection against COVID-19 and its variants thereof. Let us hope that one day in the not-so-distant future safe and effective protection will be available. Until then, we all can live in hope and do the best we can to protect ourselves and the community at large.

www.ingramcontent.com/pod-product-compliance
Lightning Source LLC
LaVergne TN
LVHW091709070526
838199LV00050B/2322